Bioactive Compounds and Cancer

Bioactive Compounds and Cancer

Editor: Chris Dalton

FOSTER ACADEMICS
www.fosteracademics.com

www.fosteracademics.com

FOSTER ACADEMICS

Cataloging-in-Publication Data

Bioactive compounds and cancer / edited by Chris Dalton.
p. cm.
Includes bibliographical references and index.
ISBN 978-1-64646-554-5
1. Cancer--Nutritional aspects. 2. Bioactive compounds. 3. Nutrition. I. Dalton, Chris.
RC268.45 .B56 2023
616.994 065 4--dc23

Foster Academics,
118-35 Queens Blvd., Suite 400,
Forest Hills, NY 11375, USA

ISBN 978-1-64646-554-5 (Hardback)

Contents

Preface

This book was inspired by the evolution of our times; to answer the curiosity of inquisitive minds. Many developments have occurred across the globe in the recent past which has transformed the progress in the field.

Natural products play an important role in pharmacotherapy, particularly in the treatment of infectious diseases and cancer. These products originate from fungi, animals and plants. These products, which include oils, fruits, nuts, whole grains and vegetables, contain modest levels of bioactive compounds, which have therapeutic potential and health-promoting properties. Major categories of bioactive compounds comprise tannins, lycopene, lignin, indoles, resveratrol, and alkaloids. Extensive researches have been conducted for exploring the therapeutic potential of bioactive compounds in heart disease, cancer, diabetes, and cardiovascular diseases. Various natural bioactive compounds are fast catching are being researched for their anti-cancer properties. They have been found to have a chemopreventive effect by altering pro-inflammatory gene expression. This book aims to shed light on some of the unexplored aspects of bioactive compounds and their use in the treatment and management of cancer. It is appropriate for students seeking detailed information in this area as well as for experts.

This book was developed from a mere concept to drafts to chapters and finally compiled together as a complete text to benefit the readers across all nations. To ensure the quality of the content we instilled two significant steps in our procedure. The first was to appoint an editorial team that would verify the data and statistics provided in the book and also select the most appropriate and valuable contributions from the plentiful contributions we received from authors worldwide. The next step was to appoint an expert of the topic as the Editor-in-Chief, who would head the project and finally make the necessary amendments and modifications to make the text reader-friendly. I was then commissioned to examine all the material to present the topics in the most comprehensible and productive format.

I would like to take this opportunity to thank all the contributing authors who were supportive enough to contribute their time and knowledge to this project. I also wish to convey my regards to my family who have been extremely supportive during the entire project.

Editor

1

Anticancer Effect of *Citrus hystrix* DC. Leaf Extract and Its Bioactive Constituents Citronellol and, Citronellal on the Triple Negative Breast Cancer MDA-MB-231 Cell Line

Yathsoeung Ho [1], Nungruthai Suphrom [2], Krai Daowtak [1], Pachuen Potup [1], Yordhathai Thongsri [1] and Kanchana Usuwanthim [1,*]

1 Cellular and Molecular Immunology Research Unit, Faculty of Allied Health Sciences, Naresuan University, Phitsanulok 65000, Thailand; yathsoeung@gmail.com (Y.H.); kraid@nu.ac.th (K.D.); pachuenp@nu.ac.th (P.P.); yordhathait@nu.ac.th (Y.T.)

2 Department of Chemistry, Faculty of Science and Center of Excellence for Innovation in Chemistry, Naresuan University, Phitsanulok 65000, Thailand; suphrom.n1@gmail.com

* Correspondence: kanchanau@nu.ac.th

Abstract: Triple negative breast cancer is one of the most aggressive breast cancer type with abilities of early metastasis and chemoresistance. The tropical plant *Citrus hystrix* DC. has been reported to promote many biological activities including anticancer. However, the effect of *C. hystrix* against triple negative breast cancer has not yet been identified. This study aimed to evaluate the anticancer properties of *C. hystrix* leaf extract and its bioactive constituents citronellol and citronellal against the triple negative breast cancer MDA-MB-231 cell line. *C. hystrix* leaves were powdered and sequentially macerated. The in vitro anticancer effects of *C. hystrix* leaf extracts, and its bioactive constituents (citronellol and citronellal) were evaluated against MDA-MB-231 cell line using cytotoxic MTT assay, cell proliferation, wound scratch migration, colony formation, cell cycle, apoptosis assay, Hoechst staining, RT-qPCR, and Western blot analysis. Results showed that crude hexane extract, citronellol, and citronellal significantly reduced cell proliferation, colony formation, and cell migration by inducing cell cycle arrest, while also inducing apoptosis in MDA-MB-231 cells through inhibition of anti-apoptotic Bcl-2 expression, leading to activation of the caspase-3-dependent pathway. This study is the first report to demonstrate the effect of *C. hystrix*, citronellol, and citronellal against triple negative breast cancer MDA-MB-231 cells.

Keywords: triple negative breast cancer; MDA-MD-231; *Citrus hystrix* DC.; leaf extract; citronellol; citronellal

1. Introduction

Triple negative breast cancer (TNBC) is a sub-type of breast cancer. TNBC is characterized by tumors that do not express estrogen receptor (ER) or progesterone receptor (PR), with immunohistochemical (IHC) staining present at less than 1% repartitioning of these receptors in the tissue and less than 10% for human epidermal receptor 2 (Her-2) [1,2]. TNBC accounts for 15–20% of invasive breast cancers in women [3] and presents a higher frequency of recurrence and lower overall survival rate compared to non-TNBC patients [4]. It is one of the most aggressive types of breast cancer due to its early metastasis and resistance to chemotherapies such as anthracyclines, taxanes, and many others [5]. Several new anticancer plant-derived molecules have been put through clinical trials [6] and some such as cabazitaxel and homoharringtonine have been approved by the FDA for use in treatment resistance [7,8]. Plant materials are now becoming increasingly recognized as a substantial source of anticancer agents and urgently require assessment for future development.

Citrus hystrix DC., also known as kaffir lime, is a tropical plant belonging to the Rutaceae family. The tree can grow up to six meters high and has double pointy oval shaped leaf, white fragrant flowers, and green to yellow ellipsoid fruits with irregular bumpy skin. Many compounds have been identified in the fruit including phenolics, flavonoids, terpenoids, alkaloids, coumarins, glycosides, saponins, tannins, hydrocarbons, and fatty acids [9–11]. In Thailand, *C. hystrix* is believed to have cancer-prevention and anti-inflammation properties and it is used as a remedy in traditional medicine [12]. *C. hystrix* has also been reported to exert potency against many types of cancers. It induced selective cytotoxicity against brain and cervical cancer cells [13], induced cell cycle arrest in lymphoma cells [14], and also suppressed cell migration and induced cell shrinkage in human pancreatic cancer cells [15]. Citronellol and citronellal are two acyclic monoterpenoids that have been identified in *C. hystrix*. They have been reported to exert many varied biological activities including anti-inflammatory and anti-microbial activities [16]. Citronellal exhibited toxicity against MCF-7 breast cancer cells [17] and reduced proliferation by inducing apoptosis in Huh7 hepatocellular carcinoma [18], while citronellol induced necroptosis of lung cancer [19]. Both molecules have also been reported to inhibit the action of multidrug resistance P-glycoprotein, which ameliorates the efficacity of drug treatments [20]. However, the effect of *C. hystrix* and its bioactive compounds citronellol and citronellal have not yet been observed on triple negative breast cancer. Here, the anticancer effects of *C. hystrix* crude extracts, citronellol, and citronellal were evaluated against the triple negative breast cancer MDA-MB-231 cell line in terms of cell proliferation, migration, cell cycle arrest and apoptosis. Findings revealed that *C. hystrix* leaf extract and its active compounds citronellol and citronellal strongly inhibited tumor cell growth and triggered apoptosis via over-expression of cleaved caspase-3 and Bax, while down-regulating the anti-apoptotic Bcl-2.

2. Results

2.1. Extraction Yields of *C. hystrix* Leaf Powder

Maceration *C. hystrix* leaf powder with hexane solvent resulted in a sticky dark green extract with yield of 1.1% (*w/w* dried powder). The following sub-sequential extractions culminated in a similar consistency of extracts with yield of 1.8% obtained using ethyl acetate and 7.6% using 95% ethanol.

2.2. Identification of Volatile Components in Crude Hexane Extract by GC-MS

Analysis of the total ionic chromatogram by GC-MS identified 45 volatile compounds from crude hexane extract. Relative amounts (%) of the compositions were calculated by peak-area normalization (Table 1). Most of the identified compounds of crude *C. hystrix* hexane extract were terpenoids (19.84%). The extract contained oxygenated monoterpenes (3.99%), hydrocarbon monoterpenes (2.19%), oxygenated sesquiterpenes (7.67%), and hydrocarbon sesquiterpenes (5.99%) as major compounds. The identification of two oxygenated monoterpenes, citronellal and citronellol, were found in leaf extract and then confirmed with authentic standards which they were observed at retention time (RT) at 10.75 min and 12.85 min, respectively (Figure S1). Other constituents comprised long-chain hydrocarbons, phytosterols, fatty acids, fatty alcohols, and vitamins.

Table 1. The identified compounds from crude hexane by GC-MS.

No.	RT (min)	R.I [1]	Identified Compounds	Classification	R.A [2] (%)
1	9.23	1100	Linalool	Monoterpene [a]	0.34
2	10.56	1146	Isopulegol	Monoterpene [a]	1.01
3	10.75	1154	Citronellal	Monoterpene [a]	0.67
4	11.46	1179	Terpinen-4-ol	Monoterpene [a]	0.29
5	11.83	1193	α-Terpineol	Monoterpene [a]	0.11
6	12.85	1229	Citronellol	Monoterpene [a]	1.42
7	14.08	1354	3,7-dimethyloct-1,7-dien-3,6-diol	Monoterpene [a]	0.15
8	16.23	1354	α-Cubebene	Sesquiterpene [b]	0.94
9	16.94	1381	α-Copaene	Sesquiterpene [b]	1.44
10	17.29	1395	β-Cubebene	Sesquiterpene [b]	0.34
11	18.08	1426	Caryophyllene	Sesquiterpene [b]	1.59
12	18.30	1435	Bicyclosequiphellandrene	Sesquiterpene [b]	0.20
13	18.93	1460	α-Humulene	Sesquiterpene [b]	0.23
14	19.47	1482	γ-Muurolene	Sesquiterpene [b]	0.12
15	20.05	1505	α-Muurolene	Sesquiterpene [b]	0.31
16	20.61	1529	δ-Cadinene	Sesquiterpene [b]	0.62
17	21.23	1555	Elemol	Sesquiterpene [a]	0.13
18	21.53	1568	Nerolidol	Sesquiterpene [a]	0.71
19	21.98	1586	Spathulenol	Sesquiterpene [a]	1.34
20	22.12	1592	Caryophyllene oxide	Sesquiterpene [a]	3.74
21	23.21	1641	Caryophylladienol	Sesquiterpene [a]	0.39
22	23.67	1661	Viridiflorene	Sesquiterpene [b]	0.20
23	24.05	1678	Caryophyllenol	Sesquiterpene [a]	1.14
24	25.90	1764	Tetradecanoic acid	Fatty acid [a]	0.34
25	26.29	1785	Alloaromadendrene oxide	Sesquiterpene [a]	0.22
26	27.63	1847	Hexahydrofarnesyl acetone	Sesquiterpene derivative	0.81
27	29.24	1927	Methyl palmitate	Fatty acid [a]	0.30
28	30.19	1976	Palmitic acid	Fatty acid [a]	6.82
29	32.79	2015	Phytol	Diterpene	0.40
30	33.30	2144	Linoleic acid	Fatty acid [a]	1.89
31	33.40	2149	(6Z),(9Z)-Pentadecadien-1-ol	Fatty acid [a]	2.39
32	44.09	2833	Supraene	Triterpene	0.31
33	44.92	2893	cis-2,6-Dimethyl-2,6-octadiene	Monoterpene [b]	2.19
34	48.24	3103	Tetracosane	Hydrocarbon	3.21
35	48.98	3139	α-Tocopherol	Vitamin	0.56
36	49.15	3147	Pentacosane	Hydrocarbon	1.03
37	50.92	3227	Campesterol	Phytosterol	0.46
38	51.73	3260	Stigmasterol	Phytosterol	1.07
39	52.86	3309	Heneicosane	Hydrocarbon	2.57
40	53.00	3350	1-Eicosanol	Fatty alcohol	0.37
41	53.27	3317	γ-Sitosterol	Phytosterol	2.90
42	53.81	3335	Lanosterol	Triterpene	2.45
43	58.99	3485	Lupenyl acetate	Triterpene	0.68
44	60.02	3510	17-Pentriacontene	Hydrocarbon	2.23
45	62.13	3556	Neophytadiene	Diterpene [b]	0.61
			Total R.A of identified compounds		51.24%
			Oxygenated monoterpenes		3.99%
			Hydrocarbon monoterpene		2.19%
			Oxygenated sesquiterpenes		7.67%
			Hydrocarbon sesquiterpenes		5.99%
			Hydrocarbons		9.04%
			Fatty acids and fatty alcohols		12.11%
			Other		10.25%

[1] Retention indices (R.I) were calculated using a homologous series of n-alkanes (C8–C32); [2] Relative amounts (R.A) were obtained by peak areas normalization; [a] Oxygenated form; [b] Hydrocarbon form.

2.3. *Cytotoxicity of Crude Extracts, Citronellol, and Citronellal*

After 24 h of treatment, half maximal inhibitory concentration (IC_{50}) values were obtained using a dose-response inhibition curve. *C. hystrix* crude extracts, citronellol, and citronellal reduced cell viability of MDA-MB-231 cells with IC_{50} of 317.63 ± 2.00 μg/mL for crude hexane extract (Figure 1a), 547.10 ± 0.90 μg/mL for crude ethyl acetate extract (Figure 1b) and IC_{50} > 1000 μg/mL for crude ethanolic extract (Figure 1c). For citronellol, IC_{50} values were 1.16 ± 0.10 nM (Figure 1d) and 1.41 ± 0.03 nM for citronellal (Figure 1e). The cytotoxicity of crude hexane extract, citronellol, and citronellal on normal cells, human monocyte-derived macrophages, were performed as the experimental model (Figure S2).

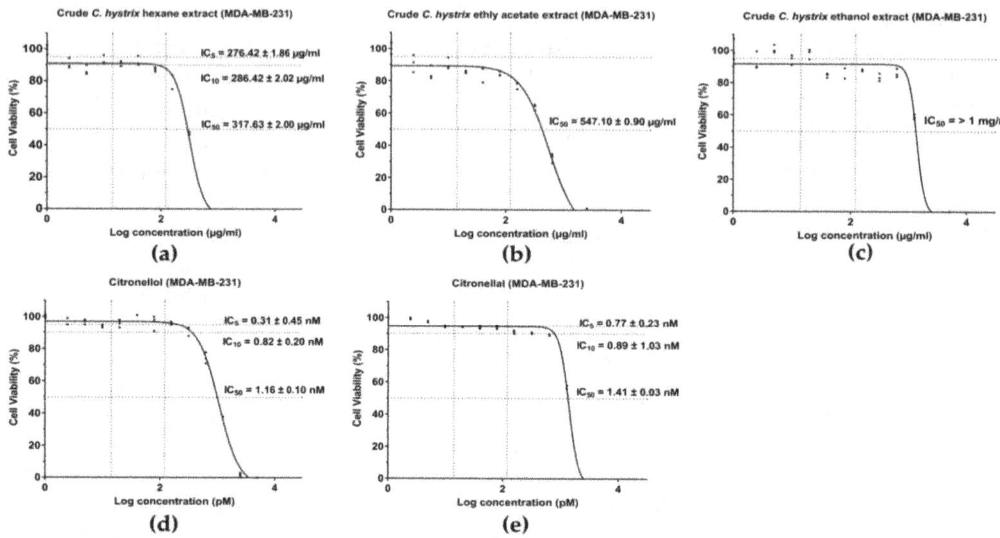

Figure 1. IC_{50} value of treatments on MDA-MB-231 cells: (**a**) Crude hexane extract, (**b**) crude ethyl acetate extract, (**c**) crude ethanolic extract, (**d**) citronellol, and (**e**) citronellal.

2.4. *Effect of Crude Hexane, Citronellol, and Citronellal on Cell Proliferation*

The cytotoxicity of crude hexane extract, citronellol and citronellal on cell proliferation rate of MDA-MB-231 cells was performed by the MTT assay. For the non-treated group, cell viability value doubled at 48 h, indicating that the cells significantly duplicated their population. By contrast, results showed that all treatment groups significantly reduced proliferation of MDA-MB-231 cells in both a dose- and time-dependent manner when compared to the non-treated group at each specific incubation time of 24 h and 48 h (Figure 2).

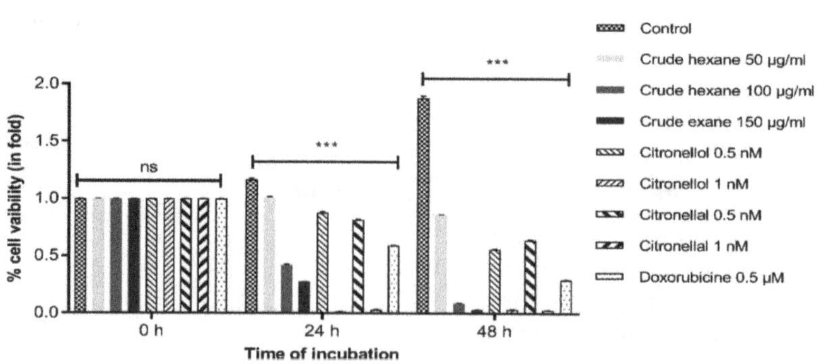

Figure 2. Crude hexane extract, citronellol, and citronellal reduced MDA-MB-231 cell proliferation at both 24 h and 48 h. Data are presented as means ± SEM. One-way ANOVA with Dunnett's multiple comparisons test was used to analyze the difference between control and treatment groups, p value < 0.05 considered significant (*** $p < 0.001$).

2.5. Crude Hexane, Citronellol, and Citronellal on Inhibited MDA-MB-231 Cell Migration

Cell migration is one of the important processes in cancer metastasis. The effects of crude hexane extract, citronellol, and citronellal on cell migration were evaluated by in vitro wound scratch migration assay. In the control group, MDA-MB-231 cells migrated to completely close the wound areas at 24 h (Figure 3). However, in the treatment groups, crude hexane extract, citronellol, and citronellal significantly reduced cell migration into wound areas at 6 h, 12 h, and 24 h in both a dose- and time-dependent manner.

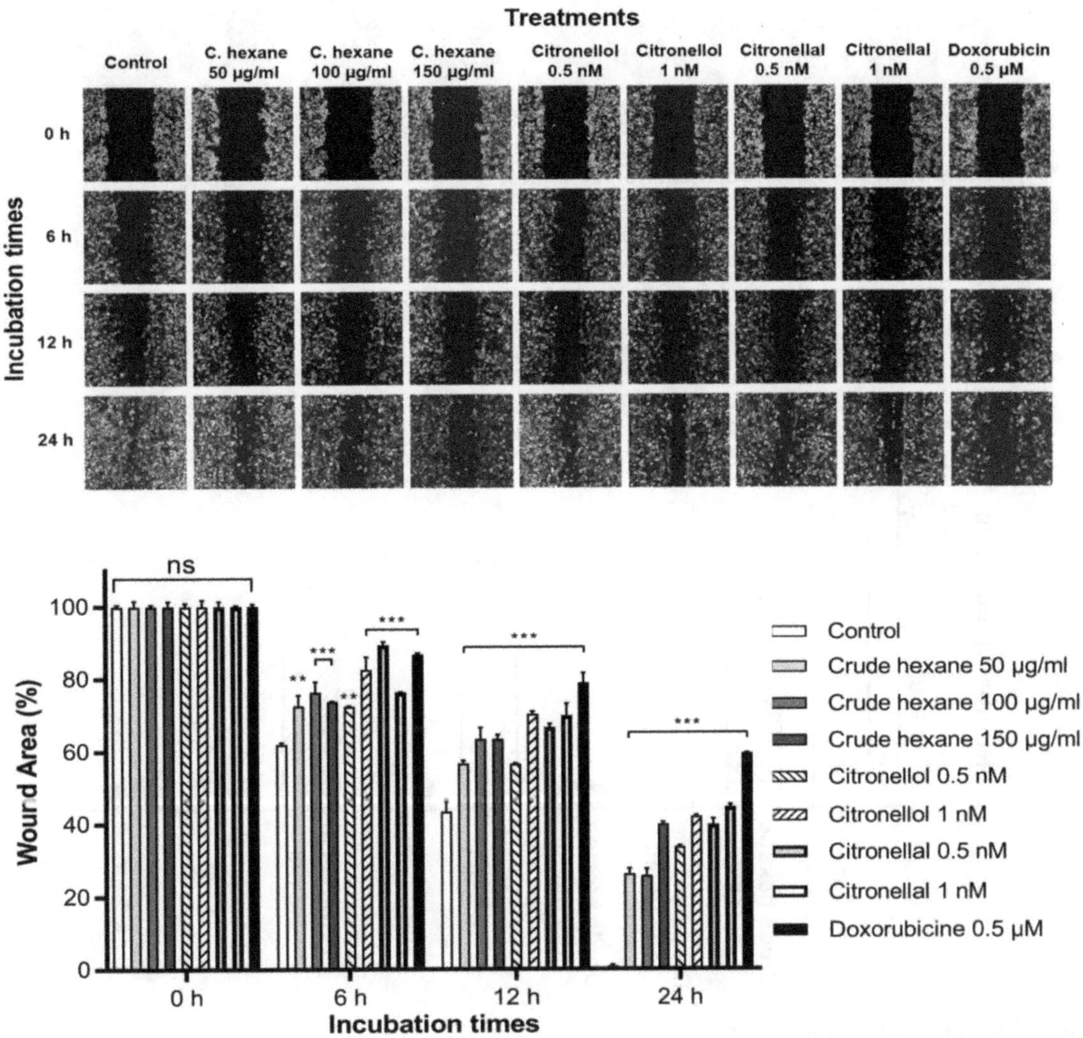

Figure 3. Cells migration into wound areas was observed under microscope at 6 h, 12 h, and 24 h. ImageJ 1.52a software was used to analyze cells migration into wound areas. Data are presented as means ± SEM. One-way ANOVA with Dunnett's multiple comparisons test was used to analyze the difference between control and treatment groups, p value < 0.05 considered significant (** $p < 0.01$, *** $p < 0.001$).

2.6. *C. hystrix* Hexane Extract, Citronellol, and Citronellal Reduced Number of Colonies Forming in MDA-MB-231 Cells

The colony forming assay was used to evaluate cell survival by studying cell growth from a single cell to form colonies in response to toxic substances. Here, colony formations of MDA-MB-231 cells under treatments by crude hexane extract, citronellol, citronellal, and doxorubicin were observed. In the treatment groups, crude hexane extract, citronellol, and citronellal significantly reduced colony formation of MDA-MB-231 cells in a dose-dependent manner, while only a few colonies were formed under treatment of doxorubicin 0.5 µM (Figure 4).

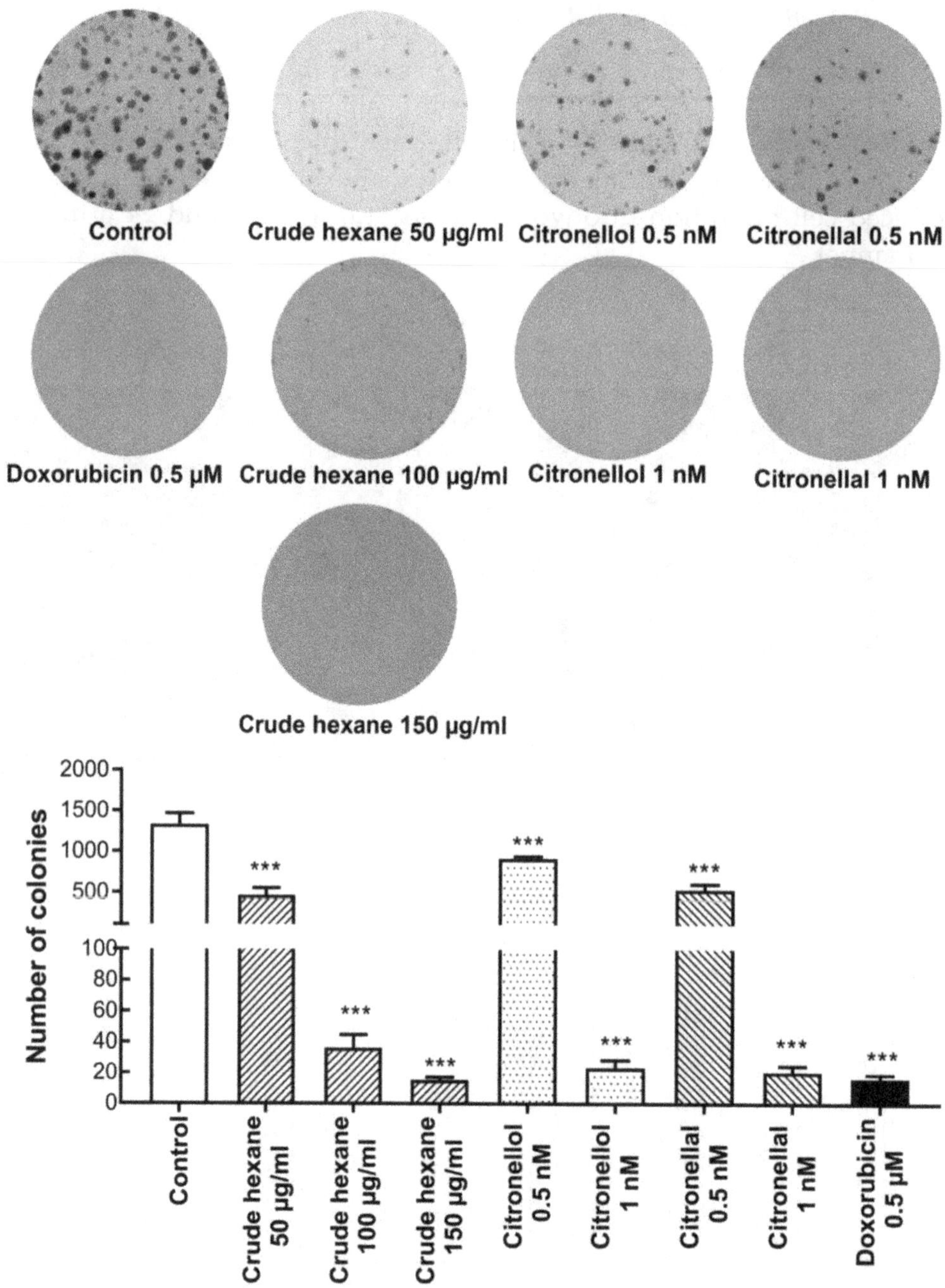

Figure 4. Colonies picture as 8-bit grayscale images under different treatments. Crude hexane, citronellol, and citronellal reduced number of MDA-MB-231 cell colonies in a dose-dependent manner. Data are presented as means ± SEM. One-way ANOVA with Dunnett's multiple comparisons test was used to analyze the difference between control and treatment groups, p value < 0.05 considered significant (*** $p < 0.001$).

2.7. Crude Hexane, Citronellol, and Citronellal Induced Cell Cycle Arrest in MDA-MB-231 Cell

Cell cycle arrest is a mechanism that cells use to prevent cell cycle progression when they encounter a toxic substance, DNA damage during DNA replication. In the treatment groups, crude hexane extract significantly induced cell cycle arrest at the G0/G1 phase when compared to the non-treated group. However, in the citronellol- and citronellal-treated groups, the cells were significantly arrested at the G2/M phase, while doxorubicin significantly induced cell cycle arrest at the G2/M phase (Figure 5).

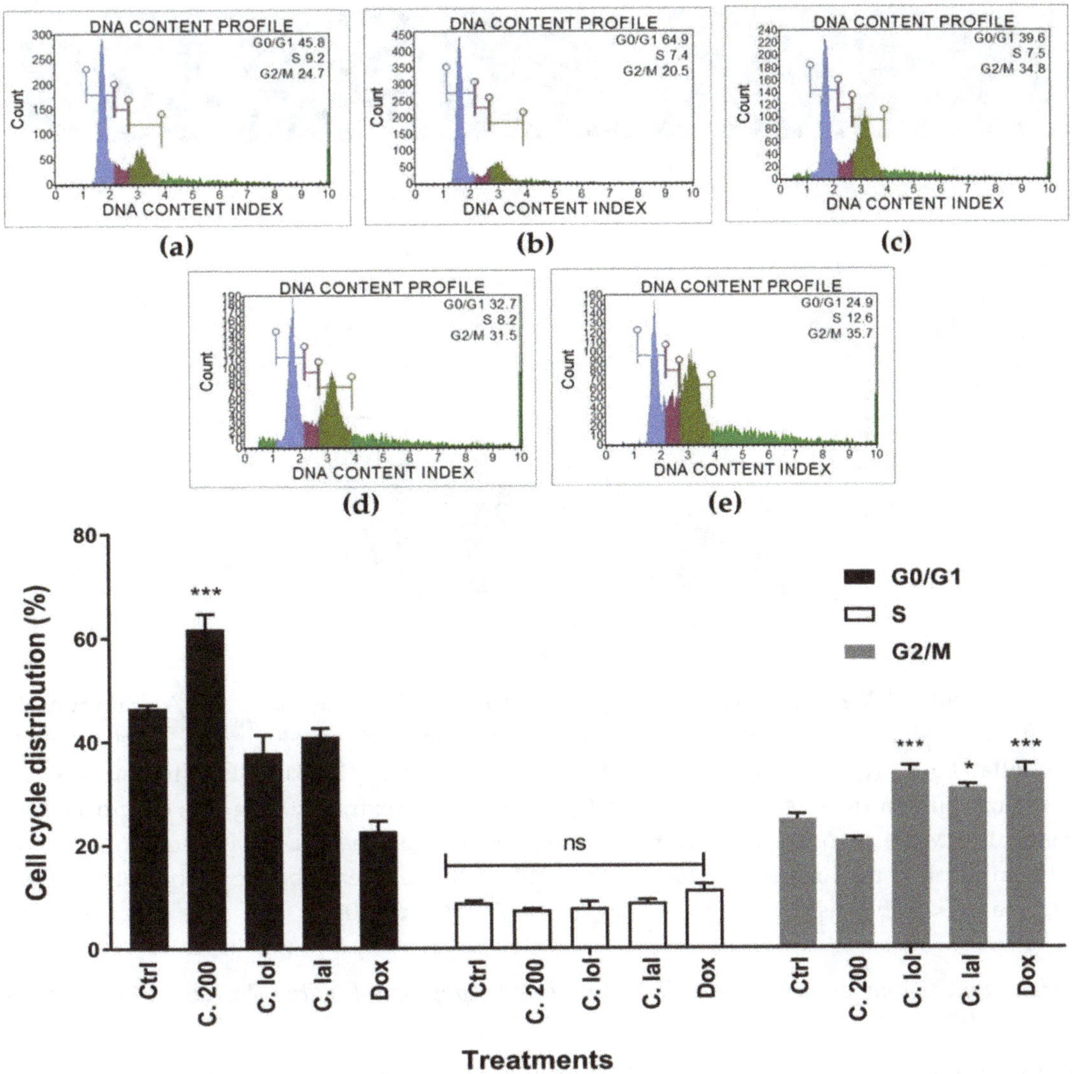

Figure 5. Cell cycle arrest induced by treatment groups on MDA-MB-231 cells. (**a**) Control (Ctrl), (**b**) crude hexane extract 200 µg/mL (C.200), (**c**) citronellol 1 nM (C. lol), (**d**) citronellal 1 nM (C. lal), (**e**) Doxorubicin 0.5 µM (Dox). Data are presented as means ± SEM. One-way ANOVA with Dunnett's multiple comparisons test was used to analyze the difference between control and treatment groups, p value < 0.05 considered significant (*** $p < 0.001$, * $p < 0.05$).

2.8. Crude Hexane, Citronellol, and Citronellal Induced Apoptosis in MDA-MB-231 Cells

Crude hexane extract, citronellol, and citronellal reduced cell proliferation and migration, while also decreasing the number of colony formations of MDA-MB-231 cells. When cells encounter toxic substances, they undergo a repair mechanism that reduces their active state. However, if the damage cannot be repaired, cell death or apoptosis results. Hoechst 33342 staining was used to confirm morphological change during apoptosis. The non-treated group showed normal nuclear cell structure; however, in the treatment groups, some condensed blue fluorescence appeared in cell nuclei indicating chromatin condensation and/or DNA fragmentation in cells treated by crude hexane extract 200 µg/mL (Figure 6b), citronellol (Figure 6c), citronellal (Figure 6d), and doxorubicin 0.5 µM (Figure 6e). Furthermore, apoptotic cells under treatments of crude hexane extract, citronellol, and citronellal for 24 h were observed using the Muse^{TM} Cell Analyser. Results revealed that a dose of 200 µg/mL crude hexane extract induced apoptosis in MDA-MB-231 cells at up to 11.02 ± 0.53% (Figure 6g) when compared to the control (Figure 6f). Similarly, citronellol at 1 nM induced cell apoptosis of 14.30 ± 0.89% (Figure 6h) with 13.92 ± 0.31% for citronellal at 1 nM (Figure 6i), while doxorubicin at 0.5 µM induced cell apoptosis of 19.02 ± 0.81% (Figure 6j).

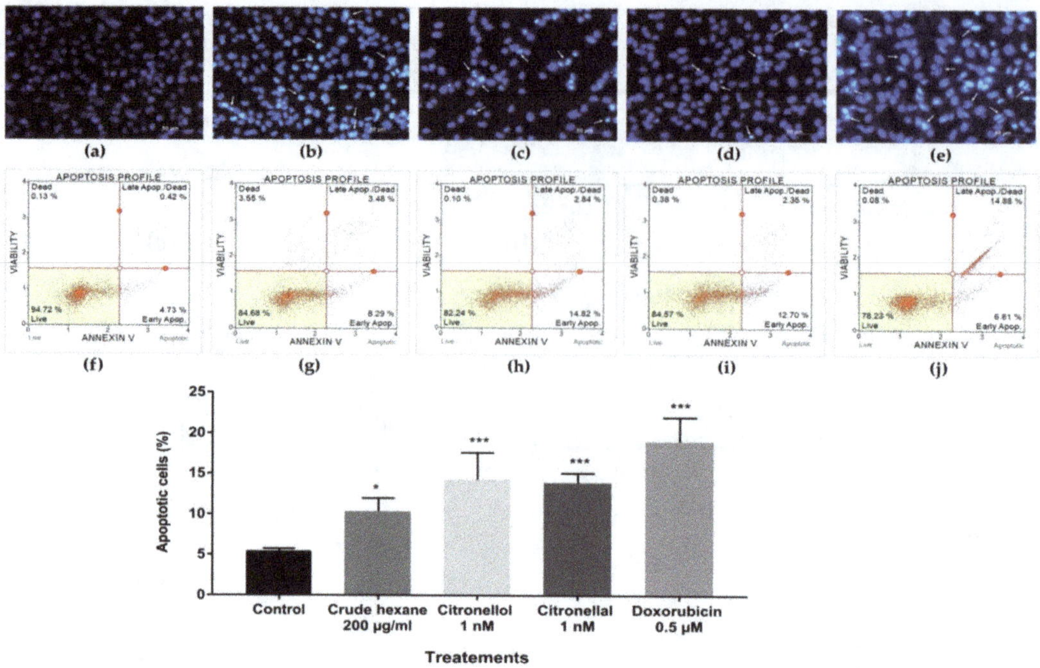

Figure 6. Hoechst 33342 staining showing chromatin condensation and DNA fragmentation in apoptotic cells under treatment of (**a**) control, (**b**) crude hexane extract 200 µg/mL, (**c**) citronellol 1 nM, (**d**) citronellal 1 nM, (**e**) doxorubicin 0.5 µM. Apoptotic MDA-MB-231 cells using Annexin-V and 7-AAD staining under treatment of (**f**) control, (**g**) crude hexane extract 200 µg/mL, (**h**) citronellol 1 nM, (**i**) citronellal 1 nM, (**j**) doxorubicin 0.5 µM. Data are presented as means ± SEM. One-way ANOVA with Dunnett's multiple comparisons test was used to analyze the difference between control and treatment groups, p value < 0.05 considered significant (* $p < 0.05$, *** $p < 0.001$).

2.9. Crude Hexane, Citronellol, and Citronellal Modulated Apoptosis-Related Proteins Gene Expression in MDA-MB-231 Cells

The expression level of apoptosis-related genes was performed using RT-qPCR to better understand cell apoptosis. Cells were treated 24 h before mRNA extraction. Results showed that the expression level of the *Bax* gene significantly increased in the treatment of crude hexane extract 200 µg/mL, citronellol 1 nM, citronellal 1 nM and doxorubicin 0.5 µM (Figure 7a). On the other hand, expression level of the *Bcl-2* gene was markedly downregulated in each treated group compared to the control (Figure 7b).

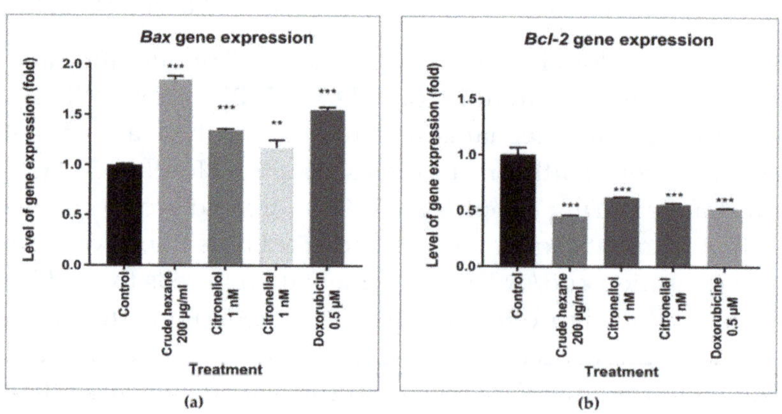

Figure 7. Alteration apoptosis-related genes expression (**a**) *Bax* and (**b**) *Bcl-2*. Data are presented as means ± SEM. One-way ANOVA was used to analyze the difference between control group and treatment groups. p value < 0.05 considered significant (** $p < 0.01$, *** $p < 0.001$).

2.10. Crude Hexane, Citronellol, and Citronellal Induced Apoptosis and DNA Fragmentation in the Cells by Inhibiting the Anti-Apoptotic Bcl-2 Protein and Activating Caspase Dependent Apoptotic Pathway

To further confirm the results, another experiment was conducted to measure the protein expression of both Bax and Bcl-2 proteins using Western blot analysis. Surprisingly, the expression of Bcl-2 protein significantly decreased after treatment by crude hexane extract 200 µg/mL, citronellol 1 nM, citronellal 1 nM, and doxorubicin 0.5 µM compared to the control group (Figure 8a), while Bax protein expression was upregulated in the same treated groups (Figure 8b). In response to the treatments, cells upregulated Bax protein expression and downregulated Bcl-2 protein expression. Alteration of Bax/Bcl-2 expression may lead to the activation of caspase-3 protein, which is an executioner in apoptosis caspase-dependent activation. To confirm this hypothesis, pro-caspase-3 and cleaved-caspase-3 protein levels were measured by Western blot analysis. Results demonstrated a significant decrease in intensities of pro-caspase-3 in the treatment groups compared to the control (Figure 8c), with significantly increase cleaved-caspase-3 protein intensity (Figure 8d).

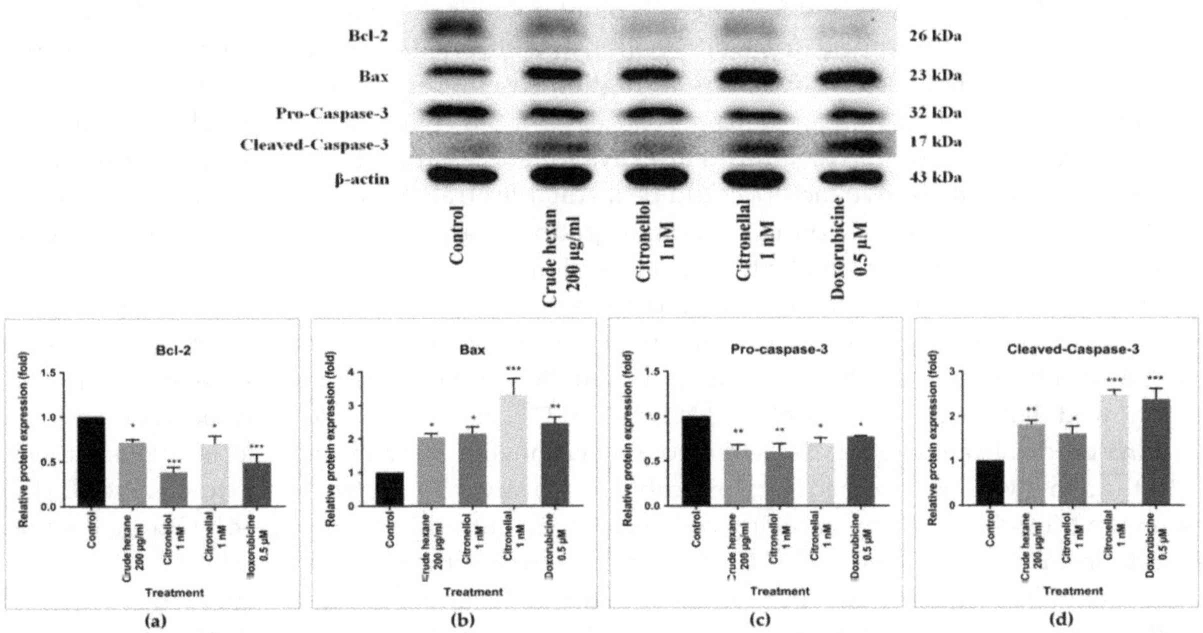

Figure 8. Western Blot analysis on: (**a**) Bcl-2 protein, (**b**) Bax protein, (**c**) Pro-Caspase-3, (**d**) Cleaved-Caspase-3. Full length of Western blot analysis (Figure S3). Data are expressed as mean ± SEM. One-way ANOVA was used to analyze the difference between control group and treatment groups, *p* value < 0.05 considered significant (* $p < 0.05$, ** $p < 0.01$, *** $p < 0.001$).

3. Discussion

C. hystrix has been reported to possess many biological activities. In this experiment, we extracted *C. hystrix* leaf by the sequential maceration method using lower polar solvent to higher polar solvent (hexane, ethyl acetate, and 95% ethanol). Higher yield was obtained from the ethanolic extract compared to crude hexane and ethyl acetate extract. The MTT assay showed that crude *C. hystrix* hexane extract had higher efficiency in reducing MDA-MB-231 cell viability compared to the two other crude extracts, while the two pure compounds showed similar toxicity on MDA-MB-231 cell viability. Moreover, TLC fingerprints of crude *C. hystrix* hexane extract showed more trace of compounds compared to other two extracts with the trace of citronellol and citronellal could be identified at similar retention factor (R_f) (Figure S4). A previous study reported that crude ethyl acetate and crude ethanolic extract showed a higher effect against HeLa cells compared to crude hexane extract [21]. Doxorubicin is an anticancer agent that is widely used in cancer treatments. It acts as an anti-topoisomerase 2, which prevents DNA from replication [22]. We used doxorubicin as a drug control in all experiments.

Crude *C. hystrix* hexane extract was selected for chemical constituent analysis by GC-MS. Results indicated that terpenoids comprised the most compounds identified from *C. hystrix* leaf extract, while citronellal (0.67%) and citronellol (1.42%) of *C. hystrix* leaf crude hexane extract from the GC chromatogram appeared at retention times of 10.75 min and 12.85 min, respectively.

We then tested the effect of crude hexane extract, citronellol, and citronellal on the proliferation of MDA-MB-231 breast cancer cells. Results showed that crude hexane extract significantly reduced cell growth rate compared to the non-treated group. Anti-proliferative effects of *C. hystrix* were also reported in previous studies on leukemic cell lines [23] and on HeLa cervical cancer cells [21], while the anti-proliferative effect on MDA-MB-231 cells was also significant under treatments of both citronellol and citronellal. A previous study reported that citronellal reduced proliferation in Huh7 hepatocellular carcinoma cells [18], while citronellol inhibited non-small cell lung carcinoma A-549 cells [24]. Further experiments were performed to support the results of pre-existing anti-proliferative effects of both crude hexane extract and the two pure compounds. Clonogenic assay was performed to mimic cancer growth from single mutated cells to form cancer cell colonies or tumor mass. In the control group, MDA-MB-231 cells grew and formed cell colonies within 15 days of incubation. However, in the treatment groups, crude hexane extract, citronellol, and citronellal significantly reduced the number of colonies and inhibited colony formation at higher doses. Bergamottin was also found to inhibit colonies forming in PANC-1 human pancreas cancer [15]. Surviving under a tough environment with highly proliferative and migrative abilities are keys for successful cancer development or metastasis. Therefore, decreasing these two factors could be a suitable strategy to prevent early metastasis of the cancer. To test this hypothesis, wound scratch migration assay was conducted to study the effects of crude hexane extract, citronellol, and citronellal on cell migration. Results indicated that the treatments groups slowed down cell migration into wound areas in a dose and time dependent manner. Cell cycle analysis and apoptosis assay were performed to better understand whether the anti-proliferative and anti-migrative effects of crude hexane extract, citronellol, and citronellal were linked to these events. Results showed that a significant number of MDA-MB-231 cancer cells were arrested at the G0/G1 phase by *C. hystrix* crude hexane extract. Cells treated with citronellol and citronellal accumulated at the G2/M phase in the same way as treatment by doxorubicin. However, *C. hystrix* leaf extract showed different effects on the Molt-4 cell line by inducing cell cycle arrest at the G2/M phase [14]. Citronellol was also reported to induce lung cancer NCI-H1299 cell cycle arrest at the G0/G1 phase [19].

Results indicated a significant number of apoptotic cells under treatments of crude hexane extract, citronellol, and citronellal, while morphological changes as chromatin condensation and swelling were seen under the treatment groups. To help define a support mechanism for cell apoptosis, the levels of genes and proteins involved were analyzed using RT-qPCR and Western blot techniques. Results proved that levels of the *Bcl-2* gene and protein expression decreased under the treatment group, while the *Bax* gene and protein expression increased in intensity. During apoptosis, cleavage of DNA by endonuclease occurs after the activation of caspase-3 [25]. Results from Western blot analysis clearly demonstrated the activation of caspase-3 through decreasing density of total caspase-3 in the treated groups compared to the control and increasing the intensity of cleaved-caspase-3 protein, indicating activation of the caspase-dependent apoptosis pathway. The induction of apoptosis in MDA-MB-231 cells by the treated groups was probably activated by the caspase-dependent apoptosis pathway through inhibition of anti-apoptotic protein Bcl-2, leading to an increase of pro-apoptotic Bax protein activity. Bax protein mediated the pore formation complex at the outer membrane of mitochondria and consequentially triggered the release of cytochrome C, leading to the activation of caspase 3 protein. The effect of doxorubicin inducing apoptosis through the caspase-dependent apoptosis pathway was also reported [22]. Bergamottin, a compound identified in *C. hystrix*, induced apoptosis in human pancreas cancer cells PANC-1 by inhibiting the Akt/mTOR signaling pathway, leading to inhibition of cell survival, proliferation, and migration [15]. However, further research is necessary to better understand the mechanism behind cell cycle arrest to reduce cell migration. Animal model experiments should also be launched to enhance drug development of *C. hystrix* leaf extract and its bioactive compounds citronellol and citronellal.

4. Materials and Methods

4.1. Chemicals and Reagents

β-Citronellol, citronellal (analytical standard grade), and doxorubicin were purchased from Sigma-Aldrich, Inc., St. Louis, MO, USA, and stored at 4 °C. Dimethyl sulphoxide (DMSO) was used to dissolve the crude extracts and doxorubicin was dissolved with deionized water.

4.2. Plant Materials and Extraction Process

C. hystrix leaf fine powder was received from Khaolaor Laboratories Co., Ltd., Nakhon Pathom, Thailand (COA no. 250818) and crude extracts were obtained using the sequential maceration method. Finely powdered leaves (500 mg) were extracted with 1000 mL of hexane and stirred continuously for 3 days at room temperature. The mixture was then filtered and evaporated using a rotary evaporator to give crude *C. hystrix* hexane extract. The maceration procedure was repeated three times. The marc was further extracted with ethyl acetate and 95% ethanol using the same procedure. The filtrates obtained were evaporated and stored at −20 °C until required for use.

4.3. Cell Culture

MDA-MB-231 cell line (ATCC® HTB-26™ATCC) was maintained in Dulbecco's Modified Eagle Medium (DMEM; Gibco™; Thermo Fisher Scientific, Inc., Waltham, MA, USA) with 10% fetal bovine serum (FBS; Gibco™; Thermo Fisher Scientific, Inc., Waltham, MA, USA) and 1% of antibiotic-antimycotic (amphotericin B, penicillin, streptomycin) (Gibco™; Thermo Fisher Scientific, Inc., Waltham, MA, USA) at 37 °C, CO_2 5%.

4.4. Human Monocyte Isolation

Human monocytes were isolated from fresh buffy coat by Ficoll-Paque™ (Sigma-Aldrich, Inc.) using the density gradient centrifugation method. Human monocyte-derived macrophages were obtained by culturing the freshly isolated monocytes in RPMI-1640 medium (Gibco™; Thermo Fisher Scientific, Inc., Waltham, MA, USA) with 10% FBS incubated at 37 °C, CO_2 5% for one week before performing the experiments. Buffy coat was obtained from the Blood Bank, Naresuan University Hospital, Phitsanulok, Thailand. Ethics approval was obtained from the Human Ethics Committee of Naresuan University (IRB no. 0945/62).

4.5. Gas Chromatography-Mass Spectrometry Analysis (GC-MS)

The analysis of volatile compounds in crude hexane extract from *C. hystrix* leaf powder was performed using a Hewlett Packard Gas Chromatograph model 6890 (Agilent Technologies, Palo Alto, CA, USA) equipped with a mass selective detector. Crude hexane extract (50 mg/mL) was prepared by dissolving in hexane and then injected into GC-MS system. Volatile compounds in sample were separated using silica capillary Hewlett Packard HP-5 (5% phenyl methyl siloxane) column (30 m × 0.25 mm i.d., 0.25 μm film thickness). High-purity helium was used as the carrier gas with constant flow rate at 13.7 mL/min. Initial injector temperature was set at 250 °C with split ratio mode at ratio 10:1 and 1 μL injector volume. The oven temperature was started at 70 °C for 3 min, then increased to 280 °C (5 °C/min) and held for 20 min. Transfer temperature was set at 280 °C and the mass detection ranges were set from 50 to 700 amu in full scan. Retention indices (RIs) were determined by analyzing a solution containing a homologous series of n-alkanes (C_8–C_{32}) under the same chromatographic conditions and then calculated as described by van Den Dool and Dec. Kratz [26]. Identification of the volatile components was performed by computer matching of their recorded mass spectra fragmentation patterns with those stored in the Wiley 7n MS spectral library. Further identification was made by comparison of their mass spectra and their RIs relative to n-alkanes with those of the National Institute of Standards and Technology (NIST) Chemistry WebBook [27,28] or with previously published data. The presence of citronellol and citronellal in the extract was also confirmed by analyzing authentic standards under the same chromatographic conditions. Relative contents of each component in the sample were also calculated based on the normalization of peak areas as the percentage of total detected volatile components.

4.6. Cell Viability MTT Assay

MDA-MB-231 cells were plated in 96-well plates at density of 10^4 cells/well and 5×10^4 for human monocyte derived macrophages cells/well. Cells were treated by various concentrations of each crude extracts, citronellol, citronellal for 24 h, and 48 h for doxorubicin. All treatments were then removed, and cells were then washed by phosphate saline buffer (PBS). Culture medium was used as vehicle control. 0.5 mg/mL of 3-(4,5-dimethylthiazol-2-yl)-2,5-diphenyl tetrazolium bromide salt (MTT) from Thermo Fischer Scientific (Waltham, MA, USA) was introduced to cells with 3 h of incubation. The MTT was discarded, and the dye was solubilized by 100 μL of DMSO. Absorbances of the dissolved tetrazolium salt was measured at 570 nm by ELISA microplate reader (PerkinElmer, Inc., Waltham, MA, USA). The IC50 value was generated by dose-response curves using GraphPad Prism 7.

4.7. Identification Effect of Crude Hexane, Citronellol, and Citronellal on Cell Proliferation

MDA-MB-231 cells were seeded at a density of 2×10^4 cells/well and treated with 50, 100, and 150 μg/mL crude hexane extract, 0.5 and 1 nM of citronellol and citronellal, and 0.5 μM doxorubicin for 24 h and 48 h. Cells treat with culture medium only was used as vehicle control. Cell viability was measured at 24 h and 48 h to represent the growth of the cells.

4.8. Clonogenic Assay

Cells were seeded at a density of 500 cells/well in 6-well plates for 24 h. Different concentrations of crude hexane extract, citronellol, citronellal, and doxorubicin were treated on cells for 24 h. Cells treated with culture medium only were used as vehicle control. Treated cells were washed by PBS and then cultured in culture medium for 10 days with medium replacement every 3 days. Cells were washed twice with PBS and fixed with 10% neutral buffer formalin for 30 min before fixing by 0.5% crystal violet for 1 h. Pictures of colonies were captured using a Canon macro lens 50 mm/f1.8 STM. The photos were converted to 8-bit greyscale images. Numbers of colonies of MDA-MB-231 cells were counted by Colony Area plugin using ImageJ 1.52a software.

4.9. Wound Scratch Migration Assay

MDA-MB-231 cells were seeded and cultured to confluence. SPLScar™ cell scraper (SPL Life Sciences, Gyeonggi-do, Korea) was used to create wound areas. Cells were washed twice by PBS to remove cell debris and floating cells before treatment with various concentrations of crude hexane extract, citronellol, citronellal, and doxorubicin. Cells treated with culture medium only were used as vehicle control. Cell migration into the wound areas was then observed under an inverted microscope (Zeiss Microscopy, Oberkochen, Germany) with objective 10× magnification. Wound closed areas were quantified by MRI_Wound_Healing_Tool plugin using ImageJ 1.52a software.

4.10. Cell Cycle Analysis

A total of 200 μg/mL crude hexane extract, 1 nM citronellol and citronellal, and 0.5 μM doxorubicin were treated with MDA-MB-231 cells for 24 h. Cells treat with culture medium only was used as vehicle control. Cells were harvested, transferred into a 1.5 mL microtube, and washed twice by cold PBS. Cells were then fixed with 1 mL of 70% ethanol for 5 h. Two hundred microliters of cell suspension (10^6 cells/mL) were washed with 250 μL of PBS and 200 μL of Muse™ cell cycle reagent and then incubated in the dark for 20 min at room temperature. The apoptotic cells were analyzed using a Muse™ cell analyzer (Merck, Darmstadt, Germany).

4.11. Apoptosis Analysis

Crude hexane extract, citronellol, citronellal, or doxorubicin were treated on MDA-MB-231 cells for 24 h. Cells treat with culture medium only was used as vehicle control. Cells were harvested and transferred into a 1.5 mL microtube and washed twice in cold PBS. Then, the cells were resuspended in 1% BSA and 100 μL of Muse™ Annexin V and dead cell reagent (Merck, Darmstadt, Germany) were added to 100 μL of cell suspension (5×10^5 cells/mL) and incubated in the dark for 20 min at room temperature. The apoptotic cells were analyzed using Muse™ cell analyzer, gated on Annexin V-FITC positive cells and 7-AAD positive cells.

4.12. Hoechst 33342 Staining

Cells were cultured on cover slides for 24 h and then treated with crude hexane extract, citronellol, citronellal, or doxorubicin for 24 h. Cells treated with culture medium only were used as vehicle control. The cells were washed twice with PBS and fixed with 4% formaldehyde for 15 min at room temperature. After washing twice with PBS, the cells were permeabilized with 0.15% Triton-X 100 for 15 min at room temperature, followed by washing twice with PBS. An aliquot of 4 μg/mL of Hoechst 33342 solution was used to stain cells for 10 min in the dark at room temperature. Then, 70% glycerol was used as an anti-fade solution. Cover slides were then mounted on the slides and sealed with nail polisher. DNA fragmented or chromatin condensed cells were observed under a fluorescence microscope (Zeiss Microscopy, Oberkochen, Germany) with objective 40× magnification.

4.13. RT-qPCR

Crude hexane extract, citronellol, citronellal, or doxorubicin were treated on MDA-MB-231 cells for 24 h. Cells treated with culture medium only were used as vehicle control. Total RNA was extracted from MDA-MB-231 cells using Ribozol™ RNA extraction reagent kits (AMRESCO, VWR Life Science, OH, USA). Briefly, cDNA synthesis was performed using Tetro cDNA synthesis kits (Bioline Reagents Ltd., London, UK). Real-time PCR was carried out using SensiFAST™ SYBR No-ROX kits (Bioline Reagents Ltd., London, UK). The initial denaturing temperature started from 95 °C at 1 min, with 45 cycles of 15 s denaturation followed by 30 s of annealing and elongation at 60 °C. The whole reaction was performed in a CFX96 Touch Real-Time PCR Detection System (Bio-Rad Laboratories, Hercules, CA, USA). Primer sequences of β-actin, Bcl-2, and Bax were obtained from previous studies and checked by the BLAST tool from the National Institute of Health (Table 2). All samples were performed in triplicate and levels of gene expression were normalized to the level of β-actin as the reference gene. The relative amount of target gene expression was calculated using $2^{-\Delta\Delta CT}$ [29].

Table 2. Primer sequences.

Target Genes	Primer Sequences	References
β-actin	Fw: 5′-AGAAAATCTGGCACCACACC-3′ Rw: 5′-CCATCTCTTGCTCGAAGTCC-3′	[30]
Bcl-2	Fw: 5′-GATGTGATGCCTCTGCGAAG-3′ Rw: 5′-CATGCTGATGTCTCTGGAATCT-3′	[31]
Bax	Fw: 5′-GGTTGTCGCCCTTTTCTA-3′ Rw: 5′-CGGAGGAAGTCCAATGTC-3′	[31]

4.14. Western Blot Analysis

Crude hexane extract, citronellol, citronellal, or doxorubicin were treated on MDA-MB-231 cells for 24 h. Cells treated with culture medium only were used as vehicle control. RIPA lysis buffer

(Sigma-Aldrich, Inc.) containing 1% of protease and phosphatase inhibitor cocktail (Sigma-Aldrich, Inc.) was used to extract total protein. Proteins from cell lysates were quantified using Pierce™ Coomassie (Bradford) protein assay kit (Thermo Fisher Scientific, Inc.) by measuring absorbance at 595 nm. An aliquot of 50 µg of total protein from cell lysates was introduced to 12% SDS-PAGE and then transferred to PDVF membranes. Five percent skim milk in TBST was used as blocking buffer for 1 h at room temperature. Primary antibody against proteins β-actin, Bcl-2, Bax, pro-caspase-3, and cleaved-caspase-3 from (Santa Cruz Biotechnology, Inc., Dallas, TX, USA) were probed on membranes (1:1000 dilution) and shaken overnight at 4 °C. After washing three times for 5 min each with TBST, the membranes were incubated with HRP-conjugated anti-mouse IgG (Santa Cruz Biotechnology) in 1% BSA-TBST (1:10,000 dilution) at room temperature for 1 h, followed by washing three times. Protein bands were detected by adding horse radish peroxidase chemiluminescence substrate and quantified by Chemi Doc XRS Imaging System (Bio-Rad Laboratories, Inc., Hercules, CA, USA).

4.15. Data Analysis

All the experiments were performed in triplicate and data were expressed as means ± SEM. One-way ANOVA with Dunnett's test was used to analyze degree of significance between controls and samples. p value < 0.05 was considered significant.

5. Conclusions

Our results demonstrated that crude *C. hystrix* hexane extract and its compounds citronellol and citronellal showed anticancer effects by inducing apoptosis in the triple negative breast cancer MDA-MB-231 cell line through inhibition of the anti-apoptotic protein Bcl-2, leading to activation of the pro-apoptotic Bax protein and inducing the downstream caspase-dependent apoptosis pathway by activating caspase-3 protein. Crude hexane extract, citronellol, and citronellal downregulated the active state of the cells and this decreased their proliferation rate and ability to migrate and survive under harsh environmental conditions (Figure 9).

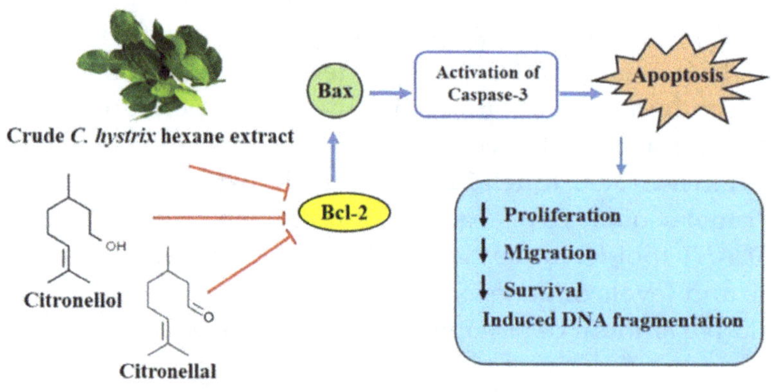

Figure 9. Inhibition of Bcl-2 protein in MDA-MB-231 cells by *C. hystrix*, citronellal, and citronellol leading to activation of caspase dependent apoptotic pathway.

Supplementary Materials
Figure S1: Total ion chromatogram of crude hexane extract, Figure S2: IC50 value of treatments on human monocyte derived macrophages, Figure S3: Full length of Western blot analysis, Figure S4: TLC fingerprints of crude *C. hystrix* hexane extract, ethyl acetate extract, ethanolic extract, and two standard compounds (citronellol and citronellal).

Author Contributions: This research was contributed by conceptualization, K.U. and N.S.; methodology, Y.H., K.U., and K.D.; validation, K.D. and Y.T.; writing—original draft preparation, Y.H.; writing—review and editing, K.U. and N.S.; visualization, P.P.; supervision, K.U.; funding acquisition, K.U.; Project administration. All authors have read and agreed to the published version of the manuscript.

Acknowledgments: Author would like to acknowledge the Royal Scholarship under Her Royal Highness Princess Maha Chakri Sirindhorn Education Project to the Kingdom of Cambodia for Yathsoeung Ho during study in Master's degree of Biomedical Sciences, Faculty of Allied Health Sciences, Naresuan University.

Abbreviations

C. hystrix	*Citrus hystrix* DC.
ER	Estrogen receptor
GC-MS	Gas chromatography-Mass spectrometry
Her-2	Human epidermal receptor 2
PR	Progesterone receptor
RA	Retention areas
RI	Retention indices
RT	Retention times
TNBC	Triple Negative Breast Cancer

References

1. Hammond, M.E.H.; Hayes, D.F.; Dowsett, M.; Allred, D.C.; Hagerty, K.L.; Badve, S.; Fitzgibbons, P.L.; Francis, G.; Goldstein, N.S.; Hayes, M.; et al. American Society of Clinical Oncology/College of American Pathologists Guideline Recommendations for Immunohistochemical Testing of Estrogen and Progesterone Receptors in Breast Cancer (Unabridged Version). *Arch. Pathol. Lab. Med.* **2010**, *134*, e48–e72. [CrossRef] [PubMed]
2. Wolff, A.C.; Hammond, M.E.H.; Hicks, D.G.; Dowsett, M.; McShane, L.M.; Allison, K.H.; Allred, D.C.; Bartlett, J.M.S.; Bilous, M.; Fitzgibbons, P.; et al. Recommendations for Human Epidermal Growth Factor Receptor 2 Testing in Breast Cancer: American Society of Clinical Oncology/College of American Pathologists Clinical Practice Guideline Update. *J. Clin. Oncol.* **2013**, *31*, 3997–4013. [CrossRef] [PubMed]
3. Garrido-Castro, A.C.; Lin, N.U.; Polyak, K. Insights into Molecular Classifications of Triple-Negative Breast Cancer: Improving Patient Selection for Treatment. *Cancer Discov.* **2019**, *9*, 176. [CrossRef]
4. Gonçalves, H., Jr.; Guerra, M.R.; Duarte Cintra, J.R.; Fayer, V.A.; Brum, I.V.; Bustamante Teixeira, M.T. Survival Study of Triple-Negative and Non-Triple-Negative Breast Cancer in a Brazilian Cohort. *Clin. Med. Insights Oncol.* **2018**, *12*. [CrossRef] [PubMed]
5. Nedeljkovic, M.; Damjanovic, A. Mechanisms of Chemotherapy Resistance in Triple-Negative Breast Cancer-How We Can Rise to the Challenge. *Cells* **2019**, *8*. [CrossRef] [PubMed]
6. Saklani, A.; Kutty, S.K. Plant-derived compounds in clinical trials. *Drug Discov. Today* **2008**, *13*, 161–171. [CrossRef]
7. Vrignaud, P.; Semiond, D.; Benning, V.; Beys, E.; Bouchard, H.; Gupta, S. Preclinical profile of cabazitaxel. *Drug Des. Dev. Ther.* **2014**, *8*, 1851–1867. [CrossRef]
8. Agouillal, K.; Hagop, M.; O'Brien, S.; Cortes, J. Homoharringtonine/omacetaxine mepesuccinate: The long and winding road to food and drug administration approval. *Clin. Lymphoma Myeloma Leuk.* **2013**, *13*, 530–533. [CrossRef]
9. Agouillal, F.; Taher, Z.M.; Moghrani, H.; Nasrallah, N.; El Enshasy, H. A Review of Genetic Taxonomy, Biomolecules Chemistry and Bioactivities of Citrus hystrix DC. *Biosci. Biotechnol. Res. Asia* **2017**, *14*, 285–305. [CrossRef]
10. Butryee, C.; Sungpuag, P.; Chitchumroonchokchai, C. Effect of processing on the flavonoid content and antioxidant capacity of Citrus hystrix leaf. *Int. J. Food Sci. Nutr.* **2009**, *60*, 162–174. [CrossRef]
11. Dilla Dertyasasa, E.; Anindito Sri Tunjung, W. Volatile Organic Compounds of Kaffir Lime (Citrus hystrix DC.) Leaves Fractions and their Potency as Traditional Medicine. *Biosci. Biotechnol. Res. Asia* **2017**, *14*, 1235–1250. [CrossRef]

12. Salguero, C.P. Kaffir lime. In *A Thai Herbal Traditional Recipes for Health and Harmony*; Barton, L., Ed.; Findhorn Press: Findhorn Forres, UK, 2003; p. 112.
13. Tunjung, W.; Cinatl, J.; Michaelis, M.; Mark Smales, C. Anti-Cancer Effect of Kaffir Lime (Citrus Hystrix DC) Leaf Extract in Cervical Cancer and Neuroblastoma Cell Lines. *Procedia Chem.* **2015**, *14*, 465–468. [CrossRef]
14. Utthawang, W.; Ampasavate, W.; Okonogi, S.; Rungrojsakul, M.; Chiampanichayakul, S.; Tima, S.; Anuchapreeda, S. Low doses of partially purified fraction of kaffir lime (Citrus hystrix DC.) leaf extract induce cell death in Molt4 cells. *J. Assoc. Med. Sci.* **2017**, *50*, 27–37. [CrossRef]
15. Sun, S.; Phrutivorapongkul, A.; Dya Fita, D.; Balachandran, C.; Awale, S. Chemical Constituents of Thai Citrus hystrix and Their Antiausterity Activity against the PANC-1 Human Pancreatic Cancer Cell Line. *J. Nat. Prod.* **2018**, *81*. [CrossRef] [PubMed]
16. Sato, A.; Asano, K.; Sato, T. The Chemical Composition of Citrus Hystrix DC (Swangi). *J. Essent. Oil Res.* **1990**, *2*, 179–183. [CrossRef]
17. Stone, S.; Vasconcellos, F.A.; Lenardao, E.; Do Amaral, R.; Jacob, R.; Leite, F. Evaluation of potential use of Cymbopogon sp. essential oils, (R)-citronellal and N-citronellylamine in cancer chemotherapy. *Int. J. Appl. Res. Nat. Prod.* **2013**, *6*, 11–15.
18. Maßberg, D.; Simon, A.; Häussinger, D.; Keitel, V.; Gisselmann, G.; Conrad, H.; Hatt, H. Monoterpene (−)-citronellal affects hepatocarcinoma cell signaling via an olfactory receptor. *Arch. Biochem. Biophys.* **2015**, *566*, 100–109. [CrossRef]
19. Yu, W.-N.; Lai, Y.-J.; Ma, J.-W.; Ho, C.-T.; Hung, S.-W.; Chen, Y.-H.; Chen, C.-T.; Kao, J.-Y.; Way, T.-D. Citronellol Induces Necroptosis of Human Lung Cancer Cells via TNF-α Pathway and Reactive Oxygen Species Accumulation. *In Vivo* **2019**, *33*, 1193–1201. [CrossRef]
20. Yoshida, N.; Koizumi, M.; Adachi, I.; Kawakami, J. Inhibition of P-glycoprotein-mediated transport by terpenoids contained in herbal medicines and natural products. *Food Chem. Toxicol.* **2006**, *44*, 2033–2039. [CrossRef]
21. Wijayanti, N.; Tunjung, W.; Setyawati, Y. Cytotoxicity and Apoptosis Induction by Kaffir Lime Leaves Extract (*Citrus hystrix* DC.) In HeLa Cells Culture (Human Cervical Cancer Cell line). *KnE Life Sci.* **2015**, *2*, 631. [CrossRef]
22. Pilco-Ferreto, N.; Calaf, G. Influence of doxorubicin on apoptosis and oxidative stress in breast cancer cell lines. *Int. J. Oncol.* **2016**, *49*. [CrossRef] [PubMed]
23. Anuchapreeda, S.; Chueahongthong, F.; Viriyaadhammaa, N.; Panyajai, P.; Anzawa, R.; Tima, S.; Ampasavate, C.; Saiai, A.; Rungrojsakul, M.; Usuki, T.; et al. Antileukemic Cell Proliferation of Active Compounds from Kaffir Lime (*Citrus hystrix*) Leaves. *Molecules* **2020**, *25*, 1300. [CrossRef] [PubMed]
24. Song, W.; Liu, X.Y.; Shi, Y. Citronellol terpenoid inhibits cancer cell proliferation and induces apoptosis in non-small cell lung carcinoma. *Lat. Am. J. Pharm.* **2015**, *34*, 1652–1657.
25. Alenzi, F. Links between apoptosis, proliferation and the cell cycle. *Br. J. Biomed. Sci.* **2004**, *61*, 99–102. [CrossRef]
26. Vandendool, H.; Kratz, P.D. A Generalization Of The Retention Index Sytsem Icluding Linear Temperature Programmed Gas-Liquid Partition Chromatography. *J. Chromatogr.* **1963**, *11*, 463–471. [CrossRef]
27. Babushok, V.I.; Linstrom, P.J.; Reed, J.J.; Zenkevich, I.G.; Brown, R.L.; Mallard, W.G.; Stein, S.E. Development of a database of gas chromatographic retention properties of organic compounds. *J. Chromatogr. A* **2007**, *1157*, 414–421. [CrossRef]
28. Linstrom, P.; Mallard, G. The NIST Chemistry WebBook: A chemical data resource on the Internet. *J. Chem. Eng. Data* **2001**, *46*. [CrossRef]
29. Razak, N.A.; Abu, N.; Ho, W.Y.; Zamberi, N.R.; Tan, S.W.; Alitheen, N.B.; Long, K.; Yeap, S.K. Cytotoxicity of eupatorin in MCF-7 and MDA-MB-231 human breast cancer cells via cell cycle arrest, anti-angiogenesis and induction of apoptosis. *Sci. Rep.* **2019**, *9*, 1514. [CrossRef]

30. Khan, S.A.; Tyagi, M.; Sharma, A.K.; Barreto, S.G.; Sirohi, B.; Ramadwar, M.; Shrikhande, S.V.; Gupta, S. Cell-type specificity of β-actin expression and its clinicopathological correlation in gastric adenocarcinoma. *World J. Gastroenterol.* **2014**, *20*, 12202–12211. [CrossRef]

31. Golestani Eimani, B.; Sanati, M.H.; Houshmand, M.; Ataei, M.; Akbarian, F.; Shakhssalim, N. Expression and prognostic significance of bcl-2 and bax in the progression and clinical outcome of transitional bladder cell carcinoma. *Cell J.* **2014**, *15*, 356–363.

2

Dereplication of Natural Products with Antimicrobial and Anticancer Activity from Brazilian Cyanobacteria

Tania Keiko Shishido [1,2,†], Rafael Vicentini Popin [1,†], Jouni Jokela [1], Matti Wahlsten [1], Marli Fatima Fiore [3], David P. Fewer [1], Lars Herfindal [4] and Kaarina Sivonen [1,*]

1 Department of Microbiology, University of Helsinki, Viikinkaari 9, FI-00014 Helsinki, Finland; tania.shishido@helsinki.fi (T.K.S.); rafael.popin@helsinki.fi (R.V.P.); jouni.jokela@helsinki.fi (J.J.); matti.wahlsten@helsinki.fi (M.W.); david.fewer@helsinki.fi (D.P.F.)
2 Institute of Biotechnology, University of Helsinki, Viikinkaari 5D, FI-00014 Helsinki, Finland
3 Center for Nuclear Energy in Agriculture, University of São Paulo, Avenida Centenário 303, 13400-970 Piracicaba, São Paulo, Brazil; fiore@cena.usp.br
4 Centre for Pharmacy, Department of Clinical Science, University of Bergen, 5020 Bergen, Norway; lars.herfindal@uib.no
* Correspondence: kaarina.sivonen@helsinki.fi
† These authors contributed equally to this work.

Abstract: Cyanobacteria are photosynthetic organisms that produce a large diversity of natural products with interesting bioactivities for biotechnological and pharmaceutical applications. Cyanobacterial extracts exhibit toxicity towards other microorganisms and cancer cells and, therefore, represent a source of potentially novel natural products for drug discovery. We tested 62 cyanobacterial strains isolated from various Brazilian biomes for antileukemic and antimicrobial activities. Extracts from 39 strains induced selective apoptosis in acute myeloid leukemia (AML) cancer cell lines. Five of these extracts also exhibited antifungal and antibacterial activities. Chemical and dereplication analyses revealed the production of nine known natural products. Natural products possibly responsible for the observed bioactivities and five unknown, chemically related chlorinated compounds present only in Brazilian cyanobacteria were illustrated in a molecular network. Our results provide new information on the vast biosynthetic potential of cyanobacteria isolated from Brazilian environments.

Keywords: natural products; mass spectrometry; leukemia; antifungal; antibacterial; cyanotoxins; *Nostoc*

Key Contribution: The molecular network constructed using mass spectrometry data indicates natural products potentially involved in anticancer and antimicrobial activities and unknown chlorinated molecules to be characterized.

---

1. Introduction

Cyanobacteria are photosynthetic bacteria commonly found in diverse aquatic and terrestrial environments [1]. They produce a large range of secondary metabolites (natural products) that are predominantly produced to gain evolutionary advantages, such as adaptation to the surrounding environment or as a defense mechanism, rather than being part of primary metabolism (i.e., growth, development, or reproduction) [2–4]. Many cyanobacterial natural products are synthesized by non-ribosomal peptide synthetases (NRPS), polyketide synthase (PKS), or hybrid NRPS-PKS (NRPS/PKS) [5]. These molecules have diverse applications in pharmacology, biotechnology, and bioenergy production [6–9].

Cyanobacterial natural products have a diverse array of biological activities and properties [10–12]. Toxins and protease inhibitors are amongst the most commonly reported [13–16]. Antibiotic activity is frequently found in cyanobacterial extracts, but the active compounds have seldom been determined [17–19]. Cyanobacteria are also a promising source of anticancer compounds [20,21]. These include the elastase inhibitor lyngbyastatin [22], the microtubulin inhibitor curacin A [23], the sodium-channel blocker kalkitoxin [24,25], and the antitumor cryptophycin [26]. Although the anticancer activity of cyanobacterial compounds has not been thoroughly investigated, some studies point to diverse implications in apoptosis [27].

Several cyanobacteria produce antileukemic compounds [21–26,28]. Approximately 80% of the cases of acute leukemia in adults in the United States are acute myeloid leukemia (AML). Over 29,000 cases of AML were recorded in Europe between 1995 and 2002 [29]. The treatment for this disease is currently based on chemotherapy, and long-term prognosis for such patients is poor [30]. The discovery and development of new drugs to treat AML are necessary due to emerging AML drug resistance and the harsh side effects of the current treatments [31]. Marine cyanobacteria are a rich source of anticancer compounds, but cyanobacteria isolated from underexplored environments are promising alternative source of drug leads for drug discovery [9,27,32,33].

Brazilian biomes are characterized by unusually high biodiversity, and new cyanobacterial taxa are frequently described from these biomes [34–39]. Strains isolated from these biomes have antimicrobial and anticancer activities [40–42]. New natural products are continuously described from cyanobacteria isolated from these habitats [40,43,44]. Metabolic profiling has increasingly been used to visualize and organize the vast chemical diversity and large repertoire of molecules synthesized by microorganisms [45]. This approach enables the assessment of groups of compounds with analogous biosynthetic origins and structures, which may facilitate the discovery of novel compounds [46].

In this study, we screened cyanobacterial isolates from Brazilian habitats for natural products and tested the antileukemic and antimicrobial activity of their culture extracts. Furthermore, we constructed a molecular network to expand the current knowledge of their chemical diversity.

2. Results

2.1. *Cyanobacterial Isolates*

A total of 62 isolates from diverse biomes from Brazil were tested for antimicrobial and anticancer activities (Table S1). A phylogenetic tree based on 16S rRNA gene was constructed in order to access the evolutionary history of these strains (Figure 1). The 62 isolates belong to 23 different genera spread among five different orders: Synechococcales, Oscillatoriales, Chroococcales, Chroococcidiopsidales, and Nostocales.

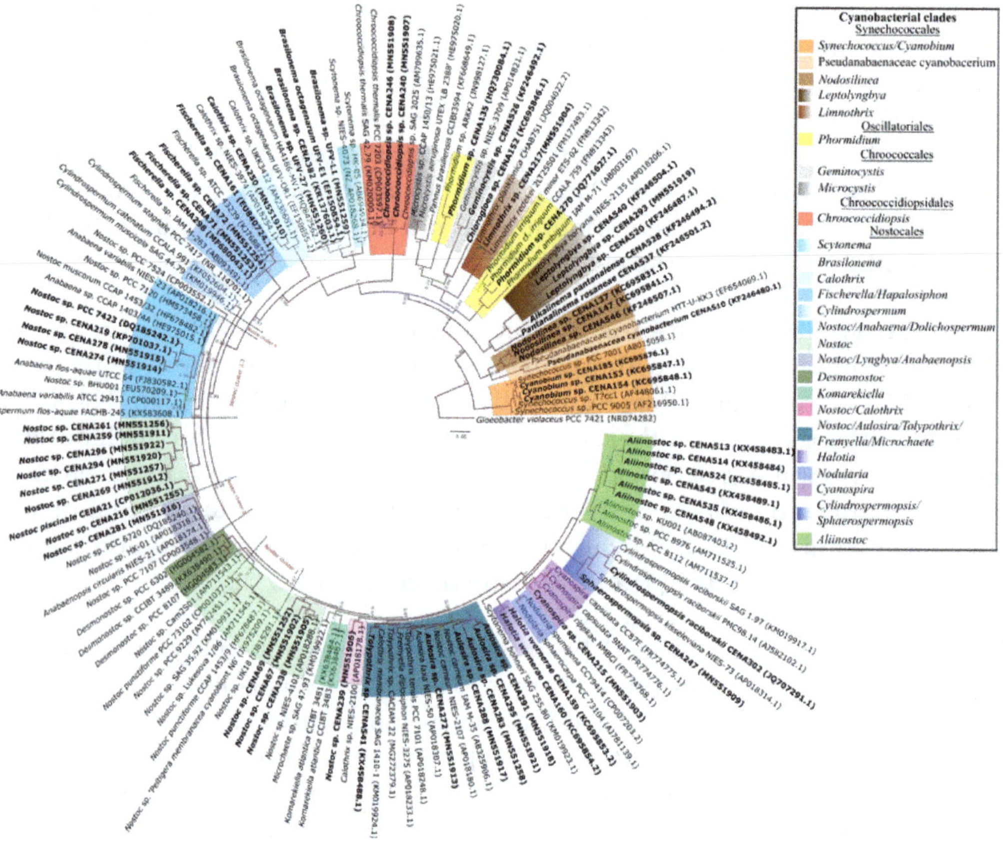

Figure 1. Evolutionary history based on 16S rRNA gene sequences of the 62 analyzed cyanobacterial strains (in bold) and 73 other strains: According to this Bayesian inference, the sequences formed diverse clades belonging to different orders. Accession numbers in NCBI are shown in parentheses.

2.2. *Bioactivity Screening*

Aqueous and organic cyanobacterial cell extracts were first tested for their cytotoxic activity against the human leukemia MOLM-13 cell line (Table S2). Two of the 62 aqueous extracts resulted in 70–90% cell death (CCIBt3594 and CENA185), while 11 were highly cytotoxic with 90–100% cell death (CENA69, 72, 161, 219, 270, 513, 514, 524, 535, 543, and 548). The organic extracts from the cyanobacteria were more potent, 13 samples induced 70–90% cell death (CENA21, 67, 137, 147, 152, 153, 154, 159, 160, 215, 216, 272, and 526), and 26 induced apoptosis in 90–100% of the cells (CCIBt3594; UFV-E1; UFV-L1; UFV-27; and CENA69, 71, 72, 135, 161, 185, 217, 219, 270, 283, 296, 298, 302, 382, 510, 513, 514, 524, 535, 541, 543, and 548). A dilution of the organic extracts to 3.99 mgDW·ml^{-1} (0.3%) revealed that two samples induced cell apoptosis in 70–90% of the cells (CENA69 and 382) and 13 samples induced apoptosis in 90–100% (CENA71, 72, 161, 185, 219, 270, 296, 298, 513, 514, 524, 535, and 548). The extracts that induced apoptosis between 70–90% of the MOLM-13 cells were diluted 10 times, and the extracts inducing over 90% cell death were diluted 10 and 100 times to further compare the cytotoxic potential. For the aqueous extracts, only *Nostoc* sp. CENA219 presented a moderate apoptosis rate (51%) at 100 times dilution. The organic extracts of *Aliinostoc* sp. CENA69 and CENA513 and *Fischerella* sp. CENA161 were highly cytotoxic (above 70%) towards MOLM-13 cells even at a concentration of 0.133 mgDW mL^{-1} (100-fold dilution).

The cyanobacterial extracts with the highest apoptosis induction of MOLM-13 cells were also tested for cytotoxicity towards the normal rat kidney epithelial NRK cell line (Table 1). By comparing the potency of normal and malignant cells, the test provided evidence for potential use as an anticancer compound. The strains *Fischerella* sp. CENA72, *Cyanobium* sp. CENA185, *Limnothrix* sp. CENA217, *Nostoc* sp. CENA296, and *Aliinostoc* sp. CENA524 showed particularly selective cytotoxicity towards MOLM-13 cells over NRK cells; these strains had an over nine-fold greater EC_{50} value for NRK than

MOLM-13 (Table 1). It is noteworthy that the organic extracts from *Cyanobium* sp. CENA185 and *Limnothrix* sp. CENA217 showed no apparent toxicity to NRK cells after 24 h (Figure S1). *Nostoc* sp. CENA69, *Fischerella* sp. CENA161, and *Aliinostoc* spp. CENA513 and CENA514 showed relatively smaller differences in cytotoxicity between the two cell lines as judged by EC_{50} values than the other strains.

Table 1. Comparison of inhibition caused by organic cyanobacterial extracts in rat kidney epithelial NRK and human leukemia MOLM-13 cell lines as measured by the area under the curve (AUC) of cells with normal nuclei and EC_{50}. See methods Section 5.3 for calculations of EC_{50} and AUC.

Cyanobacterial Strain	AUC					EC_{50}	
	NRK		MOLM-13		Ratio		
	Total Area	Std. Error	Total Area	Std. Error		NRK	MOLM-13
Nostoc sp. CENA69	63.01	2.902	26.61	4.412	2.4	0.098	0.054
Fischerella sp. CENA71 *	106.3	9.467	45.45	4.053	2.3	1.493	0.363
Fischerella sp. CENA72 *	164.4	14.78	52.32	9.073	3.1	3.129	0.201
Fischerella sp. CENA161	134.0	6.417	69.02	7.495	1.9	0.508	0.083
Cyanobium sp. CENA185	199.7	-	110.7	–	–§	>15#	1.590
Limnothrix sp. CENA217	198.6	1.033	137.7	3.028	–§	>15#	1.410
Nostoc sp. CENA296 *	172.5	15.93	96.91	4.076	1.8	11.26	1.212
Fischerella sp. CENA298	124.9	8.210	98.90	12.37	1.3	2.283	1.324
Aliinostoc sp. CENA513	129.2	6.390	53.58	5.328	2.4	0.491	0.087
Aliinostoc sp. CENA514 *	108.2	4.706	32.96	5.631	3.3	0.842	0.140
Aliinostoc sp. CENA524 *	159.6	4.367	65.36	4.124	2.4	6.012	0.620
Aliinostoc sp. CENA535	85.71	2.182	60.54	10.19	1.4	1.218	0.566

Range given due to missing data in intermediate toxicity (see Figure S1); * p-value < 0.0001 calculated using extra-sum-of-squares F test in GraphPad; # Cells were not affected with highest concentration tested. § Value could not be calculated due to a lack of activity in NRK cells.

Another method to evaluate drug selectivity for one cell over another is to calculate the area under the curve (AUC) of the dose-response curves (Table 1 and Figure S1). *Aliinostoc* sp. CENA514 has a large AUC ratio between NRK and MOLM-13 cell lines, which indicates that the concentrations needed to kill MOLM-13 AML cells will not harm nonmalignant NRK cells. The cell extract from *Nostoc* sp. CENA69 was toxic for both MOLM-13 and NRK cell lines (Figure 2 and Table 1). The low value of the half maximum effective concentration (EC_{50}) of *Nostoc* sp. CENA69 shows the high potency of this cell extract for both tested cell lines (Table 1).

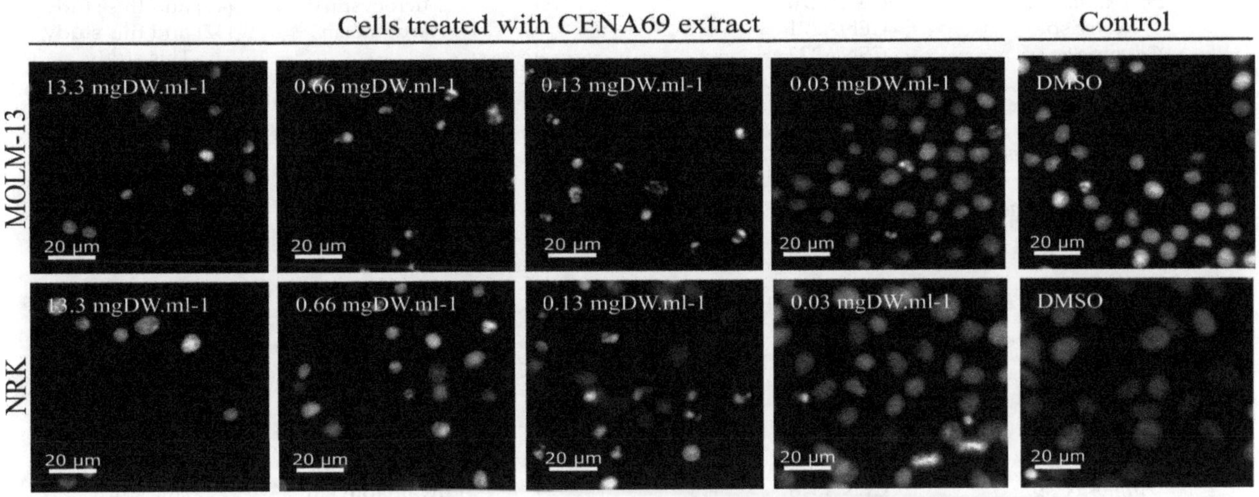

Figure 2. Cytotoxic cell extract from *Nostoc* sp. CENA69: Human leukemia MOLM-13 and rat kidney epithelial NRK cells in different concentrations of cyanobacterial organic extract (indicated as mg of dry weight (DW) of freeze-dried cell mass used per ml of cell suspension). DMSO: dimethyl sulfoxide (negative control). Note the appearance of pyknotic and hypercondenced chromatin in the cells treated with high concentration of CENA69 extract.

To identify possible antibacterial and antifungal activity, organic extracts obtained from cyanobacterial freeze-dried cells were also tested against *Staphylococcus aureus* and *Candida albicans* (Table 2, Files S1 and S2). *Fischerella* spp. CENA71, CENA72, CENA161, and CENA298 and *Aliinostoc* sp. CENA513 showed both antibacterial and antifungal activity. *Aliinostoc* spp. CENA514, CENA535, and CENA548 extracts had antifungal activity while CENA524 presented antibacterial activity.

Table 2. Summary of the antifungal (F), antibacterial (B), and anticancer (C) activities observed in the cyanobacterial crude extracts (see also Files S1 and S2). Bioactive cell extracts (+) showed inhibition zone in the antimicrobial assay and above 70% induction of apoptosis of MOLM-13 cell lines at the concentration of 13.3 mgDW mL^{-1}. Previously obtained information of the compounds produced by the studied strains are presented. Cyanobacterial extracts that induced apoptosis in less than 70% of MOLM-13 cells did not present inhibition halo in the antimicrobial assays or that were not previously described to produce a natural product were not included in this table. The use of sterile water may have influenced the susceptibility of fungal and bacterial cells.

Taxon	Strain	Activity			Compounds Detected	Reference
		F	B	C [a]		
Pannus brasiliense	CCIbt3594	–	–	+	–	This study
Nostoc piscinale	CENA21	–	–	+	–	This study
Nostoc sp.	CENA67	–	–	+ *	–	[42] and this study
Nostoc sp.	CENA69	–	–	+ *	–	[42] and this study
Fischerella sp.	CENA71	+	+	+	–	This study
Fischerella sp.	CENA72	+	+	+	–	This study
Oxynema sp.	CENA135	–	–	+ *	Microcystin, Saxitoxin	[41,42] and this study
Nodosilinea sp.	CENA137	–	–	+	–	this study
Nodosilinea sp.	CENA147	–	–	+	–	this study
Chlorogloea sp.	CENA152	–	–	+	–	this study
Cyanobium sp.	CENA153	–	–	+	Microcystin, Aeruginosin	[41,47] and this study
Cyanobium sp.	CENA154	–	–	+ *	Aeruginosin	[42,47] and this study
Halotia wernerae	CENA159	–	–	+	–	This study
Halotia wernerae	CENA160	–	–	+	–	This study
Fischerella sp.	CENA161	+	+	+	Microcystin	[48] and this study
Cyanobium sp.	CENA185	–	–	+	Microcystin	[41] and this study
Cyanospira sp.	CENA215	–	–	+	–	This study
Nostoc sp.	CENA216	–	–	+	–	This study
Limnothrix sp.	CENA217	–	–	+	–	This study
Nostoc sp.	CENA219	–	–	+	Hassallidin	[32] and this study
Phormidium sp.	CENA270	–	–	+	Microcystin	[49] and this study
Nostoc sp.	CENA271	–	–	–	Aeruginosin	[47] and this study
Gloeotrichia sp.	CENA272	–	–	+	–	This study
Calothrix sp.	CENA283	–	–	+	–	This study
Nostoc sp.	CENA296	–	–	+	–	This study
Fischerella sp.	CENA298	+	+	+	–	This study
Cylindrospermopsis raciborskii	CENA302	–	–	+	Saxitoxin	[50] and this study
Brasilonema sp.	CENA382	–	–	+	–	This study
Pseudanabaenaceae cyanobacterium	CENA510	–	–	+	–	This study
Aliinostoc sp.	CENA513	+	+	+	–	This study
Aliinostoc sp.	CENA514	+	–	+	–	This study
Aliinostoc sp.	CENA524	–	+	+	–	This study
Geminocystis sp.	CENA526	–	–	+	–	This study
Aliinostoc sp.	CENA535	+	–	+	Puwainaphycin	This study
Tolypothrix sp.	CENA541	–	–	+	–	This study
Aliinostoc sp.	CENA543	–	–	+	Nodularin, Anabaenopeptin, Pseudoaeruginosin	[11,43] and this study
Aliinostoc sp.	CENA548	+	–	+	Puwainaphycin	This study
Brasilonema octagenarum	UFV-E1	–	–	+	–	This study
Brasilonema sp.	UFV-L1	–	–	+	–	This study
Brasilonema sp.	UFV-27	–	–	+	–	This study

[a] Cytotoxic towards MOLM-13 cells (see Table 1).*Anticancer activity has also been previously observed [40].

2.3. Natural Products Produced by Brazilian Cyanobacteria

Cell extracts were analyzed using mass spectrometry, and a molecular network was constructed based on the MS/MS spectra of the detected compounds. Due to the size of the resulting network, only clusters containing potential new novel compounds detected exclusively in Brazilian cyanobacterial extracts and previously known natural products are presented in Figure 3. The complete network can be found in the Supplementary Materials (Figure S2). Cyanobacterial cell extracts from strains producing known compounds were included in the analysis to facilitate the dereplication of different compounds (Table S3). Puwainaphycins produced by *Aliinostoc* spp. CENA535 and CENA548 were detected using a dereplication tool (GNPS) (Figure S3; Table S4).

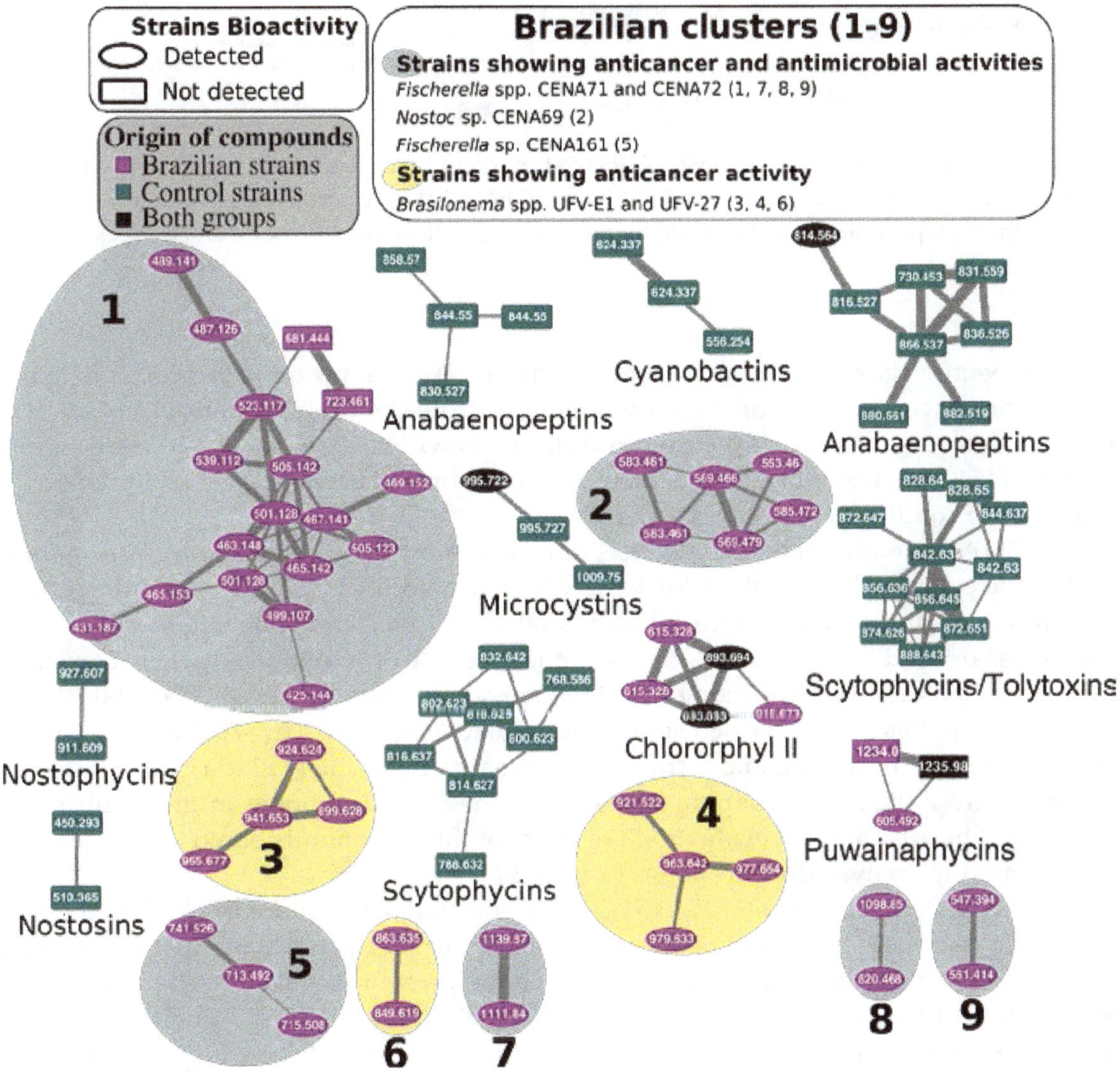

Figure 3. Molecular network of natural products in cyanobacterial extracts from Brazilian (purple) and control (green) strains: Clusters of molecules found only in the former strains are highlighted (1–9). Compound mass/charge ratios (*m/z*) are indicated in the node labels. The complete network can be found in Figure S2.

Cyanobacterial extracts that showed potent anticancer or cytotoxic activity presented novel compounds detected only in Brazilian strains (Figure 4). The chlorinated compounds (M1–5) could not be assigned in this study to any known molecule. Further information on these compounds are presented in the Supplementary Material (Figure S4, File S3).

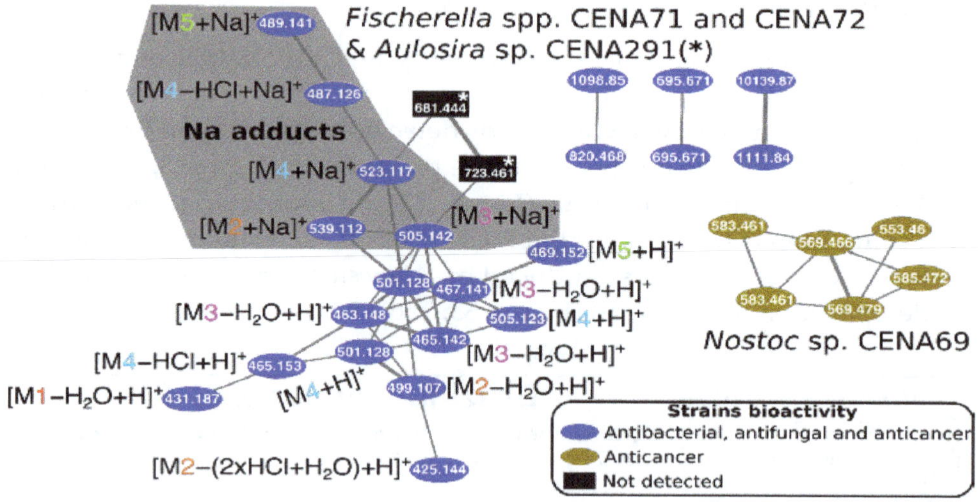

Figure 4. Cluster of compounds in cyanobacterial extracts from Brazilian strains showing potent anticancer or cytotoxic activities (except *Aulosira* sp. CENA291): Compound mass/charge ratios (*m/z*; more than one isotope ion/compound could be present) are indicated in the node labels. See also Figure S4 and File S3.

3. Discussion

There has been a recent increase in the number of studies on natural products synthesized by Brazilian cyanobacteria, particularly on toxins and protease inhibitors [43,44,51–53]. However, the diversity of these organisms and their natural products will likely expand as these ecosystems are further explored [54–56]. Therefore, strains were isolated from different biomes and their biosynthetic potential in culture conditions is discussed here.

The 16S rRNA gene phylogenetic analysis demonstrated that, while some *Nostoc* strains were distributed in the previously described *Nostoc* clusters 1, 2, and 3.3 [43], the remaining strains were located in sparse and diverse clades more closely related to other Nostocalean genera.

Previous research indicated that analysis of a broad selection of taxonomical genera of cyanobacteria would increase the possibility of detecting novel bioactive compounds [21,43]. The analysis of several strains investigated in this study revealed significant antileukemic activity (≥70%). Approximately 21% of the aqueous and 61% of the organic extracts were bioactive, in which all the cyanobacterial strains that produced hydrophilic active compounds also contained a hydrophobic antileukemic extract. The analysis measured by AUC aids in evaluating the effect of the compounds based on concentration and is a reliable method to analyze dose-response curves [57].

Cell extracts of *Cyanobium* sp. CENA154, *Nostoc* spp. CENA67 and CENA69, and *Oxynema* sp. CENA135 have previously been described as having anticancer activity against the murine colon cancer cell line CT-26 and lung carcinoma 3LL [42]. In the present work, cell extracts of these strains were similarly found to induce apoptosis of the AML cell line MOLM-13. Their organic extract is responsible for the antileukemic activity, except for *Nostoc* sp. CENA69, in which the aqueous extract also exhibited antileukemic activity at 13.3 mgDW mL^{-1} concentration. CENA69 showed a high potency to induce cell death in MOLM-13 and was further tested using normal cells (NRK), which also showed high cytotoxicity. *Fischerella* spp. CENA71 and CENA72 and *Aliinostoc* spp. CENA513, CENA514, and CENA524 produce antileukemic compound(s) with higher potency against MOLM-13 cells than normal NRK cells. A similar study that investigated extracts from Portuguese cyanobacteria also revealed effects against cancer cells but did not reduce the viability of NRK cells [58].

Among the 39 strains exhibiting high antileukemic activity, 12 of them produce previously described compounds. *Cyanobium* spp. CENA153 and CENA185, *Fischerella* sp. CENA161, *Oxynema* sp. CENA135, and *Phormidium* sp. CENA270 produce microcystins. These peptides are potent hepatotoxins due to their protein serine/threonine phosphatase inhibitor activity [59]. Hepatocytes efficiently take up microcystin and are therefore the primary target of toxicity [60]. However, high doses of microcystin can also induce oxidative stress [61]. The cellular effects of protein phosphatase inhibitors, such as microcystin and nodularin, are due to differences in uptake. These toxins do not distinguish between malignant and nonmalignant cells if microinjected into the cells [62]. Nevertheless, previous studies have shown that there is no correlation between phosphatase inhibitors and apoptogenic activity against SH-SY5Y-neuroblastoma and AML cells [58,63]. The lipopeptides hassallidin and puwainaphycin have been previously shown to have cytotoxic activity [64,65]. Aeruginosin and anabaenopeptin are protease inhibitors with no reported cytotoxic effects. Lastly, saxitoxin is a neurotoxin that is associated with cytotoxic effects on mammalian cells [66–68]. Further analysis using isolated compounds would be necessary to show which are the antileukemic compounds produced by the tested Brazilian cyanobacteria. Three of the 62 strains are likely to produce new antibacterial, antifungal, or anticancer molecules.

The construction of a molecular network was used to explore the complex variety of natural products synthesized by the analyzed cyanobacteria. Although most of the molecules are produced by both Brazilian and control strains, approximately 20% of the resulting clusters are exclusively present in the group of Brazilian strains. Compounds that had already been identified in the strains, such as microcystin-LR (*Fischerella* sp. CENA161) [48], [D-Leu[1]]microcystin-LR (*Phormidium* sp. CENA270) [49], anabaenopeptin, and nodularin (*Aliinostoc* sp. CENA543) [43], were again found here (Figure S2 and Table S4). The molecular network also highlighted molecules that are possibly related to their bioactivities, though the mass spectrometry analysis was not sufficient for identification and further isolation and characterization are necessary.

Previous studies involving 17 of the 62 strains tested here (CENA21, 67, 69, 135, 152, 153, 154, 159, 160, 185, 216, 217, 247, 271, 281, 283, and 510) reported anticancer and antimicrobial activity on other cell lines and microorganisms [41,42,47]. Thus, our analysis expands the number of strains producing known bioactive compounds, especially from the *Nostoc* and *Fischerella* genera [32,43,52]. *Nostoc* is a cosmopolitan genus of cyanobacteria that is predominantly terrestrial but is also frequently found in symbiosis with other organisms [69,70]. They are known as a prolific producer of secondary metabolites, such as peptides, polyketides, and alkaloids [71,72]. The compounds already described include microcystin (hepatotoxin) [73], nostophycin (cytotoxic activity) [74], cryptophycin (tumor inhibitor) [75], nostocyclamide (algae and bacteria growth inhibitor) [76], nostocarboline (acetylcholinesterase inhibitor) [77], nostocine A (algae and plant growth inhibitor) [78], muscoride A (antibacterial activity) [79], and cyanobacterin (cyanobacterial growth inhibitor) [80]. Nevertheless, the biosynthetic potential of *Nostoc* remains underestimated, as many compounds have not yet been identified [65]. Although *Fischerella* is comparatively less studied that *Nostoc*, several natural products have been identified, such as microcystin [43], the antitumor welwitindolinones [81], the antibacterial and antimycotic hapalindoles [82], and the antibacterial ambiguine [83].

4. Conclusions

Brazilian cyanobacteria belonging to 5 different orders and isolated from different biomes showed anticancer, antibacterial, and antifungal activity. The known compounds microcystin, saxitoxin, aeruginosin, hassallidin, nodularin, anabaenopeptin, pseudoaeruginosin, and puwainaphycin were detected by mass spectrometry analysis and a dereplication tool. Nonetheless, the biosynthetic potential of the strains remains mostly unknown as most of the molecular network could not be assigned to known natural products. Among these compounds, some were found only in Brazilian strains and could potentially be involved in the detected bioactivities. The unknown chlorinated molecules detected in extracts showing relatively high anticancer activity are promising candidates for isolation and characterization. We hypothesize that further studies with Brazilian cyanobacteria may reveal an even larger biosynthetic repertoire, as the tested strains are expected to represent just a small fraction of isolation sources in the ecosystems in the country.

5. Materials and Methods

5.1. Cyanobacterial Strains

Nostoc spp. CENA67 and CENA69 and *Fischerella* spp. CENA71 and CENA72 (No. 3–6 in Table S1) were isolated from the anthropogenic Amazon Dark Earth soils, which are highly fertile anthropogenic soils produced by native populations of Central Amazonia [84]. *Phormidium, Nodosilinea, Chlorogloea, Cyanobium,* and *Halotia* strains (No. 7–14 in Table S1) originate from Cardoso Island on the coast of the State of São Paulo. This region is covered by the Atlantic Forest, mangroves, and restingas (herbaceous vegetation) and is part of one of the most biodiverse ecosystems in the world [85]. Caatinga, the biome in which *Aulosira, Calothrix, Chroococcidiopsis, Cyanospira, Fischerella, Lyngbya, Nostoc,* and *Phormidium* strains (No. 17–43 in Table S1) were isolated, is a semiarid region with singular adapted species that is largely neglected by conservation policies in Brazil [54]. Lastly, *Alkalinema, Geminocystis, Leptolyngbya, Nodosilinea, Nostoc, Pannus,* and *Pantanalinema* strains (No. 1 and 46–59 in Table S1) were isolated from the Pantanal, which is the largest continental wetland on the planet and is colonized by unique cyanobacteria [54]. The strains are maintained in the UHCC culture collection of the University of Helsinki, Helsinki, Finland, and the culture collection of CENA/University of São Paulo, Piracicaba, São Paulo, Brazil.

5.2. DNA Extraction and Sequencing, and Phylogenetic Analyses

Total genomic DNA of the strains was extracted from 3-weeks old cultures according to the method by Fiore et al. [86]. The 16S rRNA genes were obtained by PCR using the set primer 27F-23S30R [87]. PCR products were cloned and sequenced, and the resulting reads were assembled into contigs using the Phred/Phrap/Consed package [88–90].

The evolution model GTR + I + G was selected as the best-fit model by jModelTest 2 v0.1.1 [91,92] and was therefore used for inferring the 16S rRNA phylogenetic tree. In total, 141 cyanobacterial nucleotide sequences were implemented in MrBayes v3.2.6 [93] with 5,000,000 generations.

5.3. Cyanobacterial Extracts

The Brazilian strains selected for the bioactivity assays (Table S1) were cultivated in 3 L of Z8 [94] medium (with or without 0.467 g/L of $NaNO_3$ as nitrogen source; see Table S5) under constant light of 10 ± 1 μmol m^{-2} s^{-1} at 20 ± 1 °C. Cells in exponential phase of growth (21–28 days of cultivation) were freeze-dried, and 100 mg was used for methanol extraction. To perform the extraction, 1 mL of methanol and glass beads (0.5-mm diameter, Scientific Industries INC, Bohemia, NY, USA) were added to the cell matter to be disrupted in a plastic tube using a FastPrep™-24 homogenizer (Fastprep®-24, MpBiomedicals, Irvine, CA, USA) for three times of 30 s at 6.5 m/s. The sample tubes were centrifuged at 10,000× *g* for 5 min, and the supernatant was reserved in a new tube. The extraction was repeated. The supernatant from both extractions was combined and dried using a vacuum concentrator (RVC 2–18 CDplus, Martin Christ, Osterode, Germany). Samples were resuspended in 500 μL of methanol (Sigma-Aldrich, San Luis, MO, USA) by vortexing and pipetting. Dichloromethane (Merck) and milli-Q water were added 1:1 *v/v* (500 μL:500 μL), and the samples were inverted to mix the solvents. The samples were then centrifuged at 10,000× *g* for 5 min at 20 °C. The aqueous and organic phases were collected, placed in different tubes, and left with the lid open at room temperature in a laboratory fume hood overnight. The aqueous phase was evaporated in a speed-vac (Eppendorf) at 30 °C. Dried samples were stored at −20 °C. Organic-phase extracts were resuspended in 75 μL of dimethyl sulfoxide (DMSO, Sigma-Aldrich, ≥99.9%, A.C.S. spectrophotometric grade), while the aqueous phase was resuspended in 300 μL of 25% DMSO (25 DMSO:75 milli-Q water). Samples were stored at −20 °C.

Frieze-dried cells (100 mg) were extracted twice with 1 mL of methanol and centrifuged as described above. The extracts (300 μL) were added to discs and evaporated overnight. The discs were used for antibacterial and antifungal assays. A volume of 40 μL of filtered (22 μm) extract was mixed with 160 μL of methanol to be analyzed by mass spectrometry and stored at −20 °C. Frieze-dried cells (10 to 24.3 mg) from 10 cyanobacteria (Table S3) were extracted once with 1 mL of methanol as described above, and 200 μL of the extract was filtered and reserved for mass spectrometry analysis.

5.4. Cell-Based Assay

The acute myeloid leukemia (AML) cell line MOLM-13 (ACC, 554; [95]) and rat kidney epithelial cell line NRK (ATCC, CRL-6509) were used. Aqueous (4 μL) and organic (1 μL) cyanobacterial extracts were cultured in RPMI or DMEM medium, respectively, and both were supplemented with fetal bovine serum (FBS, F7524, Sigma-Aldrich) and penicillin and streptomycin (P0781, Sigma-Aldrich). The MOLM-13 cells were maintained at concentrations between 10^5 and 8×10^5 cells/mL. NRK cells were detached by mild trypsin treatment at 70–90% confluence and reseeded at 30–50% confluence. The cells were incubated in a humified atmosphere at 37 °C and 5% CO_2. To test for cytotoxicity, extracts were added in 96-well plates (Nunclon™ Delta Surface, Thermo Scientific) and MOLM-13 cell suspensions (25–40 × 10^5 cells/mL) were added to a final volume of 0.1 mL in each well. NRK cells were seeded in wells the day before the experiment (7–8 × 10^4 cells/mL) and left overnight to attach. Fresh medium containing the cyanobacterial cell extracts were added to the wells. Both cell lines were incubated at 37 °C for 24 h before the cells were fixed by adding 100 μL of 3.7% formaldehyde in phosphate-buffered saline buffer, pH 7.4. The DNA-specific dye Hoechst 33342 (0.01 mg/mL) was then added. Plates were kept at 4 °C overnight, and nuclear morphology was assessed as previously described [96] using a Zeiss Axio Vert.a1 microscope. In brief, we scrutinized Hoechst-stained nuclei and scored them as normal or abnormal. Normal nuclei were moderately stained and bean-shaped, whereas nuclei from dead (apoptotic or necrotic) cells were typically hypercondensed, fragmented, and not bean-shaped. See Figure 2 and Reference [96] for examples and details. The numbers of normal and abnormal nuclei were used to determine the percentage of cell death. At least 100 cells were counted to determine cytotoxicity.

The extracts were first screened for cytotoxic potential, and based on the cytotoxic potential of those inducing more than 50% cell death (50–70%, 70–90%, and above 90%), dilutions series were made to estimate EC_{50} values. All extracts were tested in duplicates. EC_{50} values were calculated, and dose-response curves were created using the nonlinear regression function of GraphPad Prism 8 (GraphPad Software, La Jolla, CA, USA). The program was also employed for calculating p-value using the extra-sum-of-squares F test.

5.5. Antifungal and Antibacterial Assays

The activity of crude extracts obtained from Brazilian cyanobacteria were tested for antifungal (*Candida albicans* HAMBI484) and antibacterial (*Staphylococcus aureus* HAMBI66) activities. The antifungal test was performed as previously described [32]. PDA and BHI media were used for the growth and activity assay of *Candida albicans* HAMBI484 (at 35 °C) and *Staphylococcus aureus* HAMBI66 (at 37 °C), respectively. Microbial cells grown overnight on solid media were added to sterile water in a sterile tube, and turbidity was measured at 530 nm to approximately McFarland 0.5. The *S. aureus* HAMBI66 inoculum (800 μL) was spread onto BHI plates and dried for 30 min in sterile conditions. *C. albicans* HAMBI484 inoculum was spread using a sterile swab. The discs containing dry cyanobacterial cell extracts were added to the plates and incubated at 35 °C or 37 °C overnight, after which the inhibitions zones were measured. Nystatin (25 μg) and kanamycin (1000 μg, Abtek biological) were used as positive controls against *C. albicans* HAMBI484 and *S. aureus* HAMBI66, respectively.

5.6. Liquid Chromatography-Mass Spectrometry (LC-MS)

Samples were injected into an Acquity UPLC system (Waters, Manchester, UK) equipped with a Kinetex® C8 100 LC Column (50 × 2.1 mm, 1.7 μm, 100 Å). The UPLC was operated with a flow-rate of 0.3 mL/min in gradient mode at a temperature of 40 °C. Solvents used in the gradient were A: 0.1% formic acid in water and B: 0.1% formic acid in acetonitrile/isopropanol (1:1). The initial conditions of the linear gradient were A: 95% and B: 5% and the conditions were changed to A: 0% and B: 100%

in 5 min. The injection volume was 0.5 μL. Mass spectra were recorded with a Waters Synapt G2-Si mass spectrometer (Waters, Manchester, UK). Measurements were performed using positive and negative electrospray ionization (ESI) in resolution mode. Precursor ions were scanned in the range from *m/z* 400 to 2000 and productions from *m/z* 50 to 2000. MS analyses were performed with scan times of 0.1 s and MS/MS analyses with scan times of 0.2 s. The capillary voltage was 1.5 kV (2.0 kV in negative ionization), source temperature was 120 °C, sampling cone was 40.0, source offset was 80.0, desolvation temperature was 600 °C, desolvation gas flow was 1000 L/h, and nebulizer gas flow was 6.5 Bar. Leucine-encephalin was used as a lock mass, and calibration was performed with sodium formate and Ultramark 1621.

5.7. Molecular Network

The data obtained with LC-MS was converted to mzXML using MSConvert [97]. A molecular network was obtained using the GNPS: Global Natural Products Social Molecular Network website [98]. The data was filtered, peaks with + or −17 Da of the precursor were removed, and peaks throughout the spectrum other than the top six +/−50 Da were filtered out. The data were then clustered with MS-Cluster with a parent mass tolerance of 0.2 Da and a MS/MS fragment ion tolerance of 0.2 Da to create consensus spectra. Consensus spectra that contained less than two spectra were discarded. A network was then created where edges were filtered to have a cosine score above 0.7 and more than six matched peaks. Further edges between two nodes were kept in the network only if each of the nodes appeared in each other's respective top 10 most similar nodes. The spectra in the network were then searched against the GNPS spectral libraries. The library spectra were filtered in the same manner as the input data. All matches kept between network spectra and library spectra were required to have a score above 0.7 and at least six matched peaks.

The *in silico* peptidic natural product dereplicator tool from the GNPS website was used to search for potential known compounds produced by Brazilian cyanobacteria. The precursor and fragment ion mass tolerance selected was 0.02 Da, and a search for analogs was performed (VarQuest).

5.8. Data Availability Statement

The 16S rRNA or 16S-23S rRNA sequence accession numbers in NCBI are *Nostoc* spp. CENA67 (MN551902), CENA69 (MN551252), CENA216 (MN551255), CENA238 (MN551905), CENA239 (MN551906), CENA259 (MN551911), CENA261 (MN551256), CENA269 (MN551912), CENA271 (MN551257), CENA274 (MN551914), CENA278 (MN551915), CENA281 (MN551916), and CENA294 (MN551920); *Leptolyngbya* CENA293 (MN551919); *Fischerella* spp. CENA71 (MN551253) and CENA 72 (MN551254); *Cyanospira* sp. CENA215 (MN551903); *Limnothrix* sp. CENA217 (MN551904); *Chroococcidiopsis* spp. CENA240 (MN551907) and CENA246 (MN551908); *Sphaerospermopsis* sp. CENA247 (MN551909); *Calothrix* sp. CENA250 (MN551910); *Aulosira* spp. CENA272 (MN551913), CENA283 (MN551258), CENA288 (MN551917), CENA291 (MN551918), and CENA295 (MN551921); Nostocales CENA296 (MN551922); and *Brasilonema* spp. UFV-L1 (MN551259) and UFV-27 (MN551260).

Supplementary Materials
Figure S1: Dose-response curves of the selected cyanobacterial extracts on NRK (Blue) and MOLM-13 (red) cell lines: These were the basis for estimating EC_{50} values, Figure S2: Complete molecular networking of cyanobacterial extracts from Brazilian (purple) and control (green) strains: Known compounds are indicated (see also Tables S3 and S4). Node numbers represent mass/charge ratios (*m/z*), Figure S3: MS/MS spectra of puwainaphycins identified in *Aliinostoc* sp: CENA535 using the dereplication tool (GNPS). See Table S4 for further information, Figure S4: Spectra of potentially new compounds produced only by Brazilian strains (see also Figure 4 and File S3), Table S1: List of Brazilian cyanobacterial isolates tested for the synthesis of anticancer and antimicrobial compounds: The accession number of their 16S rRNA sequences and the habitat, site, city, and state from where the samples were collected are indicated, Table S2: Human leukemia MOLM-13 cells apoptosis caused by crude extracts of aqueous and organic cyanobacterial cell extracts (average of two parallel measurements indicated in %). Dilutions (0.3×, 0.1×, and 0.01×) are indicated in the table, and samples not tested in different dilutions are indicated with (−). Red color indicates high amounts of apoptotic cells, and green indicates high amounts of

normal cells. The error (Er) indicates the difference value of the average with one of the duplicates, Table S3: List of cyanobacteria used as a control in the LC-MS analysis to compare the previously discovered compounds with the molecules produced by Brazilian strains, Table S4: Dereplicator analysis of Brazilian cyanobacteria cell extracts. Predicted compounds are organized by p-value (cutoff of 10^{-11}); FDR cutoff of 15%. Compounds found in previous studies are in bold, File S1: Pictures of the antifungal activity essays using *Candida albicans* HAMBI484: The use of sterile water may have influenced the susceptibility of the fungal cells, File S2: Pictures of the antibacterial activity essays using *Staphylococcus aureus* HAMBI66: The use of sterile water may have influenced in the susceptibility of the bacterial cells, File S3: Retention times of chlorinated compounds detected in *Fischerella* sp. CENA72, Table S5: Culture media used for the cultivation of the strains: The addition of nitrogen refers to 0.467 g/L of $NaNO_3$.

Author Contributions: Conceptualization, T.K.S., L.H., M.W., J.J., D.P.F., M.F.F., and K.S.; methodology, T.K.S., R.V.P., L.H., and M.W.; formal analysis, T.K.S., R.V.P., L.H., M.W., J.J., and D.P.F.; writing—original draft preparation, T.K.S. and R.V.P.; writing—review and editing, T.K.S., R.V.P., L.H., M.W., J.J., D.P.F., M.F.F., and K.S.; supervision, L.H., J.J., D.P.F., and K.S.; project administration, K.S.; funding acquisition, L.H., K.S, and M.F.F. All authors have read and agreed to the published version of the manuscript.

Acknowledgments: We thank Lyudmila Saari for maintaining and handling the cyanobacteria strains.

References

1. Stanier, R.Y.; Bazine, G.C. Phototrophic Prokaryotes: The Cyanobacteria. *Annu. Rev. Microbiol.* **1977**, *31*, 225–274. [CrossRef]
2. Carmichael, W.W. Cyanobacteria secondary metabolites-the cyanotoxins. *J. Appl. Microbiol.* **1992**, *72*, 445–459. [CrossRef]
3. Bohlin, L.; Göransson, U.; Alsmark, C.; Wedén, C.; Backlund, A. Natural products in modern life science. *Phytochem. Rev.* **2010**, *9*, 279–301. [CrossRef]
4. Dias, D.A.; Urban, S.; Roessner, U. A historical overview of natural products in drug discovery. *Metabolites* **2012**, *2*, 303–336. [CrossRef] [PubMed]
5. Welker, M.; Von Döhren, H. Cyanobacterial peptides—Nature's own combinatorial biosynthesis. *FEMS Microbiol. Rev.* **2006**, *30*, 530–563. [CrossRef] [PubMed]
6. Burja, A.M.; Banaigs, B.; Abou-Mansour, E.; Grant Burgess, J.; Wright, P.C. Marine cyanobacteria—A prolific source of natural products. *Tetrahedron* **2001**, *57*, 9347–9377. [CrossRef]
7. Ehrenreich, I.M.; Waterbury, J.B.; Webb, E.A. Distribution and Diversity of Natural Product Genes in Marine and Freshwater Cyanobacterial Cultures and Genomes. *Appl. Environ. Microbiol.* **2005**, *71*, 7401–7413. [CrossRef] [PubMed]
8. Angermayr, S.A.; Hellingwerf, K.J.; Lindblad, P.; Teixeira de Mattos, M.J. Energy biotechnology with cyanobacteria. *Curr. Opin. Biotechnol.* **2009**, *20*, 257–263. [CrossRef]
9. Kehr, J.-C.; Gatte Picchi, D.; Dittmann, E. Natural product biosyntheses in cyanobacteria: A treasure trove of unique enzymes. *Beilstein J. Org. Chem.* **2011**, *7*, 1622–1635. [CrossRef]
10. Marahiel, M.A.; Stachelhaus, T.; Mootz, H.D. Modular peptide synthetases involved in nonribosomal peptide synthesis. *Chem. Rev.* **1997**, *97*, 2651–2674. [CrossRef]
11. Finking, R.; Marahiel, M.A. Biosynthesis of Nonribosomal Peptides. *Annu. Rev. Microbiol.* **2004**, *58*, 453–488. [CrossRef] [PubMed]
12. Sieber, S.A.; Marahiel, M.A. Molecular mechanisms underlying nonribosomal peptide synthesis: Approaches to new antibiotics. *Chem. Rev.* **2005**, *105*, 715–738. [CrossRef] [PubMed]
13. Fujii, K.; Harada, K.; Suzuki, M.; Kondo, F.; Ikai, Y.; Oka, H.; Carmichael, W.W.; Sivonen, K. Occurrence of novel cyclic peptides together with microcystins from toxic cyanobacteria, Anabaena species. In *Harmful and Toxic Algal Blooms*; Intergovernmental Oceanographic Commission of UNESCO: Paris, France, 1996; pp. 559–562.

14. Moffitt, M.C.; Neilan, B.A. Characterization of the nodularin synthetase gene cluster and proposed theory of the evolution of cyanobacterial hepatotoxins. *Appl. Environ. Microbiol.* **2004**, *70*, 6353–6362. [CrossRef] [PubMed]
15. Rouhiainen, L.; Paulin, L.; Suomalainen, S.; Hyytiäinen, H.; Buikema, W.; Haselkorn, R.; Sivonen, K. Genes encoding synthetases of cyclic depsipeptides, anabaenopeptilides, in *Anabaena* strain 90. *Mol. Microbiol.* **2000**, *37*, 156–167. [CrossRef] [PubMed]
16. Fewer, D.P.; Jokela, J.; Rouhiainen, L.; Wahlsten, M.; Koskenniemi, K.; Stal, L.J.; Sivonen, K. The non-ribosomal assembly and frequent occurrence of the protease inhibitors spumigins in the bloom-forming cyanobacterium *Nodularia spumigena*. *Mol. Microbiol.* **2009**, *73*, 924–937. [CrossRef]
17. Biondi, N.; Tredici, M.R.; Taton, A.; Wilmotte, A.; Hodgson, D.A.; Losi, D.; Marinelli, F. Cyanobacteria from benthic mats of Antarctic lakes as a source of new bioactivities. *J. Appl. Microbiol.* **2008**, *105*, 105–115. [CrossRef]
18. Kreitlow, S.; Mundt, S.; Lindequist, U. Cyanobacteria—A potential source of new biologically active substances. *J. Biotechnol.* **1999**, *70*, 61–63. [CrossRef]
19. Singh, R.K.; Tiwari, S.P.; Rai, A.K.; Mohapatra, T.M. Cyanobacteria: An emerging source for drug discovery. *J. Antibiot.* **2011**, *64*, 401–412. [CrossRef]
20. Felczykowska, A.; Pawlik, A.; Mazur-Marzec, H.; Toruńska-Sitarz, A.; Narajczyk, M.; Richert, M.; Węgrzyn, G.; Herman-Antosiewicz, A. Selective inhibition of cancer cells' proliferation by compounds included in extracts from Baltic Sea cyanobacteria. *Toxicon* **2015**, *108*, 1–10. [CrossRef]
21. Humisto, A.; Herfindal, L.; Jokela, J.; Karkman, A.; Bjørnstad, R.; Choudhury, R.R.; Sivonen, K. Cyanobacteria as a source for novel anti-leukemic compounds. *Curr. Pharm. Biotechnol.* **2016**, *17*, 78–91. [CrossRef]
22. Taori, K.; Matthew, S.; Rocca, J.R.; Paul, V.J.; Luesch, H. Lyngbyastatins 5–7, Potent elastase inhibitors from floridian marine cyanobacteria, *Lyngbya* spp. *J. Nat. Prod.* **2007**, *70*, 1593–1600. [CrossRef] [PubMed]
23. Gerwick, W.H.; Proteau, P.J.; Nagle, D.G.; Hamel, E.; Blokhin, A.; Slate, D.L. Structure of Curacin A, a novel antimitotic, antiproliferative and brine shrimp toxic natural product from the marine cyanobacterium *Lyngbya majuscula*. *J. Org. Chem.* **1994**, *59*, 1243–1245. [CrossRef]
24. Berman, F.W.; Gerwick, W.H.; Murray, T.F. Antillatoxin and kalkitoxin, ichthyotoxins from the tropical cyanobacterium *Lyngbya majuscula*, induce distinct temporal patterns of NMDA receptor-mediated neurotoxicity. *Toxicon* **1999**, *37*, 1645–1648. [CrossRef]
25. Wu, M.; Okino, T.; Nogle, L.M.; Marquez, B.L.; Williamson, R.T.; Sitachitta, N.; Berman, F.W.; Murray, T.F.; McGough, K.; Jacobs, R.; et al. Structure, synthesis, and biological properties of kalkitoxin, a novel neurotoxin from the marine cyanobacterium *Lyngbya majuscula*. *J. Am. Chem. Soc.* **2000**, *122*, 12041–12042. [CrossRef]
26. Trimurtulu, G.; Ohtani, I.; Patterson, G.M.L.; Moore, R.E.; Corbett, T.H.; Valeriote, F.A.; Demchik, L. Total structures of cryptophycins, potent antitumor depsipeptides from the blue-green alga *Nostoc* sp. strain GSV 224. *J. Am. Chem. Soc.* **1994**, *116*, 4729–4737. [CrossRef]
27. Costa, M.; Costa-Rodrigues, J.; Fernandes, M.H.; Barros, P.; Vasconcelos, V.; Martins, R. Marine cyanobacteria compounds with anticancer properties: A review on the implication of apoptosis. *Mar. Drugs* **2012**, *10*, 2181–2207. [CrossRef]
28. Liu, L.; Herfindal, L.; Jokela, J.; Shishido, T.; Wahlsten, M.; Døskeland, S.; Sivonen, K. Cyanobacteria from terrestrial and marine sources contain apoptogens able to overcome chemoresistance in acute myeloid leukemia cells. *Mar. Drugs* **2014**, *12*, 2036–2053. [CrossRef]
29. Visser, O.; Trama, A.; Maynadié, M.; Stiller, C.; Marcos-Gragera, R.; De Angelis, R.; Mallone, S.; Tereanu, C.; Allemani, C.; Ricardi, U.; et al. Incidence, survival and prevalence of myeloid malignancies in Europe. *Eur. J. Cancer* **2012**, *48*, 3257–3266. [CrossRef]
30. Rowe, J.M. AML in 2016: Where we are now? *Best Pract. Res. Clin. Haematol.* **2016**, *29*, 315–319. [CrossRef]
31. Housman, G.; Byler, S.; Heerboth, S.; Lapinska, K.; Longacre, M.; Snyder, N.; Sarkar, S. Drug resistance in cancer: An overview. *Cancers* **2014**, *6*, 1769–1792. [CrossRef]
32. Shishido, T.; Humisto, A.; Jokela, J.; Liu, L.; Wahlsten, M.; Tamrakar, A.; Fewer, D.; Permi, P.; Andreote, A.; Fiore, M.; et al. Antifungal compounds from cyanobacteria. *Mar. Drugs* **2015**, *13*, 2124–2140. [CrossRef] [PubMed]
33. Leao, T.; Castelão, G.; Korobeynikov, A.; Monroe, E.A.; Podell, S.; Glukhov, E.; Allen, E.E.; Gerwick, W.H.; Gerwick, L. Comparative genomics uncovers the prolific and distinctive metabolic potential of the cyanobacterial genus *Moorea*. *Proc. Natl. Acad. Sci. USA* **2017**, *114*, 3198–3203. [CrossRef] [PubMed]

34. Vaz, M.G.M.V.; Genuario, D.B.; Andreote, A.P.D.; Malone, C.F.S.; Sant'Anna, C.L.; Barbiero, L.; Fiore, M.F. *Pantanalinema* gen. nov. and *Alkalinema* gen. nov.: Novel pseudanabaenacean genera (Cyanobacteria) isolated from saline-alkaline lakes. *Int. J. Syst. Evol. Microbiol.* **2015**, *65*, 298–308. [CrossRef] [PubMed]
35. Martins, M.D.; Branco, L.H.Z. *Potamolinea* gen. nov. (Oscillatoriales, Cyanobacteria): A phylogenetically and ecologically coherent cyanobacterial genus. *Int. J. Syst. Evol. Microbiol.* **2016**, *66*, 3632–3641. [CrossRef] [PubMed]
36. Genuário, D.B.; de Souza, W.R.; Monteiro, R.T.R.; Sant'Anna, C.L.; Melo, I.S. *Amazoninema* gen. nov., (Synechococcales, Pseudanabaenaceae) a novel cyanobacteria genus from Brazilian Amazonian rivers. *Int. J. Syst. Evol. Microbiol.* **2018**, *68*, 2249–2257. [CrossRef] [PubMed]
37. Caires, T.A.; de Mattos Lyra, G.; Hentschke, G.S.; de Gusmão Pedrini, A.; Sant'Anna, C.L.; de Castro Nunes, J.M. *Neolyngbya* gen. nov. (Cyanobacteria, Oscillatoriaceae): A new filamentous benthic marine taxon widely distributed along the Brazilian coast. *Mol. Phylogenet. Evol.* **2018**, *120*, 196–211. [CrossRef]
38. Myers, N.; Mittermeier, R.A.; Mittermeier, C.G.; da Fonseca, G.A.B.; Kent, J. Biodiversity hotspots for conservation priorities. *Nature* **2000**, *403*, 853–858. [CrossRef]
39. Rigonato, J.; Gama, W.A.; Alvarenga, D.O.; Branco, L.H.Z.; Brandini, F.P.; Genuário, D.B.; Fiore, M.F. *Aliterella atlantica* gen. nov., sp. nov., and *Aliterella antarctica* sp. nov., novel members of coccoid Cyanobacteria. *Int. J. Syst. Evol. Microbiol.* **2016**, *66*, 2853–2861. [CrossRef]
40. Sanz, M.; Andreote, A.; Fiore, M.; Dörr, F.; Pinto, E. Structural characterization of new peptide variants produced by cyanobacteria from the Brazilian Atlantic coastal forest using liquid chromatography coupled to quadrupole time-of-flight tandem mass spectrometry. *Mar. Drugs* **2015**, *13*, 3892–3919. [CrossRef]
41. Silva, C.S.P.; Genuário, D.B.; Vaz, M.G.M.V.; Fiore, M.F. Phylogeny of culturable cyanobacteria from Brazilian mangroves. *Syst. Appl. Microbiol.* **2014**, *37*, 100–112. [CrossRef]
42. Silva-Stenico, M.E.; Kaneno, R.; Zambuzi, F.A.; Vaz, M.G.M.V.; Alvarenga, D.O.; Fiore, M.F. Natural products from cyanobacteria with antimicrobial and antitumor activity. *Curr. Pharm. Biotechnol.* **2013**, *14*, 820–828. [CrossRef] [PubMed]
43. Jokela, J.; Heinilä, L.M.P.; Shishido, T.K.; Wahlsten, M.; Fewer, D.P.; Fiore, M.F.; Wang, H.; Haapaniemi, E.; Permi, P.; Sivonen, K. Production of high amounts of hepatotoxin nodularin and new protease inhibitors pseudospumigins by the Brazilian benthic *Nostoc* sp. CENA543. *Front. Microbiol.* **2017**, *8*, 1963. [CrossRef] [PubMed]
44. Sanz, M.; Salinas, R.K.; Pinto, E. Namalides B and C and spumigins k–n from the cultured freshwater cyanobacterium *Sphaerospermopsis torques-reginae*. *J. Nat. Prod.* **2017**, *80*, 2492–2501. [CrossRef] [PubMed]
45. Nguyen, D.D.; Melnik, A.V.; Koyama, N.; Lu, X.; Schorn, M.; Fang, J.; Aguinaldo, K.; Lincecum, T.L.; Ghequire, M.G.K.; Carrion, V.J.; et al. Indexing the *Pseudomonas* specialized metabolome enabled the discovery of poaeamide B and the bananamides. *Nat. Microbiol.* **2016**, *2*, 16197. [CrossRef]
46. Watrous, J.; Roach, P.; Alexandrov, T.; Heath, B.S.; Yang, J.Y.; Kersten, R.D.; van der Voort, M.; Pogliano, K.; Gross, H.; Raaijmakers, J.M.; et al. Mass spectral molecular networking of living microbial colonies. *Proc. Natl. Acad. Sci. USA* **2012**, *109*, E1743–E1752. [CrossRef]
47. Silva-Stenico, M.E.; Rigonato, J.; Leal, M.G.; Vaz, M.G.M.V.; Andreote, A.P.D.; Fiore, M.F. Non-ribosomal halogenated protease inhibitors from cyanobacterial isolates as attractive drug targets. *Curr. Med. Chem.* **2012**, *19*, 5205–5213. [CrossRef]
48. Fiore, M.F.; Genuário, D.B.; da Silva, C.S.P.; Shishido, T.K.; Moraes, L.A.B.; Neto, R.C.; Silva-Stenico, M.E. Microcystin production by a freshwater spring cyanobacterium of the genus *Fischerella*. *Toxicon* **2009**, *53*, 754–761. [CrossRef]
49. Shishido, T.; Kaasalainen, U.; Fewer, D.P.; Rouhiainen, L.; Jokela, J.; Wahlsten, M.; Fiore, M.; Yunes, J.; Rikkinen, J.; Sivonen, K. Convergent evolution of [D-Leucine1] microcystin-LR in taxonomically disparate cyanobacteria. *BMC Evol. Biol.* **2013**, *13*, 86. [CrossRef]
50. Hoff-Risseti, C.; Dörr, F.A.; Schaker, P.D.C.; Pinto, E.; Werner, V.R.; Fiore, M.F. Cylindrospermopsin and saxitoxin synthetase genes in *Cylindrospermopsis raciborskii* strains from Brazilian freshwater. *PLoS ONE* **2013**, *8*, e74238. [CrossRef]
51. Shishido, T.K.; Jokela, J.; Fewer, D.P.; Wahlsten, M.; Fiore, M.F.; Sivonen, K. Simultaneous production of anabaenopeptins and namalides by the cyanobacterium *Nostoc* sp. CENA543. *ACS Chem. Biol.* **2017**, *12*, 2746–2755. [CrossRef]

52. Heck, K.; Alvarenga, D.O.; Shishido, T.K.; Varani, A.M.; Dörr, F.A.; Pinto, E.; Rouhiainen, L.; Jokela, J.; Sivonen, K.; Fiore, M.F. Biosynthesis of microcystin hepatotoxins in the cyanobacterial genus *Fischerella*. *Toxicon* **2018**, *141*, 43–50. [CrossRef] [PubMed]
53. Lima, S.T.; Alvarenga, D.O.; Etchegaray, A.; Fewer, D.P.; Jokela, J.; Varani, A.M.; Sanz, M.; Dörr, F.A.; Pinto, E.; Sivonen, K.; et al. Genetic organization of anabaenopeptin and spumigin biosynthetic gene clusters in the cyanobacterium *Sphaerospermopsis torques-reginae* ITEP-024. *ACS Chem. Biol.* **2017**, *12*, 769–778. [CrossRef] [PubMed]
54. Costa, N.B.; Kolman, M.A.; Giani, A. Cyanobacteria diversity in alkaline saline lakes in the Brazilian Pantanal wetland: A polyphasic approach. *J. Plankton Res.* **2016**, *38*, 1389–1403. [CrossRef]
55. Genuário, D.B.; Vaz, M.G.M.V.; de Melo, I.S. Phylogenetic insights into the diversity of homocytous cyanobacteria from Amazonian rivers. *Mol. Phylogenet. Evol.* **2017**, *116*, 120–135. [CrossRef]
56. Genuário, D.B.; Vaz, M.G.M.V.; Santos, S.N.; Kavamura, V.N.; Melo, I.S. Cyanobacteria from Brazilian extreme environments. In *Microbial Diversity in the Genomic Era*; Elsevier: Amsterdam, The Netherlands, 2019; pp. 265–284. ISBN 978-0-12-814849-5.
57. Jang, I.S.; Neto, E.C.; Guinney, J.; Friend, S.H.; Margolin, A.A. Systematic assessment of analytical methods for drug sensitivity prediction from cancer cell line data. *Pac. Symp. Biocomput.* **2014**, 63–74. [CrossRef]
58. Selheim, F.; Herfindal, L.; Martins, R.; Vasconcelos, V.; Døskeland, S.O. Neuro-apoptogenic and blood platelet targeting toxins in benthic marine cyanobacteria from the Portuguese coast. *Aquat. Toxicol.* **2005**, *74*, 294–306. [CrossRef]
59. Campos, A.; Vasconcelos, V. Molecular mechanisms of microcystin toxicity in animal cells. *Int. J. Mol.* **2010**, *11*, 268–287. [CrossRef]
60. Fischer, W.J.; Altheimer, S.; Cattori, V.; Meier, P.J.; Dietrich, D.R.; Hagenbuch, B. Organic anion transporting polypeptides expressed in liver and brain mediate uptake of microcystin. *Toxicol. Appl. Pharmacol.* **2005**, *203*, 257–263. [CrossRef]
61. Botha, N.; Gehringer, M.M.; Downing, T.G.; van de Venter, M.; Shephard, E.G. The role of microcystin-LR in the induction of apoptosis and oxidative stress in CaCo2 cells. *Toxicon* **2004**, *43*, 85–92. [CrossRef]
62. Fladmark, K.; Brustugun, O.; Hovland, R.; Bøe, R.; Gjertsen, B.; Zhivotovsky, B.; Døskeland, S. Ultrarapid caspase-3 dependent apoptosis induction by serine/threonine phosphatase inhibitors. *Cell Death Differ.* **1999**, *6*, 1099–1108. [CrossRef]
63. Oftedal, L.; Skjærven, K.H.; Coyne, R.T.; Edvardsen, B.; Rohrlack, T.; Skulberg, O.M.; Døskeland, S.O.; Herfindal, L. The apoptosis-inducing activity towards leukemia and lymphoma cells in a cyanobacterial culture collection is not associated with mouse bioassay toxicity. *J. Ind. Microbiol. Biotechnol.* **2011**, *38*, 489–501. [CrossRef] [PubMed]
64. Neuhof, T.; Dieckmann, R.; von Hans, D.; Preussel, K.; Seibold, M.; Schmieder, P. Lipopeptides Having Pharmaceutical Activity. WO2006092313A1, 8 September 2006.
65. Hrouzek, P.; Kuzma, M.; Černý, J.; Novák, P.; Fišer, R.; Šimek, P.; Lukešová, A.; Kopecký, J. The cyanobacterial cyclic lipopeptides puwainaphycins f/g are inducing necrosis via cell membrane permeabilization and subsequent unusual actin relocalization. *Chem. Res. Toxicol.* **2012**, *25*, 1203–1211. [CrossRef] [PubMed]
66. Welker, M.; Dittmann, E.; von Döhren, H. Cyanobacteria as a source of natural products. In *Methods in Enzymology*; Elsevier: Amsterdam, The Netherlands, 2012; Volume 517, pp. 23–46. ISBN 978-0-12-404634-4.
67. Zhou, Z.; Tang, X.; Chen, H.; Wang, Y. Comparative studies of saxitoxin (STX)-induced cytotoxicity in Neuro-2a and RTG-2 cell lines: An explanation with respect to changes in ROS. *Chemosphere* **2018**, *192*, 66–74. [CrossRef] [PubMed]
68. Melegari, S.P.; de Carvalho Pinto, C.R.S.; Moukha, S.; Creppy, E.E.; Matias, W.G. Evaluation of cytotoxicity and cell death induced in vitro by saxitoxin in mammalian cells. *J Toxicol. Environ. Health Part A* **2015**, *78*, 1189–1200. [CrossRef]
69. Dodds, W.K.; Gudder, D.A.; Mollenhauer, D. The ecology of *Nostoc*. *J. Appl. Phycol.* **1995**, *31*, 2–18. [CrossRef]
70. Liaimer, A.; Jensen, J.B.; Dittmann, E. A genetic and chemical perspective on symbiotic recruitment of cyanobacteria of the genus *Nostoc* into the host plant *Blasia pusilla* L. *Front. Microbiol.* **2016**, *7*. [CrossRef]
71. Kobayashi, A.; Kajiyama, S. Secondary metabolites of cyanobacteria *Nostoc* sp. *Chin. J. Oceanol. Limnol.* **1998**, *16*, 109–117. [CrossRef]
72. Dittmann, E.; Gugger, M.; Sivonen, K.; Fewer, D.P. Natural product biosynthetic diversity and comparative genomics of the cyanobacteria. *Trends Microbiol.* **2015**, *23*, 642–652. [CrossRef]

73. Oksanen, I.; Jokela, J.; Fewer, D.P.; Wahlsten, M.; Rikkinen, J.; Sivonen, K. Discovery of rare and highly toxic microcystins from lichen-associated cyanobacterium *Nostoc* sp. Strain IO-102-I. *Appl. Environ. Microbiol.* **2004**, *70*, 5756–5763. [CrossRef]
74. Fujii, K.; Sivonen, K.; Kashiwagi, T.; Hirayama, K.; Harada, K. Nostophycin, a novel cyclic peptide from the toxic cyanobacterium *Nostoc* sp. 152. *J. Org. Chem.* **1999**, *64*, 5777–5782. [CrossRef]
75. Subbaraju, G.V.; Golakoti, T.; Patterson, G.M.L.; Moore, R.E. Three new cryptophycins from *Nostoc* sp. GSV 224. *J. Nat. Prod.* **1997**, *60*, 302–305. [CrossRef] [PubMed]
76. Jüttner, F.; Todorova, A.K.; Walch, N.; von Philipsborn, W. Nostocyclamide M: A cyanobacterial cyclic peptide with allelopathic activity from *Nostoc* 31. *Phytochemistry* **2001**, *57*, 613–619. [CrossRef]
77. Becher, P.G.; Beuchat, J.; Gademann, K.; Jüttner, F. Nostocarboline: Isolation and synthesis of a new cholinesterase inhibitor from *Nostoc* 78-12A. *J. Nat. Prod.* **2005**, *68*, 1793–1795. [CrossRef] [PubMed]
78. Hirata, K.; Yoshitomi, S.; Dwi, S.; Iwabe, O.; Mahakhant, A.; Polchai, J.; Miyamoto, K. Bioactivities of nostocine a produced by a freshwater cyanobacterium *Nostoc spongiaeforme* TISTR 8169. *J. Biosci. Bioeng.* **2003**, *95*, 512–517. [CrossRef]
79. Nagatsu, A.; Kajitani, H.; Sakakibara, J. Muscoride A: A new oxazole peptide alkaloid from freshwater cyanobacterium *Nostoc muscorum*. *Tetrahedron Lett.* **1995**, *36*, 4097–4100. [CrossRef]
80. Gromov, B.V.; Vepritskiy, A.A.; Titova, N.N.; Mamkayeva, K.A.; Alexandrova, O.V. Production of the antibiotic cyanobacterin LU-1 by *Nostoc linckia* CALU 892 (cyanobacterium). *J. Appl. Phycol.* **1991**, *3*, 55–59. [CrossRef]
81. Jimenez, J.I.; Huber, U.; Moore, R.E.; Patterson, G.M.L. Oxidized welwitindolinones from terrestrial *Fischerella* spp. *J. Nat. Prod.* **1999**, *62*, 569–572. [CrossRef]
82. Cagide, E.; Becher, P.G.; Louzao, M.C.; Espiña, B.; Vieytes, M.R.; Jüttner, F.; Botana, L.M. Hapalindoles from the cyanobacterium *Fischerella*: Potential sodium channel modulators. *Chem. Res. Toxicol.* **2014**, *27*, 1696–1706. [CrossRef]
83. Mo, S.; Krunic, A.; Chlipala, G.; Orjala, J. Antimicrobial ambiguine isonitriles from the cyanobacterium *Fischerella ambigua*. *J. Nat. Prod.* **2009**, *72*, 894–899. [CrossRef]
84. Glaser, B. Prehistorically modified soils of central Amazonia: A model for sustainable agriculture in the twenty-first century. *Philos. Trans. R. Soc. Lond. B Biol. Sci.* **2007**, *362*, 187–196. [CrossRef]
85. Pupin, B.; Nahas, E. Microbial populations and activities of mangrove, restinga and Atlantic forest soils from Cardoso Island, Brazil. *J. Appl. Microbiol.* **2014**, *116*, 851–864. [CrossRef] [PubMed]
86. Fiore, M.F.; Moon, D.H.; Tsai, S.M.; Lee, H.; Trevors, J.T. Miniprep DNA isolation from unicellular and filamentous cyanobacteria. *J. Microbiol. Methods* **2000**, *39*, 159–169. [CrossRef]
87. Taton, A.; Grubisic, S.; Brambilla, E.; De Wit, R.; Wilmotte, A. Cyanobacterial diversity in natural and artificial microbial mats of Lake Fryxell (McMurdo Dry Valleys, Antarctica): A morphological and molecular approach. *Appl. Environ. Microbiol.* **2003**, *69*, 5157–5169. [CrossRef] [PubMed]
88. Ewing, B.; Green, P. Base-calling of automated sequencer traces using phred. II. Error probabilities. *Genome Res.* **1998**, *8*, 186–194. [CrossRef] [PubMed]
89. Ewing, B.; Hillier, L.; Wendl, M.C.; Green, P. Base-calling of automated sequencer traces using phred. I. Accuracy assessment. *Genome Res.* **1998**, *8*, 175–185. [CrossRef]
90. Gordon, D.; Abajian, C.; Green, P. Consed: A graphical tool for sequence finishing. *Genome Res.* **1998**, *8*, 195–202. [CrossRef]
91. Darriba, D.; Taboada, G.L.; Doallo, R.; Posada, D. jModelTest 2: More models, new heuristics and parallel computing. *Nat. Methods* **2012**, *9*, 772. [CrossRef]
92. Guindon, S.; Gascuel, O. A simple, fast, and accurate algorithm to estimate large phylogenies by maximum likelihood. *Syst. Biol.* **2003**, *52*, 696–704. [CrossRef]
93. Ronquist, F.; Teslenko, M.; van der Mark, P.; Ayres, D.L.; Darling, A.; Höhna, S.; Larget, B.; Liu, L.; Suchard, M.A.; Huelsenbeck, J.P. MrBayes 3.2: Efficient bayesian phylogenetic inference and model choice across a large model space. *Syst. Biol.* **2012**, *61*, 539–542. [CrossRef]
94. Kotai, J. *Instructions for Preparation of Modified Nutrient Solution Z8 for Algae*; Norwegian Institute for Water Research: Oslo, Norway, 1972.
95. Matsuo, Y.; MacLeod, R.; Uphoff, C.; Drexler, H.; Nishizaki, C.; Katayama, Y.; Kimura, G.; Fujii, N.; Omoto, E.; Harada, M.; et al. Two acute monocytic leukemia (AML-M5a) cell lines (MOLM-13 and MOLM-14) with

interclonal phenotypic heterogeneity showing MLL-AF9 fusion resulting from an occult chromosome insertion, ins(11;9)(q23;p22p23). *Leukemia* **1997**, *11*, 1469–1477. [CrossRef]

96. Oftedal, L.; Selheim, F.; Wahlsten, M.; Sivonen, K.; Døskeland, S.O.; Herfindal, L. Marine Benthic Cyanobacteria contain apoptosis-inducing activity synergizing with daunorubicin to kill leukemia cells, but not cardiomyocytes. *Mar. Drugs* **2010**, *8*, 2659–2672. [CrossRef] [PubMed]
97. Chambers, M.C.; Maclean, B.; Burke, R.; Amodei, D.; Ruderman, D.L.; Neumann, S.; Gatto, L.; Fischer, B.; Pratt, B.; Egertson, J.; et al. A cross-platform toolkit for mass spectrometry and proteomics. *Nat. Biotechnol.* **2012**, *30*, 918–920. [CrossRef] [PubMed]
98. Wang, M.; Carver, J.J.; Phelan, V.V.; Sanchez, L.M.; Garg, N.; Peng, Y.; Nguyen, D.D.; Watrous, J.; Kapono, C.A.; Luzzatto-Knaan, T.; et al. Sharing and community curation of mass spectrometry data with Global Natural Products Social Molecular Networking. *Nat. Biotechnol.* **2016**, *34*, 828–837. [CrossRef] [PubMed]

3

Targeting Glycolysis with Epigallocatechin-3-Gallate Enhances the Efficacy of Chemotherapeutics in Pancreatic Cancer Cells and Xenografts

Ran Wei [1,2], Robert M. Hackman [2], Yuefei Wang [1] and Gerardo G. Mackenzie [2,3,*]

1 Tea Science Institute, Zhejiang University, Hangzhou 310058, China; wran@ucdavis.edu (R.W.); zdcy@zju.edu.cn (Y.W.)
2 Department of Nutrition, University of California, Davis, CA 95616, USA; rmhackman@ucdavis.edu
3 Davis Comprehensive Cancer Center, University of California, Sacramento, CA 95817, USA
* Correspondence: ggmackenzie@ucdavis.edu

Abstract: Pancreatic cancer is a complex disease, in need of new therapeutic approaches. In this study, we explored the effect and mechanism of action of epigallocatechin-3-gallate (EGCG), a major polyphenol in green tea, alone and in combination with current chemotherapeutics on pancreatic cancer cell growth, focusing on glycolysis metabolism. Moreover, we investigated whether EGCG's effect is dependent on its ability to induce reactive oxygen species (ROS). EGCG reduced pancreatic cancer cell growth in a concentration-dependent manner and the growth inhibition effect was further enhanced under glucose deprivation conditions. Mechanistically, EGCG induced ROS levels concentration-dependently. EGCG affected glycolysis by suppressing the extracellular acidification rate through the reduction of the activity and levels of the glycolytic enzymes phosphofructokinase and pyruvate kinase. Cotreatment with catalase abrogated EGCG's effect on phosphofructokinase and pyruvate kinase. Furthermore, EGCG sensitized gemcitabine to inhibit pancreatic cancer cell growth in vitro and in vivo. EGCG and gemcitabine, given alone, reduced pancreatic tumor xenograft growth by 40% and 52%, respectively, whereas the EGCG/gemcitabine combination reduced tumor growth by 67%. EGCG enhanced gemcitabine's effect on apoptosis, cell proliferation, cell cycle and further suppressed phosphofructokinase and pyruvate kinase levels. In conclusion, EGCG is a strong combination partner of gemcitabine reducing pancreatic cancer cell growth by suppressing glycolysis.

Keywords: pancreatic cancer; epigallocatechin-3-gallate (EGCG); gemcitabine; glycolysis; ROS; phosphofructokinase

---

1. Introduction

Pancreatic cancer is one of the top five causes of cancer-related death in the United States, with an overall five-year survival rate of approximately eight percent [1]. While surgery, which offers the only realistic hope, is a viable option in a limited number of patients, current radiation therapy and chemotherapy regimens offer no significant clinical benefit [2]. For example, gemcitabine is an antimetabolite recognized as the current standard of care for unresectable locally advanced or metastatic pancreatic cancer, but its therapeutic effect for patients is limited [3]. Thus, an urgent need exists for new ways to combat pancreatic cancer, with the exploration of novel therapeutic strategies being a critical component.

Deregulated energy metabolism is recognized as one of the hallmarks of cancer [4]. Unlike normal cells, tumor cells prefer to rely on aerobic glycolysis to produce energy and to obtain intermediate metabolites that can then be directed to other biosynthetic pathways that promote tumor growth [5,6]. Moreover, the higher glycolytic rate in cancer cells has been shown to correlate to chemotherapeutic resistance [7]. Therefore, targeting tumor glycolysis remains attractive for therapeutic interventions, not only as a main target, but also for its ability to sensitize cancer cells to chemotherapeutics.

Epigallocatechin-3-gallate (EGCG), the most active polyphenol component found in green tea, presents several anticancer properties [8–10]. Accumulating evidence, including a previous study by our group, has shown that EGCG can inhibit cancer cell growth by modulating metabolic pathways [11–13]. An important consideration when exploring EGCG's mechanism of action is that in the presence of oxygen, EGCG undergoes auto-oxidation to generate reactive oxygen species (ROS) [14]. Since cancer cells are more susceptible to an increase in ROS levels [15], this has been proposed as a potential mechanism of action for the inhibitory cell growth effect by EGCG. However, to date, whether the glycolytic pathway is modulated by EGCG in pancreatic cancer, and whether it is ROS-dependent is not completely elucidated.

In the present study, we explored the effect and mechanism of action of EGCG alone and in combination with current chemotherapeutics on pancreatic cancer cell growth, focusing on glycolysis metabolism involved in pancreatic cancer cell growth, and investigated whether it is dependent on the ability of EGCG to induce ROS. Our results show that EGCG strongly reduced pancreatic cancer cell growth by suppressing glycolysis in a ROS-dependent manner. Moreover, EGCG enhanced the anticancer effect of gemcitabine in vitro and in vivo by inhibiting glycolysis and affecting cell kinetics.

2. Results

2.1. EGCG Affects Glycolysis in Pancreatic Cancer Cells

We initially evaluated the efficacy of EGCG on pancreatic cancer cells in culture. For this purpose, we treated multiple human pancreatic cancer cells with or without increasing concentrations of EGCG (20–100 μM) for 72 h. In parallel, we also compared the effect of EGCG in human pancreatic cancer cells to that of human pancreatic normal epithelial cells (HPNE). EGCG reduced human pancreatic cancer cell growth in a concentration-dependent manner. Of note, EGCG reduced cell growth more potently in human pancreatic cancer cells compared to HPNE cells. For instance, at 72 h, EGCG 80 μM reduced MIA PaCa-2 and Panc-1 cell growth by 84% and 64% ($p < 0.05$), respectively. In contrast, EGCG at 80 μM for 72 h had significantly less effect on the HPNE cells, reducing cell growth by only 24% (Figure 1A).

Given that alterations in cancer cell metabolism can lead to an inhibition of cell growth [16], and because EGCG has been shown to affect glycolysis in other tumor types [11–13], we evaluated the effect of EGCG on glucose metabolism in two human pancreatic cancer cells and one murine pancreatic cancer cell line (KPC). We assessed the impact of EGCG on glycolysis by measuring the extracellular acidification rate (ECAR) in the MIA PaCa-2, Panc-1, and KPC cell lines. After 24 h of treatment, EGCG strongly reduced ECAR in all three cell lines, revealing an inhibitory effect of EGCG on glycolysis (Figure 1B and Figure S1).

Next, we determined the effect of EGCG on pancreatic cancer cell growth under the conditions of either glucose deprivation or treatment with 2-Deoxy-D-glucose (2-DG), a glucose analog. As shown in Figure 1C, the reduction in cell growth induced by EGCG was enhanced under glucose deprivation or 2-DG treatment. For example, 2-DG alone reduced the cell growth rate by 5%, 27%, and 8% in Panc-1, MIA PaCa-2, and KPC cells, respectively, whereas when combined with EGCG, the cell growth was reduced by 71%, 58%, and 89%, respectively ($p < 0.01$; Figure 1C). Moreover, EGCG treatment reduced ATP levels concentration-dependently (Figure 1D). Treatment with EGCG at 40 μM for 24 h reduced ATP levels in Panc-1 and MIA PaCa-2 cells by 35% and 32%, respectively ($p < 0.01$ for both, Figure 1D).

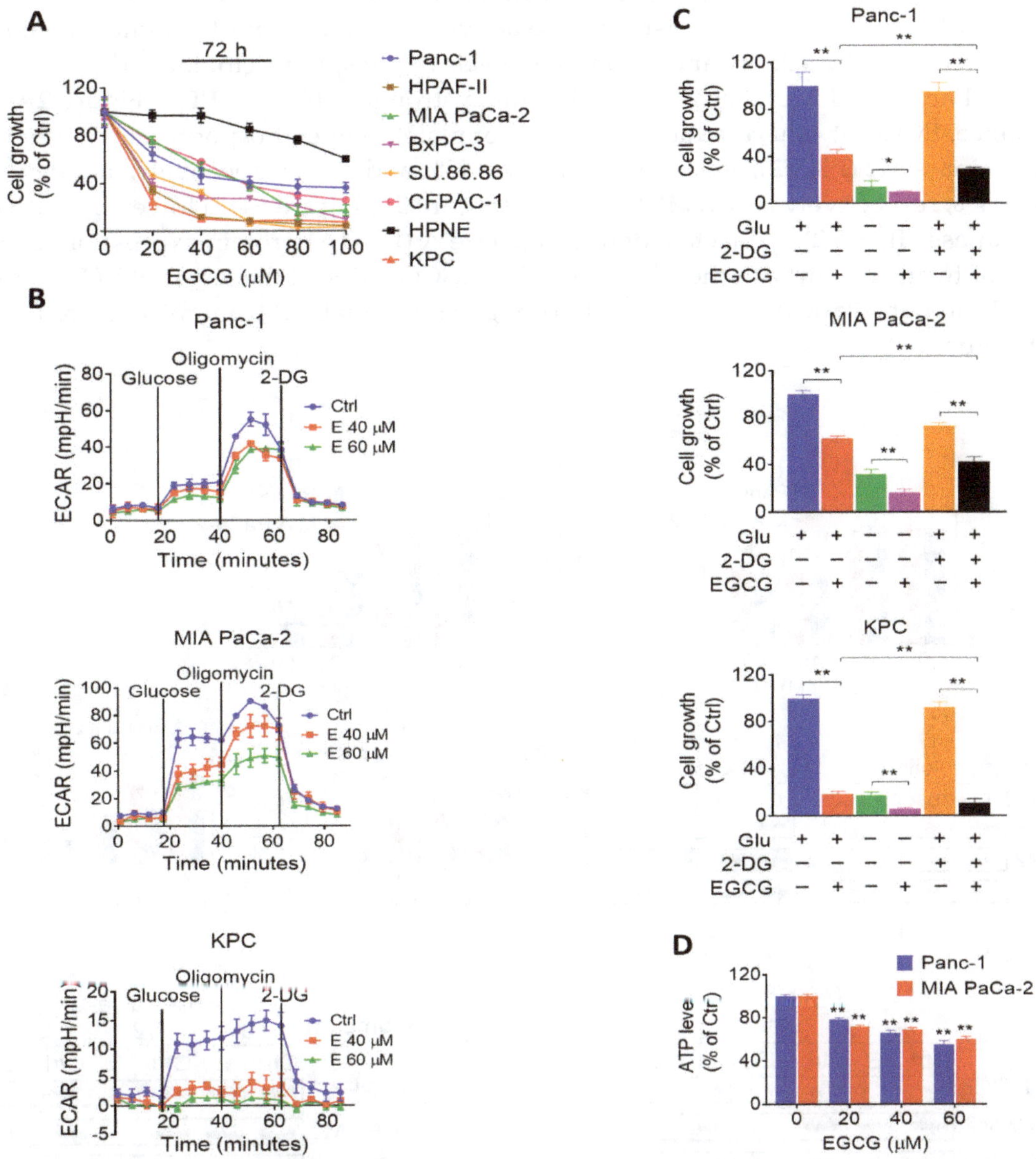

Figure 1. Epigallocatechin-3-gallate (EGCG) inhibits pancreatic cancer cell growth through glycolysis suppression. (**A**) EGCG inhibits human pancreatic cancer cell growth in a concentration-dependent manner. Cell growth was determined in Panc-1, MIA PaCa-2, HPAF-II, BxPC-3, SU-86.86, CFPAC-1, and KPC pancreatic cancer cells, and in the human pancreatic normal epithelial (HPNE) cells after treatment with increasing EGCG concentrations for 72 h. Results are expressed as a percentage of control. (**B**) EGCG suppresses glycolysis capacity in Panc-1, MIA PaCa-2, and KPC cells after 24 h. Glucose (25 mM), Oligomycin (1 μM) and 2-Deoxy-D-glucose (2-DG) (75 mM) were injected and the extracellular acidification rate (ECAR) of live cells was monitored during the experimental period. Results are presented as the mean ± SD of ECAR. (**C**) Cell growth was measured in Panc-1, MIA PaCa-2, and KPC cells treated with or without EGCG (40 μM) under glucose deprivation or 2-DG (10 mM) treatment condition. Results are expressed as a percentage of control. * $p < 0.05$, ** $p < 0.01$ vs. control. (**D**) EGCG reduced ATP levels in Panc-1 and MIA PaCa-2 cells after 24 h. Results are expressed as a percentage of control. * $p < 0.05$, ** $p < 0.01$ vs. control.

2.2. EGCG Inhibits Glycolysis through Suppressing Rate-Limiting Enzymes

Given the effect of EGCG on glycolysis, we evaluated whether EGCG could affect any particular step in the glycolytic pathway by measuring the activity and levels of glycolytic enzymes. EGCG treatment reduced both the activity and expression levels of phosphofructokinase (PFK) and pyruvate kinase (PK) in Panc-1 and MIA PaCa-2 cells, having a stronger effect on PFK (Figure 2A–C, Figure S5). For instance, EGCG at 40 μM reduced the levels of platelet-type phosphofructokinase (PFKP) and the pyruvate kinase M2 (PKM2), an isoform of PK, by 65% and 49%, respectively, in Panc-1 cells, and by 57% and 34%, respectively in MIA PaCa-2 cells (Figure 2B, Figure S4). However, EGCG failed to reduce hexokinases II (HK2) and lactate dehydrogenase A (LDHA) protein expression levels (Figure S2, Figure S12). In agreement with the in vitro results, EGCG reduced the levels of PFKP and PKM2 ($p < 0.01$ for both) in pancreatic tumor xenograft homogenates, obtained from mice treated with EGCG (Figure 2D, Figure S6).

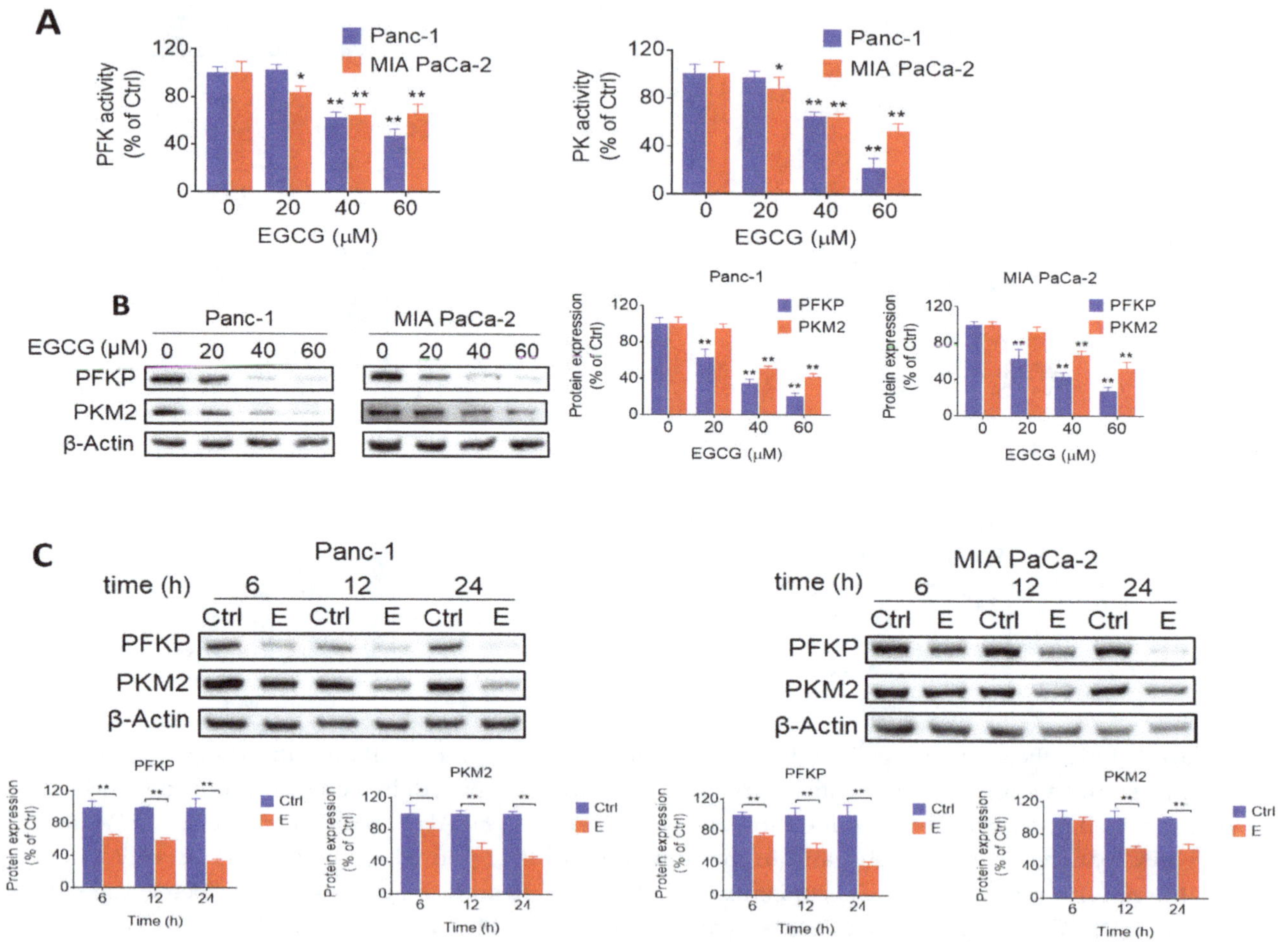

Figure 2. *Cont.*

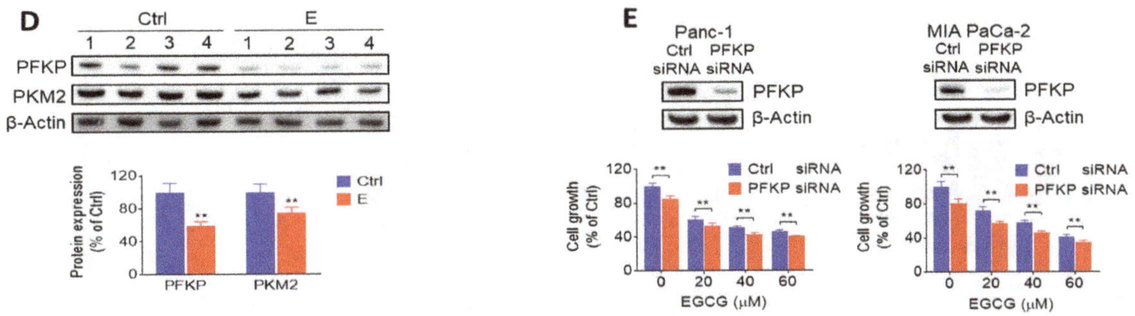

Figure 2. EGCG inhibits glycolysis through suppressing rate-limiting enzyme activity and expression. (**A**) Phosphofructokinase (PFK) and pyruvate kinase (PK) activities were determined in Panc-1 and MIA PaCa-2 cells after treatment with EGCG for 24 h. Results are expressed as a percentage of control. * $p < 0.05$, ** $p < 0.01$ vs. control. (**B**) Immunoblots for platelet-type phosphofructokinase (PFKP) and pyruvate kinase M2 (PKM2) in total cell protein extracts from Panc-1 and MIA PaCa-2 cells treated with escalating concentrations of EGCG, as indicated, for 24 h. Loading control: β-Actin. Bands were quantified and results are expressed as a percentage of control. * $p < 0.05$, ** $p < 0.01$ vs. control. (**C**) EGCG (40 μM) inhibited PFKP and PKM2 protein expression in a time-dependent manner in Panc-1 and MIA PaCa-2 cells. Results are expressed as percentage of control and presented as the mean ± SD. * $p < 0.05$, ** $p < 0.01$ vs. control. (**D**) Immunoblots of PFKP, PKM2 expression on tumor tissue from control- and EGCG-treated (10mg/kg/d) mice. Results are expressed as a percentage of control. * $p < 0.05$, ** $p < 0.01$ vs. control. (**E**) Effect of silencing PFKP on EGCG-induced cell growth reduction. Panc-1 and MIA PaCa-2 cells were transfected with either control or PFKP siRNA. After transfection, cells were treated with EGCG for 72 h and cell growth was evaluated. Results are expressed as percentage of control; * $p < 0.05$, ** $p < 0.01$ vs. control. Immunoblots to verify PFKP silencing were performed on whole cell extracts obtained from these cells (top panel).

To confirm the role of PFKP on EGCG-induced cell growth inhibition, we silenced PFKP in Panc-1 and MIA PaCa-2 cells. Knocking-down PFKP reduced Panc-1 and MIA PaCa-2 cell growth by 15% and 19%, respectively. In Panc-1 and MIA PaCa-2 cells transfected with nonspecific siRNA, EGCG 40 μM decreased the number of viable cells by 49% and 42%, whereas in PFKP-silenced cells, EGCG reduced cell growth by 57% and 54% in Panc-1 and MIA PaCa-2 cells, respectively (Figure 2E, Figure S6). Taken together, these findings indicate that silencing PFKP function has a slight additive effect on the growth inhibitory response of EGCG in both cell lines, and suggest that regulating glycolysis represents an important mechanism of EGCG in inhibiting pancreatic cancer cell growth.

2.3. EGCG Affects the Glycolytic Pathway in Pancreatic Cancer Cells through a ROS-Dependent Manner

Because EGCG and other polyphenols have been shown to undergo rapid oxidization to generate free radicals in the presence of oxygen [17], we evaluated the ability of EGCG to induce reactive oxygen species (ROS) in pancreatic cancer cells. Compared to the control, treatment with EGCG significantly increased ROS levels concentration-dependently, as determined with the general probe 2′,7′-Dichlorodihydrofluorescein diacetate (H2DCFDA). For example, EGCG at 40 μM increased ROS levels by 1.4- and 1.6-fold in Panc-1 and MIA PaCa-2 cells, respectively ($p < 0.01$ for both; Figure 3A).

Next, we determined the levels of hydrogen peroxide (H_2O_2) using the Amplex™ Red indicator probe. EGCG strongly increased H_2O_2 levels in pancreatic cancer cells. Compared to controls, EGCG at 40 μM increased H_2O_2 levels by 1.5- and 1.9-fold in Panc-1 and MIA PaCa-2 cells, respectively (Figure 3B). In both cell lines, cotreatment with catalase significantly abrogated the increase in H_2O_2 levels induced by EGCG (Figure 3B). Moreover, EGCG increased the levels of mitochondria superoxide anion in a concentration and time-dependent manner in both Panc-1 and MIA PaCa-2 cells (Figure 3C).

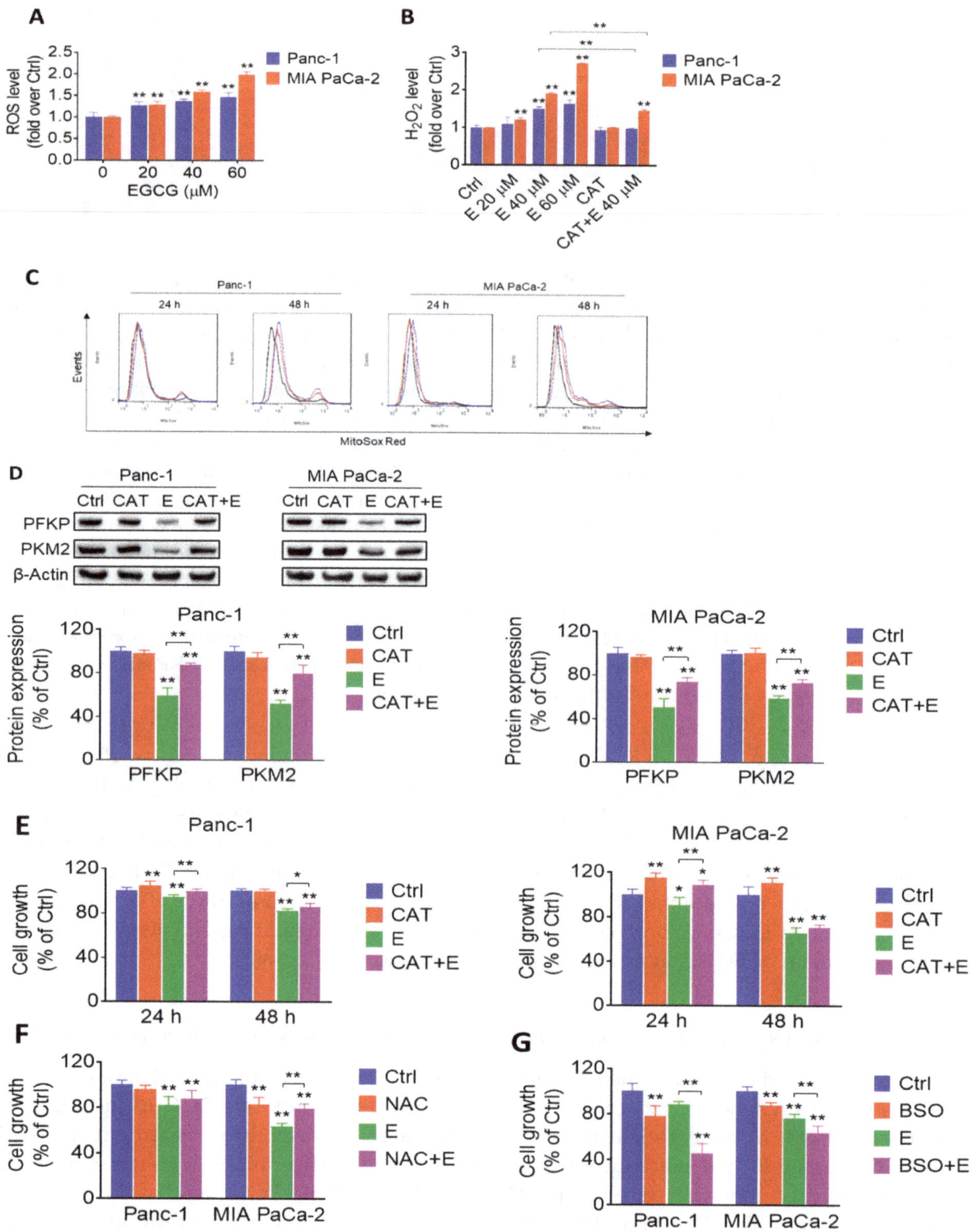

Figure 3. EGCG affects the glycolytic pathway in pancreatic cancer through a reactive oxygen species (ROS)-dependent manner. (**A**) 2′,7′-Dichlorodihydrofluorescein diacetate (H2DCFDA) fluorescence was measured in Panc-1 and MIA PaCa-2 cells treated without (control) or with EGCG at various concentration for 24 h. Results are expressed as fold change of control. * $p < 0.05$, ** $p < 0.01$ vs. control. (**B**) Amplex^{TM} Red was used to evaluate the levels of hydrogen peroxide level released by Panc-1 and MIA PaCa-2 cells. Results are expressed as fold change of control. * $p < 0.05$, ** $p < 0.01$ vs. control.

(**C**) EGCG induces a concentration- and time-dependent increase in mitochondrial superoxide anion levels. The levels of superoxide anion in the mitochondria were determined by flow cytometry using the MitoSOX-Red fluorescent probe. Black, red and blue lines represent control, EGCG 40 μM, and EGCG 60 μM groups, respectively. (**D**) The reduction in the expression levels of PFKP and PKM2 triggered by EGCG (E) was reversed by catalase (CAT). Immunoblots for PFKP and PKM2 in total cell protein extracts from Panc-1 and MIA PaCa-2 cells treated with 40 μM EGCG (E), 1500 U/mL catalase (CAT) or both, for 12 h. Loading control: β-Actin. Bands were quantified and results are expressed as a percentage of control. * $p < 0.05$, ** $p < 0.01$ vs. control. (**E**) Catalase (CAT) partly ameliorated the cell growth inhibitory effect induced by EGCG (E). Cells were treated with 40 μM EGCG (E), 1500 U/mL CAT or both, for 24 h or 48 h. Results are expressed as a percentage of control. * $p < 0.05$, ** $p < 0.01$ vs. control. (**F**) N-Acetyl-L-Cysteine (NAC) partly reversed cell inhibition effect of EGCG after 48 h. Cells were treated with 40 μM EGCG (E), 5 mM NAC or both for 48 h. Results are expressed as percentage of control. * $p < 0.05$, ** $p < 0.01$ vs. control. (**G**) L-Buthionine Sulfoximine (BSO) further aggravated cell inhibition effect of EGCG after 24 h. Cells were treated with 40 μM EGCG (E), 1 mM BSO or both for 24 h. Results are expressed as a percentage of control. * $p < 0.05$, ** $p < 0.01$ vs. control.

To elucidate whether the effect of EGCG on glycolysis is mediated through the increase in ROS, Panc-1 and MIA PaCa-2 cells were incubated with or without EGCG at 40 μM in the presence or absence of catalase for 12 h. In both cell lines, catalase mostly abrogated the inhibitory effect of EGCG on PFKP and PKM2, suggesting that the effect of EGCG on glycolytic enzymes is dependent on the ability of EGCG to induce ROS (Figure 3D, Figure S7).

However, catalase could only, in part, prevent the reduction in pancreatic cancer cell growth induced by EGCG (Figure 3E). Somewhat similar results were obtained when cotreating with N-Acetyl-L-Cysteine (NAC) (Figure 3F). In contrast, treatment with L-Buthionine Sulfoximine (BSO), an inhibitor of glutamylcysteine synthetase, strongly enhanced the reduction in cell growth induced by EGCG in both cell lines (Figure 3G). For example, in Panc-1 cells at 24 h, BSO and EGCG alone reduced cell growth by 22% and 12%, respectively, and by 54% when combined. These results suggest that EGCG reduces pancreatic cancer growth, partly, through an ROS-dependent mechanism.

2.4. EGCG Sensitizes Pancreatic Cancer Cells to Gemcitabine In Vitro

Because chemotherapeutics often display limited effects, show resistance, and cause side-effects, we evaluated whether EGCG would represent a useful partner in combination with commonly used drugs. For this purpose, we treated Panc-1 and MIA PaCa-2 cells with EGCG alone or in combination with gemcitabine, Abraxane®, 5-Fluorouracil, irinotecan, or oxaliplatin, five commonly used chemotherapeutics in pancreatic cancer patients, for 72 h and analyzed their combination index (CI) by means of the Chou–Talalay method. In both Panc-1 and MIA PaCa-2 cells, EGCG strongly synergized with gemcitabine (Figure 4 and Table S1). For example, in Panc-1 cells, the CI of all tested groups, except one, showed synergistic effects. In MIA PaCa-2 cells, the CI effects between EGCG and gemcitabine were also indicative of a strong additive effect (Figure 4). The combination effect of EGCG with the other four chemotherapeutics tested presented effects that were more variable with some showing an additive effect (Figure 4 and Table S1).

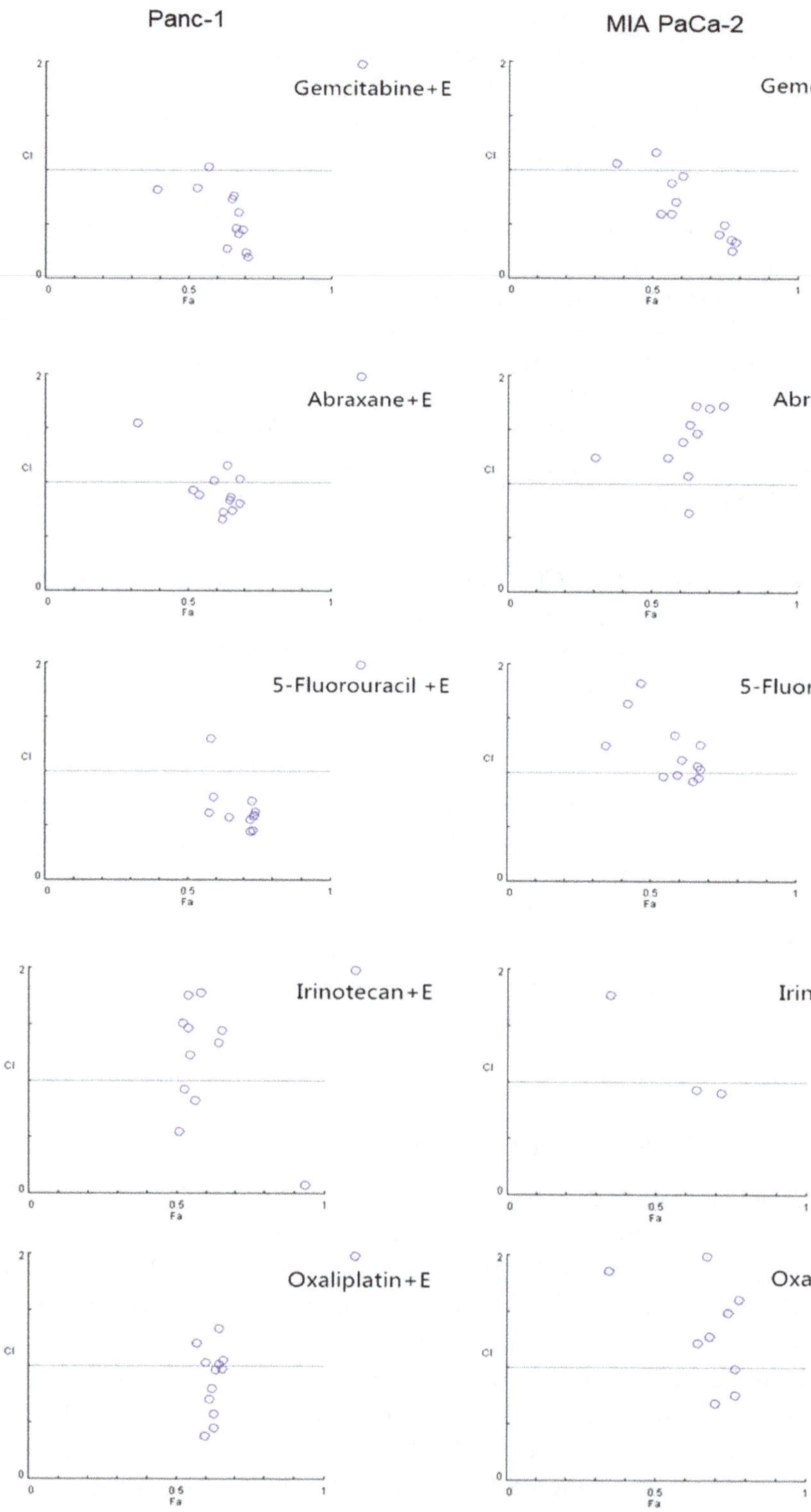

Figure 4. EGCG enhances the cell growth inhibitory effect of gemcitabine in pancreatic cancer cells. Combination index (CI) plots of EGCG (20, 40, 60 μM) in combination with gemcitabine (1, 10, 20 and 40 nM), abraxane (1, 10, 20 and 40 nM), 5 Fluorouracil (1, 10, 20 and 40 μM), irrinotecan (1, 10, 20 and 40 μM), and oxialiplatin (1, 10, 20 and 40 μM) in Panc-1 (left) and MIA PaCa-2 (right) cells. Drug interactions were quantitatively determined using the Chou–Talalay method, and CI < 1, =1, and >1 indicates synergism, additive and antagonism effect, respectively. Of note, the CI value dots depicted are based on concentrations of EGCG and the chemotherapeutic drugs shown on Table S1.

2.5. EGCG Enhances the Anticancer Effect of Gemcitabine in Pancreatic Cancer Xenografts through a Strong Cytokinetic Effect

Next, we evaluated whether EGCG could enhance the chemotherapeutic effect of gemcitabine in vivo. For this purpose, murine pancreatic cancer KPC cells were injected subcutaneously into immunocompetent mice, which gave rise to exponentially growing tumors. Once the tumors reached ~300 mm^3, the mice were treated either with EGCG (10 mg/kg) suspended in phosphate buffered saline (PBS) pH 7.4 given intraperitoneally (I.P.) once daily, gemcitabine (100 mg/kg) given I.P. twice per week, or both drugs. On day 16 of treatment, EGCG and gemcitabine, given as single agents, reduced tumor weight by 40% and 52%, respectively, compared to vehicle-treated controls ($p < 0.05$ and $p < 0.01$). In combination, EGCG plus gemcitabine reduced tumor weight by 67%, compared to controls ($p < 0.01$). Of note, the effect of the EGCG plus gemcitabine combination was significantly different from that of gemcitabine alone ($p < 0.05$; Figure 5A). Importantly, the drug combination was well tolerated by the mice, as indicated by the comparable mean body weight of the experimental groups throughout the treatment period (Figure 5B).

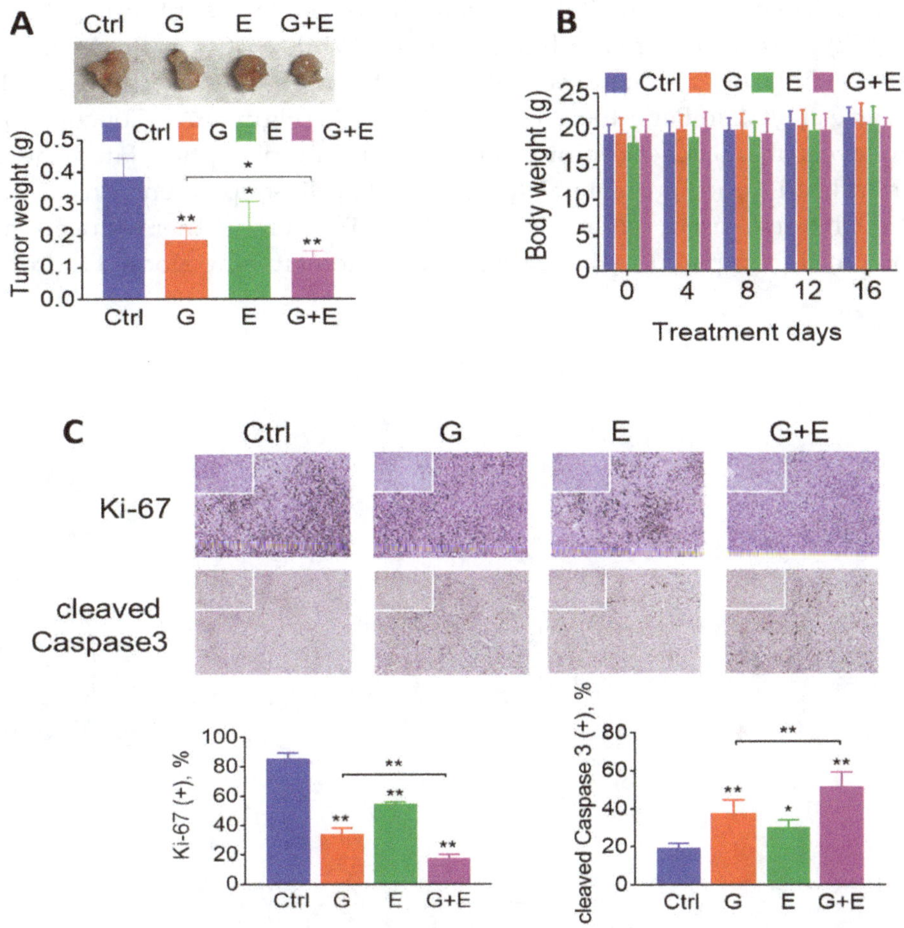

Figure 5. EGCG enhances the anticancer effect of gemcitabine in pancreatic cancer xenografts. (**A**) EGCG (E) promoted tumor weight lost with gemcitabine (G). Results are presented as the mean ± SD. * $p < 0.05$, ** $p < 0.01$ vs. control. (**B**) Mice body weight during treatment days for control, gemcitabine-treated groups (G), EGCG-treated groups (E), and the combination (G + E). Results are presented as the mean ± SD. (**C**) Immunostaining of the cell proliferation marker Ki-67 and of cleaved Caspase 3 were performed on KPC tumor sections and photographs were taken at 100× magnification. Representative images are shown. The consecutive section was stained with isotype Immunoglobulin G (IgG) as negative staining control and it is shown in the upper left corner. Results were expressed as percent of positive (+) cells ± SD per 100x field. * $p < 0.05$, ** $p < 0.01$ vs. control.

Because EGCG has been shown to be hepatotoxic at higher doses [18], and to further evaluate the safety of EGCG plus gemcitabine, we performed an acute toxicity study and determined the levels of multiple liver enzymes and kidney markers. After 16 days of EGCG plus gemcitabine treatment, liver and kidney function markers (including activity of Alanine Transaminase, Alkaline Phosphatase, Aspartate Transaminase, and the levels of blood urea nitrogen, creatinine, etc.) were in the normal range (Table S2). Consistent with the efficacy study, the mean body weights were comparable between the groups (Figure S3).

To investigate the mechanism by which EGCG plus gemcitabine reduced tumor growth, we determined cell proliferation (Ki-67 expression), and apoptosis (cleaved Caspase 3 expression) levels by immunohistochemistry in tumor tissue sections from control and EGCG plus/minus gemcitabine-treated mice (Figure 5C). Compared to controls, EGCG alone and EGCG plus gemcitabine inhibited cell proliferation (Ki-67 positive cells) by 45% and 83% in the KPC xenografts, respectively ($p < 0.01$, Figure 5C). In addition, EGCG increased the percentage of cleaved Caspase 3 positive cells by 1.6-fold when given alone and by 2.7-fold when given in combination ($p < 0.01$, Figure 5C).

In vitro, we determined the effect of EGCG and gemcitabine on cell cycle progression and cell death by apoptosis. As expected, gemcitabine, an inhibitor of DNA synthesis [19], strongly induced Synthesis/Gap2 (S/G2) phase arrest after 48 h of treatment. While EGCG at 40 μM only slightly arrested cell cycle progression, it strongly enhanced the effect of gemcitabine, with the combination further blocking the cell cycle at S/G2 in Panc-1 and MIA PaCa-2 cells (Figure 6A). Concomitant with cell cycle arrest, expression levels of S/G2 checkpoint proteins, including phosphorylated checkpoint kinases 1 (p-Chk1), phosphorylated tumor protein p53 (p-p53), and cyclin-dependent kinase (cdk) inhibitor p21 Waf1/Cip1 (p21) further increased, while cdc2 and CyclinB1 were further reduced in the EGCG plus gemcitabine-treated cells compared to those treated with gemcitabine alone (Figure 6B, Figure S8).

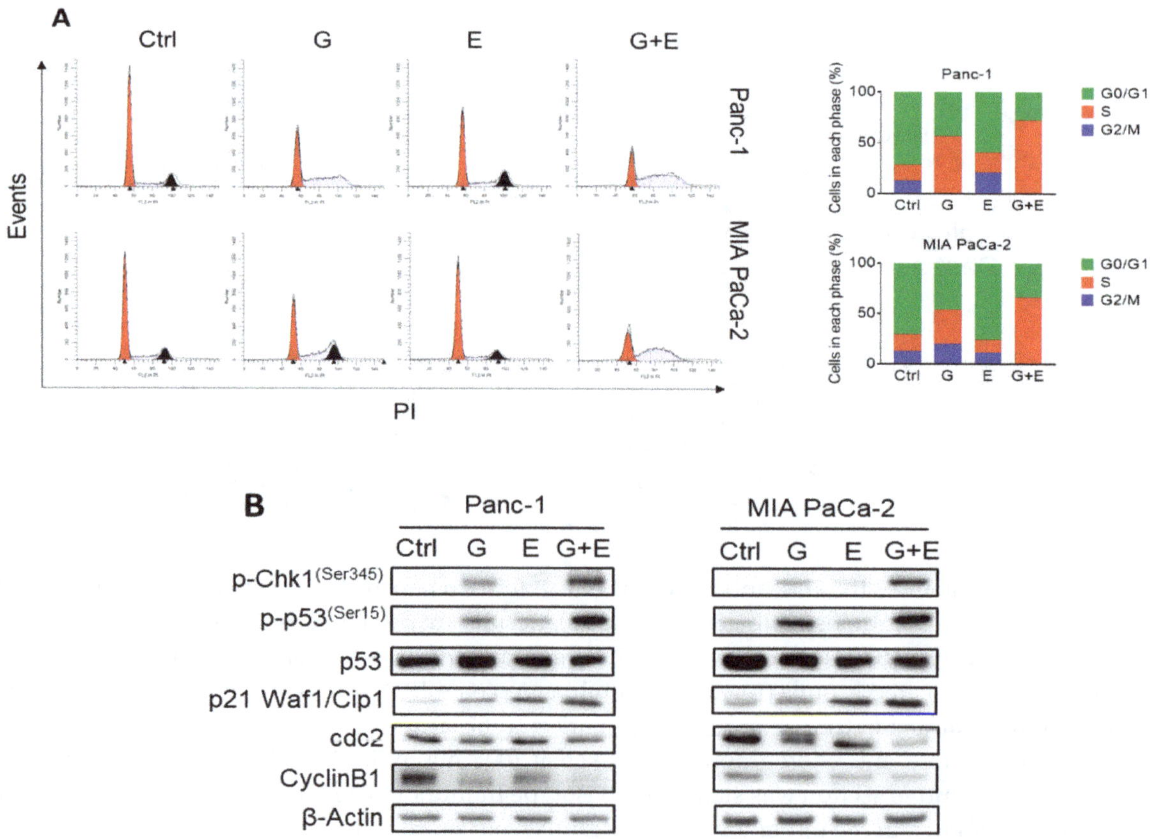

Figure 6. *Cont.*

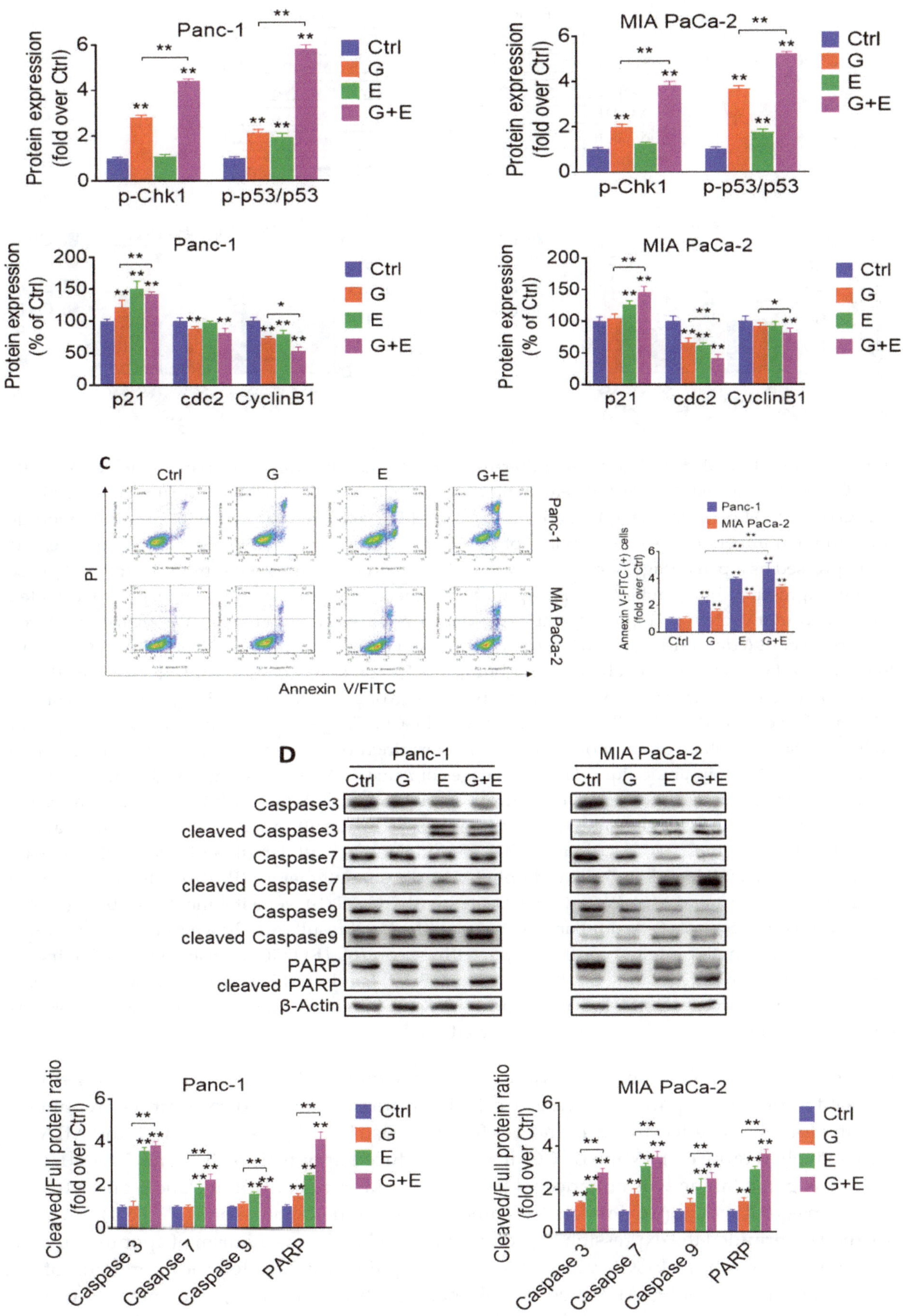

Figure 6. *Cont.*

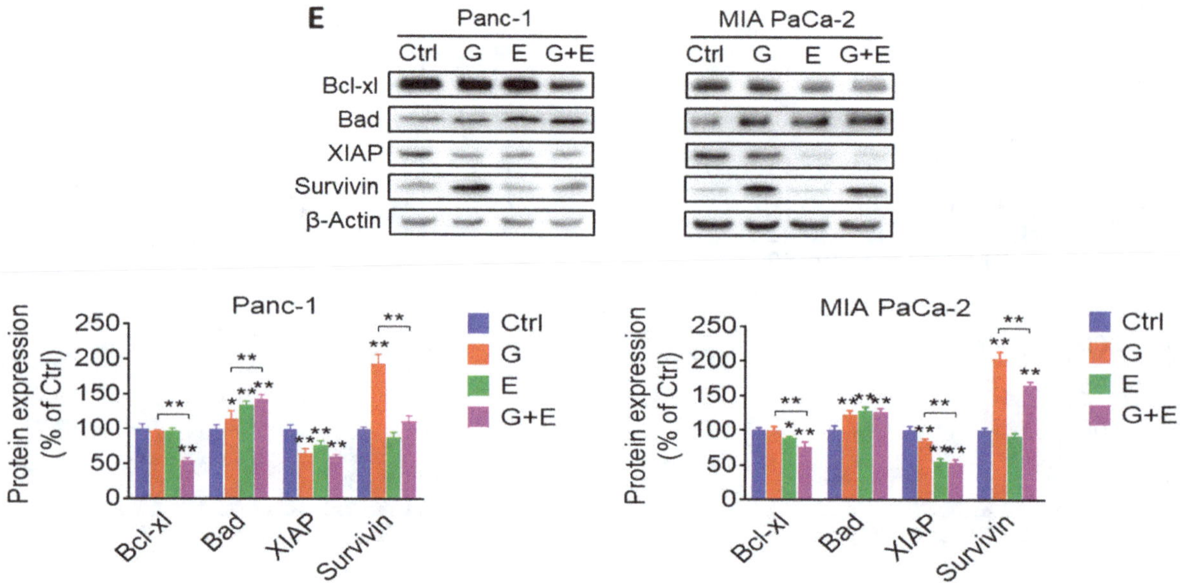

Figure 6. EGCG and gemcitabine together further affected cell kinetic in pancreatic cancer cells. (**A**) EGCG (E) enhanced the effect of gemcitabine (G) on the cell cycle. Following treatment with 40 μM EGCG (E), 20 nM gemcitabine (G), or both (G + E) for 48 h, cells were stained with propidium iodide (PI) and the number of cells in each phase of the cell cycle was measured by flow cytometry. Results are expressed as a percentage of control. (**B**) EGCG (E) and gemcitabine (G) modulated S/G2 phase protein expression. Immunoblots for phosphorylated checkpoint kinases 1 (p-Chk1), phosphorylated and total tumor protein p53 (p53), cyclin-dependent kinase (cdk) inhibitor p21 Waf1/Cip1 (p21), cell division cycle 2 (cdc2) and Cyclin B1 in total cell protein extracts from Panc-1 and MIA PaCa-2 cells treated with EGCG (E), gemcitabine (G), or both (G + E), for 48 h. Loading control: β-Actin. Bands were quantified and results are expressed as a percentage of control. * $p < 0.05$, ** $p < 0.01$ vs. control. (**C**) Panc-1 and MIA PaCa-2 cells were treated with EGCG (E), gemcitabine (G), or both (G + E) for 48 h, and the percentage of apoptotic cells were determined by flow cytometry using dual staining (Annexin V and propipium iodide). The percentages of Annexin V (+) cells was calculated, and results are expressed as the fold-increase over control. Co-treatment with EGCG (E) further increased the apoptosis rate induced by gemcitabine (G) alone after 48 h. Results are expressed as percentage of control. * $p < 0.05$, ** $p < 0.01$ vs. control. (**D**) Immunoblots for full length and cleaved Caspases 3, 7 and 9 as well as full length and cleaved poly (ADP-ribose) polymerase (PARP) in total cell protein extracts from Panc-1 and MIA PaCa-2 cells treated with EGCG (E), gemcitabine (G), or both (G + E) for 48 h. Loading control: β-Actin. Bands were quantified and results are shown as the ratio between the cleaved/full length protein; * $p < 0.05$, ** $p < 0.01$ vs. control. (**E**) EGCG sensitized gemcitabine on apoptosis induction by regulating B-cell lymphoma 2 (Bcl-2) family and Inhibitors of apoptosis proteins (IAP) family protein expression in Panc-1 and MIA PaCa-2 cells after 48 h. Results are expressed as percentage of control. * $p < 0.05$, ** $p < 0.01$ vs. control.

Besides blocking cell cycle progression and consistent with the in vivo results, gemcitabine also induced apoptosis in pancreatic cancer cells in culture. Compared to controls, treatment with gemcitabine for 48 h resulted in a 2.4- and 1.6-fold increase in apoptosis in Panc-1 and MIA PaCa-2 cells, respectively (Figure 6C). While EGCG at 40 μM induced apoptosis by 3.9- and 2.7-fold, the effect of EGCG plus gemcitabine was enhanced 4.7- and 3.4-fold over control in Panc-1 and MIA PaCa-2 cells, a response that was approximately two times that of gemcitabine alone ($p < 0.01$).

We then determined the expression of proteins involved in the mechanism of apoptosis by Western blot. Compared to controls, EGCG plus gemcitabine significantly affected the expression of cleaved Caspase 3, 7, 9, cleaved poly (ADP-ribose) polymerase (PARP), proapoptotic member of the Bcl-2 family protein Bad, antiapoptotic member of the Bcl-2 family protein Bcl-xl, and X-linked inhibitor of apoptosis protein (XIAP) levels, but not survivin (Figure 6D,E and Figure S9). Of note, no additive effect was observed on the expression of cleaved Caspase 3, 7, 9, Bad, Bcl-xl, or XIAP between EGCG plus gemcitabine and EGCG alone (Figure 6E, Figure S10), suggesting that the effect of the combination is most likely being driven by EGCG.

2.6. *EGCG Plus Gemcitabine Further Inhibits Glycolysis*

Given that EGCG strongly affected the glycolytic pathway, we evaluated whether combining EGCG with gemcitabine would lead to any additional glycolysis inhibitory effect. For this purpose, we determined the activity and levels of glycolytic enzymes in Panc-1 and MIA PaCa-2 cells, treated with EGCG and gemcitabine alone or in combination. The activity and levels of PFK and PK were significantly reduced compared to controls and gemcitabine alone groups. However, the effect of the combination group was not significant compared to the EGCG group (Figure 7A,B and Figure S11).

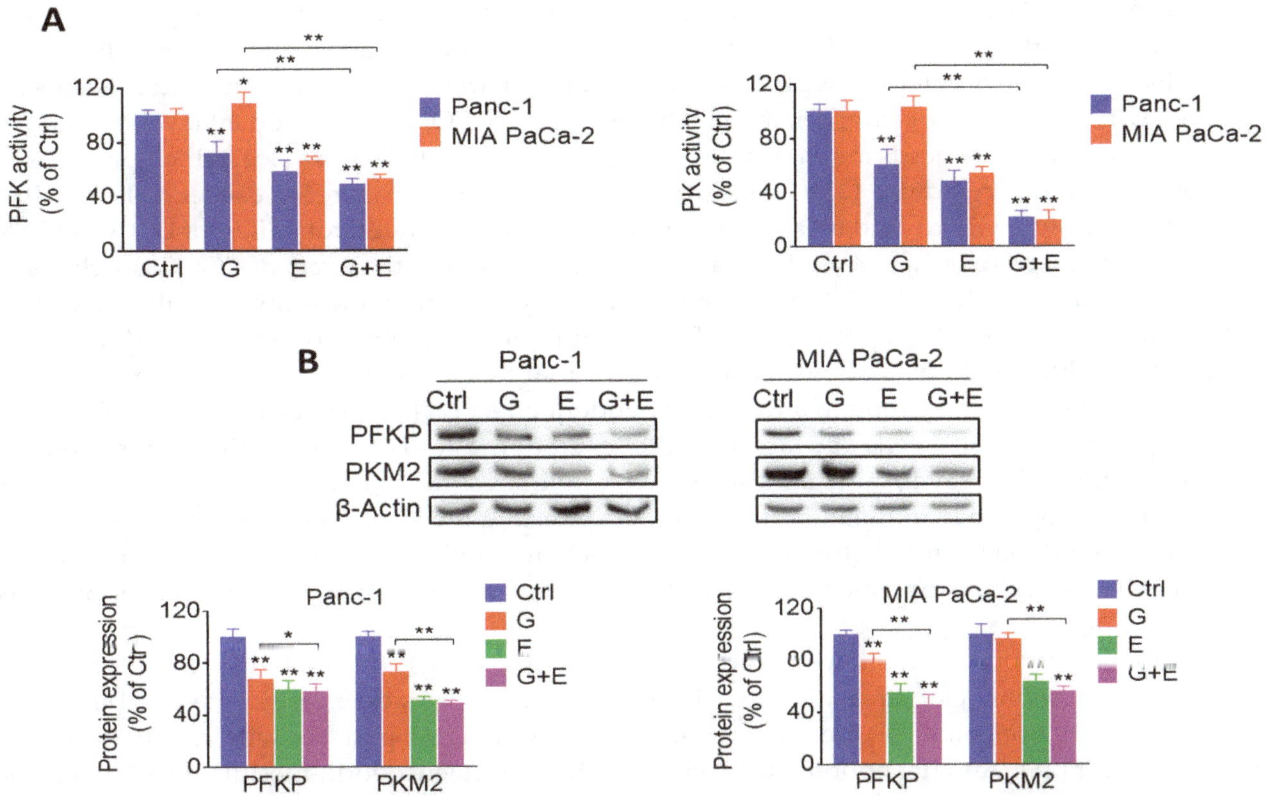

Figure 7. EGCG plus gemcitabine inhibit glycolysis. (**A**) The activity of PFK and PK was determined in Panc-1 and MIA PaCa-2 cells treated with 40 μM EGCG (E), 20 nM gemcitabine (G), or both (G + E) for 24 h. Results are expressed as a percentage of control. * $p < 0.05$, ** $p < 0.01$ vs. control. (**B**) Immunoblots for PFKP and PKM2 in total cell protein extracts from Panc-1 and MIA PaCa-2 cells treated with EGCG (E), gemcitabine (G), or both (G + E) for 12 h. Loading control: β-Actin. Bands were quantified and results are expressed as a percentage of control. * $p < 0.05$, ** $p < 0.01$ vs. control.

3. Discussion

Pancreatic cancer continues to be a significant health problem around the world. Given the lack of effective treatments that can meaningfully prolong a patient's life, an active search for agents that have additive or synergistic effect with chemotherapeutic drugs is critical in order to enhance their efficacy. In this study, we show that EGCG sensitizes pancreatic cancer cells to gemcitabine by suppressing glycolysis.

Our work identified the glycolytic pathway as one of the major signaling mechanisms involved in eliciting the growth inhibitory effect of EGCG. Glycolysis supports cell growth by rapidly generating ATP and metabolic intermediates for other biosynthetic pathways. A high rate of glycolysis is characteristic of cancer cells, even in the presence of sufficient oxygen [20]. EGCG strongly inhibited the glycolytic rate in pancreatic cancer cells by affecting the activity and expression of PFK and PK, two essential rate-limiting enzymes involved in glycolysis. The finding that glucose deprivation or 2-DG treatment enhances the growth inhibition effect of EGCG indicates that glycolysis is related to pancreatic cancer cell growth.

PFK catalyzes the first irreversible reaction of glycolysis and is usually highly expressed in tumor tissues. The platelet isoform of PFK, PFKP, functions as an important mediator in cancer cell proliferation and metastasis [21,22]. On the other hand, PKM2, an isoform of PK, is involved in regulating cell growth and metastasis [23]. Our results showed that EGCG decreased the enzyme activity and protein expression of PFK and PK in vitro and in vivo, but not HK2 or LDHA. Of note, silencing PFKP had a slight additive effect on the growth inhibitory effect of EGCG, suggesting that regulating glycolysis represents an important mechanism of EGCG in inhibiting pancreatic cancer cell growth. These results are consistent with other studies that also report inhibition of growth through the suppression of glycolysis by EGCG, such as in breast and hepatocellular cancer cell models [11,12].

The induction of oxidative stress plays a significant role in the effect of many anticancer agents [24]. Compared with normal cells, cancer cells exhibit higher levels of ROS and antioxidant levels to maintain redox homeostasis. Cancer cells are thus more susceptible to oxidative stress [15], which precedes the induction of apoptotic cell death [25]. EGCG induced ROS levels in pancreatic cancer cells in culture, consistent with its known pro-oxidant activity [26]. Interestingly, the inhibitory effect of EGCG on PFKP and PKM2 levels was mostly reversed by catalase, suggesting that the effect of EGCG on glycolytic processes is ROS-dependent. However, catalase only partly prevented the growth inhibition effect of EGCG, indicating that the ROS produced by EGCG could only explain part of the growth inhibitory effect by EGCG. Interestingly, we have recently shown that EGCG inhibits the protein kinase B (PKB, also known as Akt) pathway though a ROS-independent effect [27]. Thus, the effect of EGCG on the growth of pancreatic cancer cells appears to be the result of the sum of EGCG's ROS-dependent and independent effects. Moreover, the significance of oxidative stress in the reduction of cell growth can be further evidenced by two manipulations of the system affecting the levels of glutathione. Pretreatment with BSO, which depletes intracellular glutathione, strongly enhanced the growth inhibitory effect of EGCG. Alternatively, supplementing the cells with NAC attenuated the growth inhibitory effect of EGCG.

A common practice in the clinic is to administer multiple drugs concomitantly to cancer patients to help enhance a beneficial effect at lower doses while reducing side effects. The combination of gemcitabine with Abraxane® is the most widely used regimen for patients with newly diagnosed pancreatic cancer [28]. Another option is the combined therapy of leucovorin-modulated 5-Fluorouracil (5-FU), irinotecan, and oxaliplatin (FOLFIRINOX). Unfortunately, this regimen is given only to patients that can tolerate its toxicity, which includes a higher degree of neutropenia, diarrhea, and sensory neuropathy [29]. In this work, we explored whether EGCG could enhance the anticancer efficacy of the Food and Drug Administration (FDA)-approved drugs mentioned above. EGCG successfully enhanced the cell growth inhibition effect of gemcitabine in vitro and in vivo. Importantly, EGCG plus gemcitabine, at their effective doses, appeared to be safe to mice, being well tolerated and showing no signs of liver toxicity. As an analog of deoxycytidine, gemcitabine enters the cells, embeds into DNA, inhibits DNA synthesis, and induces cell cycle arrest. EGCG enhanced gemcitabine's suppression of cell growth through the inhibition of cell proliferation, the arrest of the cell cycle, and the induction of apoptosis through activation of execution Caspases [30], modulation of Bcl-2, and inhibition of apoptosis protein families. Mechanistically, the two agents together showed an additive effect of inhibiting glycolysis in pancreatic cancer cells. Of note, additional studies in complementary preclinical pancreatic cancer models are needed to validate the anti-tumor effect of EGCG with gemcitabine and advance the preclinical development of this drug combination. In summary, these results suggest the possibility to utilize EGCG as a useful adjuvant drug with gemcitabine to inhibit pancreatic cancer by further modulating cell kinetics and suppressing glycolysis.

4. Materials and Methods

4.1. Chemicals and Reagents

EGCG (≥98% purity) was purchased from Tocris (Minneapolis, MN, USA). 3-(4,5-dimethylthiazol-2-yl)-2,5-diphenyltetrazolium bromide (MTT) (≥97.5%), D-(+)-Glucose (≥99.5%), Oligomycin (≥90%), 2-Deoxy-D-glucose (≥99%), Irinotecan hydrochloride, Oxaliplatin, Catalase, *N*-Acetyl-L-cysteine (≥99%), DL-Buthionine-sulfoximine (≥99%), RIPA lysis buffer, Halt Protease Inhibitor Cocktail, Phosphatase Inhibitor Cocktail, and the following kits: Phosphofructokinase Activity Colorimetric assay and Pyruvate Kinase Activity assay were purchased from MilliporeSigma (St. Louis, MO, USA). Seahorse XF24 Extracellular Flux assay kits were purchased from Agilent (Santa Clara, CA, USA). CellTiter-Glo® reagent and rATP were purchased from Promega (Madison, WI, USA). PFKP siRNA plasmid was purchased from Santa Cruz Biotechnology (Dallas, TX, USA). Gemcitabine-HCL (>99%) was purchased from BIOTANG (Waltham, MA, USA). 5-Fluorouracil (≥99%) was purchased from Alfa Aesar (Haverhill, MA, USA). Annexin V-FITC conjugate, propidium iodide (PI), 2′,7′-dichlorodihydrofluorescein diacetate (H2DCFDA), Amplex® Red Hydrogen Peroxide kit, MitoSOX™ Red Mitochondrial Superoxide Indicator, Lipofectamine™ 3000 Transfection reagent, and SuperSignal™ West Dura Extended Duration Substrate were purchased from ThermoFisher Scientific (Waltham, MA, USA). Antibodies for Western blot were purchased from Cell Signaling Technology (Danvers, MA, USA). Bradford protein assay reagent, 30% (*w*/*v*) Acrylamide/Bis Solution, 4xLaemmli sample buffer, and Immun-Blot® PVDF Membranes were purchased from Bio-Rad (Hercules, CA, USA).

4.2. Cell Culture

Human pancreatic cancer cell lines (BxPC-3, HPAF-II, CFPAC-1, Su.86.86, Panc-1 and MIA PaCa-2), and human pancreatic normal epithelial (HPNE) cells were sourced from the American Type Culture Collection (Manassas, VA, USA). FC1245 cells (KPC, murine pancreatic cancer cells) were a gift from Dr. David Tuveson (Cold Spring Harbor Laboratory, Cold Spring Harbor, NY, USA). All cell lines were grown as monolayers in a specific medium under conditions suggested by the vendor. Although these cells lines were not authenticated in our lab, they were characterized by cell morphology and growth rate, and cultured in our laboratory less than six months after being received. We also routinely test for mycoplasma contamination in all cell lines every three months.

4.3. Cell Viability

Following the treatment with EGCG or the various chemotherapeutic drugs for 72 h, the reduction of 3-(4,5-dimethylthiazol-2-yl)-2,5-diphenyltetrazolium bromide dye (MTT) was determined according to the manufacture's protocol (MilliporeSigma, St. Louis, MO, USA).

4.4. Cellular Glycolytic Rate Measurements

The cellular glycolytic rate, represented as the extracellular acidification rate (ECAR), was measured using a Seahorse XF24 Extracellular Flux Analyzer (Agilent, Santa Clara, CA, USA). Briefly, Panc-1 and MIA PaCa-2 cells, plated on XF24 cell culture plates, were incubated with the agents for 24 h, and then assayed with a glycolytic stress test kit, following the manufacturer's instruction (Agilent, Santa Clara, CA, USA).

4.5. Cellular ATP Levels

Cells, plated in white 96-well plates, were treated with test drugs for 24 h. After treatment, ATP levels were measured with the CellTiter-Glo® reagent, following the manufacturer's protocol (Promega, Madison, WI, USA). A standard curve was generated using escalating concentrations of ATP.

4.6. *Glycolysis-Related Enzymes Activity*

Cells were seeded into the 6-well plates overnight and treated with EGCG for 24 h. Following the incubation, cells were collected, washed with cold PBS, and homogenized. After centrifugation, the supernatant was collected and used to measure the phosphofructokinase (PFK) and pyruvate kinase (PK) enzyme activities following the manufacturer's protocol (MilliporeSigma, Saint Louis, MO, USA). Protein concentration was determined using the Bradford protein assay.

4.7. *Gene Silencing*

Cells were plated in 6-well plates overnight, and transiently transfected with PFKP siRNA or nonspecific control siRNA for several hours using Lipofectamine™ 3000 reagent according to the manufacturer's instructions (ThermoFisher Scientific, Waltham, MA, USA). Following transfection, cells were replated and treated with EGCG for up to 72 h and cell viability was tested. The gene silencing efficiency was determined by immunoblotting.

4.8. *Determination of ROS Levels*

After treatment with EGCG for 24 h, cells were incubated with 10 μM H2DCFDA for 30 min at 37 °C and their fluorescence intensity was analyzed using a Synergy H1 microplate reader (Biotek, Winooski, VT, USA). Hydrogen peroxide (H_2O_2) levels were detected using an Amplex™ Red hydrogen peroxide kit according to the manufacturer's instruction (ThermoFisher Scientific, Waltham, MA, USA).

4.9. *Mitochondrial Superoxide Level Analysis*

After treatment with EGCG for 24 or 48 h, cells were collected and incubated with 5 μM MitoSOX™ Red mitochondrial superoxide probe at 37 °C for 30 min. The fluorescence intensity was determined by FACScan flow cytometry (Becton Dickinson, San Jose, CA, USA) and results were analyzed with FlowJo software (v7.6, Tree Star, Inc., Ashland, OR, USA).

4.10. *Cell Apoptosis*

After cells were treated with the test agents in 6-well plates, they were trypsinized and stained with Annexin V-FITC (100× dilution) and PI (0.5 μg/mL) for 15 min. Annexin V-FITC and PI fluorescence intensities were analyzed by FACScan (Becton Dickinson, San Jose, CA, USA). Annexin V (+)/PI (-) cells are apoptotic cells, Annexin V (+)/ PI (+) cells have undergone secondary necrosis, and Annexin V (-)/ PI (+) cells are necrotic cells. Results were analyzed by using FlowJo software.

4.11. *Cell Cycle Analysis*

Cells were seeded in 6-well plates and treated for 48 h. After each treatment, cells were trypsinized and fixed in 70% (*v*/*v*) ethanol overnight, stained with PI (50 μg/mL) and RNase A (10 mg/mL) for 15 min, and subjected to flow cytometric analysis (Becton Dickinson, San Jose, CA, USA).

4.12. *Western Blot*

Whole cell protein lysates were prepared, and electrophoresis and electroblotting were performed as previously described [31]. Membranes were probed overnight with the following primary antibodies (1:1000 dilution) from Cell Signaling Technology (Danvers, MA, USA): PFKP (Cat #8164), PKM2 (Cat #4053), HK2 (Cat #2867), LDHA (Cat #3582), phospho-Chk1 (Ser345) (Cat #2348), phospho-p53 (Ser15) (Cat #9286), p53 (Cat #2527), p21 Waf1/Cip1 (Cat #2947), cdc2 (Cat #28439), Cyclin B1 (Cat #12231), Caspase-3 (Cat #14220), Caspase-7 (Cat #12827), Caspase-9 (Cat #9508), and PARP (Cat #9542). β-Actin (Cat #8457) was used at the same time as a loading control. After incubation for 60 min at room temperature in the presence of the secondary antibody (HRP-conjugated; 1:5000 dilution), the conjugates were developed and visualized using a Molecular Imager FX™ System (BioRad; Hercules, CA, USA).

4.13. Animal Studies

All animal studies were approved by the Institutional Animal Care and Use Committee at the University of California, Davis (protocol # 20716; approved on September 6, 2018). For the efficacy study, C57BL/6J mice (4–6 weeks) were bilaterally, s.c injected with 0.3×10^6 KPC cells/tumor suspended in 0.1 mL sterile PBS. When KPC cells reached palpable tumor size (~300 mm^3), mice (n = 5/group) were divided randomly into four groups. Mice were either given vehicle, EGCG 10 mg/kg, 7x/week by intraperitoneal injection (I.P.) injections, gemcitabine 100 mg/kg, 2x/week by i.p injections, or EGCG in combination with gemcitabine at the above doses. The dose of EGCG was based on our previous studies [11,27]. Mice were treated for 16 days. Tumor size and body weight were measured every two days, and tumor size was determined by the equation length × width × (length + width/2) × 0.56, in millimeters [32]. At the end of the study, animals were euthanized by carbon dioxide asphyxiation, and tumor weights measured. Tumor and liver tissues were collected for analysis. For the drug combination toxicity study, C57BL/6J mice (n = 4/group) were treated either with PBS (vehicle control), or EGCG 10 mg/kg, 7x/week by i.p injections, in combination with gemcitabine 100 mg/kg, 2x/week by i.p injections. On day 16, mice were euthanized, blood was drawn, serum was collected, and a liver-kidney function panel was performed.

4.14. Immunohistochemistry

Immunohistochemical staining for for Ki-67 (Cat #12202) and cleaved Caspase-3 (Cat #9661, both from Cell Signaling Technology, Danvers, MA, USA) was performed as previously described [33]. Briefly, paraffin-embedded sections (5 µm thick) were deparaffinized and rehydrated, followed by antigen retrieval performed by microwave-heating in 0.01 M citrate buffer (pH 6.0). 3% H_2O_2 was used to block endogenous peroxidase activity for 10 min at room temperature. Slides were blocked for 60 min with serum, and incubated with primary antibody overnight at 4 °C. The following morning, slides were washed thrice with PBS, and then incubated with the biotinylated secondary antibody and the streptavidin-biotin complex (Invitrogen, Carlsbad, CA, USA) for 1 h of each at room temperature. After washing with PBS three times, slides were stained with 3,3′-Diaminobenzidine tetrahydrochloride hydrate (DAB) solution, and then counterstained with hematoxylin. Images were taken at 100× magnification. At least five fields per sample were scored and analyzed using Image J software (v1.46, NIH, Bethesda, MD, USA).

4.15. Statistical Analysis

Data were obtained from at least three independent biological experiments and results expressed as mean ± SD. One-way analysis of variance (ANOVA) and the Duncan test were used to analyze differences among multiple groups. *T*-tests were performed to compare the difference between two groups. $p < 0.05$ was regarded as being statistically significant.

5. Conclusions

EGCG strongly suppresses glycolysis through the inhibition of PFK, an effect that is ROS-dependent. In addition, EGCG presents a strong additive effect when combined with gemcitabine in pancreatic xenografts by further inhibiting glycolysis and affecting cell kinetics. Although additional studies to validate the above findings in complemmentary preclinical models of pancreatic cancer are warranted, our results suggest that EGCG is a useful combination partner of gemcitabine in pancreatic cancer treatment.

Supplementary Materials
Figure S1: EGCG reduced cell glycolysis, glycolytic capacity and glycolytic reserve in Panc-1, MIA PaCa-2 and KPC cells. Figure S2: Effect of EGCG on HK2 and LDHA protein expression. Table S1: Cell growth combination effects of EGCG with various chemotherapeutics in MIA PaCa-2 and Panc-1 cells. Table S2: Serum levels of multiple biochemical enzymes and markers of liver and kidney function for control and EGCG plus gemcitabine the end of the treatment period. Figure S3: Mice body weight progression for control and gemcitabine+EGCG

treated groups. Figure S4. Western blot images with molecular weight for PFKP and PKM2 shown in Figure 2B. Figure S5. Western blot images with molecular weight for PFKP and PKM2 shown in Figure 2C. Figure S6. Western blot images with molecular weight for PFKP and PKM2 shown in Figures 2D and 2E. Figure S7. Western blot images with molecular weight for PFKP and PKM2 shown in Figure 3D. Figure S8. Western blot images with molecular weight for p-Chk1, p53, p21, cdc2 and CyclinB1 shown in Figure 6B. Figure S9. Western blot images with molecular weight for Caspase 3, Caspase 7, Caspase 9 and PARP shown in Figure 6D. Figure S10. Western blot images with molecular weight for Bcl-xl, Bad, XIAP, Survivin shown in Figure 6E. Figure S11. Western blot images with molecular weight for PFKP and PKM2 shown in Figure 7B. Figure S12. Western blot images with molecular weight for HK2 and LDHA shown in Figure S2.

Author Contributions: Conceptualization, R.W. and G.G.M.; methodology, R.W. and G.G.M.; validation, R.W.; formal analysis, R.W.; investigation, R.W.; resources, G.G.M.; data curation, R.W.; writing—original draft preparation, R.W.; writing—review and editing, R.W., R.M.H., Y.W. and G.G.M.; supervision, G.G.M.; project administration, G.G.M.; funding acquisition, G.G.M.

References

1. Aier, I.; Semwal, R.; Sharma, A.; Varadwaj, P.K. A systematic assessment of statistics, risk factors, and underlying features involved in pancreatic cancer. *Cancer Epidemiol.* **2019**, *58*, 104–110. [CrossRef] [PubMed]
2. Kleeff, J.; Korc, M.; Apte, M.; La Vecchia, C.; Johnson, C.D.; Biankin, A.V.; Neale, R.E.; Tempero, M.; Tuveson, D.A.; Hruban, R.H.; et al. Pancreatic cancer. *Nat. Rev. Dis. Primers* **2016**, *2*. [CrossRef] [PubMed]
3. Von Hoff, D.D.; Ervin, T.; Arena, F.P.; Chiorean, E.G.; Infante, J.; Moore, M.; Seay, T.; Tjulandin, S.A.; Ma, W.W.; Saleh, M.N.; et al. Increased survival in pancreatic cancer with nab-paclitaxel plus gemcitabine. *N. Engl. J. Med.* **2013**, *369*, 1691–1703. [CrossRef] [PubMed]
4. Li, Z.; Zhang, H. Reprogramming of glucose, fatty acid and amino acid metabolism for cancer progression. *Cell Mol. Life Sci.* **2016**, *73*, 377–392. [CrossRef] [PubMed]
5. Dhup, S.; Dadhich, R.K.; Porporato, P.E.; Sonveaux, P. Multiple biological activities of lactic acid in cancer: Influences on tumor growth, angiogenesis and metastasis. *Curr. Pharm. Des.* **2012**, *18*, 1319–1330. [CrossRef] [PubMed]
6. Liberti, M.V.; Locasale, J.W. The warburg effect: How does it benefit cancer cells? *Trends Biochem. Sci.* **2016**, *41*, 211–218. [CrossRef] [PubMed]
7. Bhattacharya, B.; Mohd Omar, M.F.; Soong, R. The warburg effect and drug resistance. *Br. J. Pharmacol.* **2016**, *173*, 970–979. [CrossRef]
8. Lewis, K.A.; Jordan, H.R.; Tollefsbol, T.O. Effects of SAHA and EGCG on growth potentiation of triple-negative breast cancer cells. *Cancers* **2018**, *11*, 23. [CrossRef]
9. Du, G.J.; Zhang, Z.Y.; Wen, X.D.; Yu, C.H.; Calway, T.; Yuan, C.S.; Wang, C.Z. Epigallocatechin Gallate (EGCG) Is the most effective cancer chemopreventive polyphenol in green tea. *Nutrients* **2012**, *4*, 1679–1691. [CrossRef]
10. Wang, Y.K.; Chen, W.C.; Lai, Y.H.; Chen, Y.H.; Wu, M.T.; Kuo, C.T.; Wang, Y.Y.; Yuan, S.S.F.; Liu, Y.P.; Wu, I.C. Influence of tea consumption on the development of second esophageal neoplasm in patients with head and neck cancer. *Cancers* **2019**, *11*, 387. [CrossRef]
11. Wei, R.; Mao, L.; Xu, P.; Zheng, X.; Hackman, R.M.; Mackenzie, G.G.; Wang, Y. Suppressing glucose metabolism with epigallocatechin-3-gallate (EGCG) reduces breast cancer cell growth in preclinical models. *Food Funct.* **2018**, *9*, 5682–5696. [CrossRef] [PubMed]
12. Li, S.; Wu, L.; Feng, J.; Li, J.; Liu, T.; Zhang, R.; Xu, S.; Cheng, K.; Zhou, Y.; Zhou, S.; et al. In vitro and in vivo study of epigallocatechin-3-gallate-induced apoptosis in aerobic glycolytic hepatocellular carcinoma cells involving inhibition of phosphofructokinase activity. *Sci. Rep.* **2016**, *6*, e28479. [CrossRef] [PubMed]
13. Gao, F.; Li, M.; Liu, W.B.; Zhou, Z.S.; Zhang, R.; Li, J.L.; Zhou, K.C. Epigallocatechin gallate inhibits human tongue carcinoma cells via HK2mediated glycolysis. *Oncol. Rep.* **2015**, *33*, 1533–1539. [CrossRef] [PubMed]
14. Long, L.H.; Clement, M.V.; Halliwell, B. Artifacts in cell culture: Rapid generation of hydrogen peroxide on addition of (-)-epigallocatechin, (-)-epigallocatechin gallate, (+)-catechin, and quercetin to commonly used cell culture media. *Biochem. Biophys. Res. Commun.* **2000**, *273*, 50–53. [CrossRef]
15. Sullivan, L.B.; Chandel, N.S. Mitochondrial reactive oxygen species and cancer. *Cancer Metab.* **2014**, *2*, e17. [CrossRef]
16. Villa, E.; Ricci, J.E. How does metabolism affect cell death in cancer? *Febs. J.* **2016**, *283*, 2653–2660. [CrossRef]

17. Wei, Y.; Chen, P.; Ling, T.; Wang, Y.; Dong, R.; Zhang, C.; Zhang, L.; Han, M.; Wang, D.; Wan, X.; et al. Certain (-)-epigallocatechin-3-gallate (EGCG) auto-oxidation products (EAOPs) retain the cytotoxic activities of EGCG. *Food Chem.* **2016**, *204*, 218–226. [CrossRef]
18. Lambert, J.D.; Kennett, M.J.; Sang, S.; Reuhl, K.R.; Ju, J.; Yang, C.S. Hepatotoxicity of high oral dose (-)-epigallocatechin-3-gallate in mice. *Food Chem. Toxicol.* **2010**, *48*, 409–416. [CrossRef]
19. Mini, E.; Nobili, S.; Caciagli, B.; Landini, I.; Mazzei, T. Cellular pharmacology of gemcitabine. *Ann. Oncol.* **2006**, *17*, 7–12. [CrossRef]
20. Yu, L.; Chen, X.; Wang, L.; Chen, S. The sweet trap in tumors: Aerobic glycolysis and potential targets for therapy. *Oncotarget* **2016**, *7*, 38908–38926. [CrossRef]
21. Lee, J.H.; Liu, R.; Li, J.; Zhang, C.; Wang, Y.; Cai, Q.; Qian, X.; Xia, Y.; Zheng, Y.; Piao, Y.; et al. Stabilization of phosphofructokinase 1 platelet isoform by AKT promotes tumorigenesis. *Nat. Commun.* **2017**, *8*, e949. [CrossRef] [PubMed]
22. Lang, L.; Chemmalakuzhy, R.; Shay, C.; Teng, Y. PFKP signaling at a glance: An emerging mediator of cancer cell metabolism. *Adv. Exp. Med. Biol.* **2019**, *1134*, 243–258. [CrossRef] [PubMed]
23. Azoitei, N.; Becher, A.; Steinestel, K.; Rouhi, A.; Diepold, K.; Genze, F.; Simmet, T.; Seufferlein, T. PKM2 promotes tumor angiogenesis by regulating HIF-1alpha through NF-kappaB activation. *Mol. Cancer* **2016**, *15*, e3. [CrossRef] [PubMed]
24. Sun, Y.; Huang, L.Q.; Mackenzie, G.G.; Rigas, B. Oxidative stress mediates through apoptosis the anticancer effect of phospho-nonsteroidal anti-Inflammatory drugs: Implications for the role of oxidative stress in the action of anticancer agents. *J. Pharmacol. Exp. Ther.* **2011**, *338*, 775–783. [CrossRef] [PubMed]
25. Hegedus, C.; Kovacs, K.; Polgar, Z.; Regdon, Z.; Szabo, E.; Robaszkiewicz, A.; Forman, H.J.; Martner, A.; Virag, L. Redox control of cancer cell destruction. *Redox. Biol.* **2018**, *16*, 59–74. [CrossRef] [PubMed]
26. Qanungo, S.; Das, M.; Haldar, S.; Basu, A. Epigallocatechin-3-gallate induces mitochondrial membrane depolarization and caspase-dependent apoptosis in pancreatic cancer cells. *Carcinogenesis* **2005**, *26*, 958–967. [CrossRef] [PubMed]
27. Wei, R.; Penso, N.E.C.; Hackman, R.M.; Wang, Y.; Mackenzie, G.G. Epigallocatechin-3-gallate (EGCG) suppresses pancreatic cancer cell growth, invasion, and migration partly through the inhibition of Akt pathway and epithelial-mesenchymal transition: Enhanced efficacy when combined with gemcitabine. *Nutrients* **2019**, *11*, 1856. [CrossRef]
28. Frese, K.K.; Neesse, A.; Cook, N.; Bapiro, T.E.; Lolkema, M.P.; Jodrell, D.I.; Tuveson, D.A. nab-Paclitaxel potentiates gemcitabine activity by reducing cytidine deaminase levels in a mouse model of pancreatic cancer. *Cancer Discov.* **2012**, *2*, 260–269. [CrossRef]
29. Conroy, T.; Desseigne, F.; Ychou, M.; Bouche, O.; Guimbaud, R.; Becouarn, Y.; Adenis, A.; Raoul, J.L.; Gourgou-Bourgade, S.; de la Fouchardiere, C.; et al. FOLFIRINOX versus gemcitabine for metastatic pancreatic cancer. *N. Engl. J. Med.* **2011**, *364*, 1817–1825. [CrossRef]
30. Shi, Y. Mechanisms of caspase activation and inhibition during apoptosis. *Mol. Cell* **2002**, *9*, 459–470. [CrossRef]
31. Mallangada, N.A.; Vargas, J.M.; Thomas, S.; DiGiovanni, M.G.; Vaeth, B.M.; Nemesure, M.D.; Wang, R.X.; LaComb, J.F.; Williams, J.L.; Golub, L.M.; et al. A novel tricarbonylmethane agent (CMC2.24) reduces human pancreatic tumor growth in mice by targeting Ras. *Mol. Carcinogen.* **2018**, *57*, 1130–1143. [CrossRef] [PubMed]
32. Mackenzie, G.G.; Huang, L.; Alston, N.; Ouyang, N.; Vrankova, K.; Mattheolabakis, G.; Constantinides, P.P.; Rigas, B. Targeting mitochondrial STAT3 with the novel phospho-valproic acid (MDC-1112) inhibits pancreatic cancer growth in mice. *PLoS ONE* **2013**, *8*, e61532. [CrossRef] [PubMed]
33. Bartels, L.E.; Mattheolabakis, G.; Vaeth, B.M.; LaComb, J.F.; Wang, R.; Zhi, J.; Komninou, D.; Rigas, B.; Mackenzie, G.G. The novel agent phospho-glycerol-ibuprofen-amide (MDC-330) inhibits glioblastoma growth in mice: An effect mediated by cyclin D1. *Carcinogenesis* **2016**, *37*, 420–429. [CrossRef] [PubMed]

4

Honokiol: A Review of Its Anticancer Potential and Mechanisms

Chon Phin Ong, Wai Leong Lee, Yin Quan Tang * and Wei Hsum Yap *

School of Biosciences, Faculty of Health and Medical Sciences, Taylor's University Lakeside Campus, No. 1, Jalan Taylor's, Subang Jaya 47500, Malaysia; chonphin96@gmail.com (C.P.O.); leewl0108@gmail.com (W.L.L.)
* Correspondence: yinquan.tang@taylors.edu.my (Y.Q.T.); weihsum.yap@taylors.edu.my (W.H.Y.)

Abstract: Cancer is characterised by uncontrolled cell division and abnormal cell growth, which is largely caused by a variety of gene mutations. There are continuous efforts being made to develop effective cancer treatments as resistance to current anticancer drugs has been on the rise. Natural products represent a promising source in the search for anticancer treatments as they possess unique chemical structures and combinations of compounds that may be effective against cancer with a minimal toxicity profile or few side effects compared to standard anticancer therapy. Extensive research on natural products has shown that bioactive natural compounds target multiple cellular processes and pathways involved in cancer progression. In this review, we discuss honokiol, a plant bioactive compound that originates mainly from the *Magnolia* species. Various studies have proven that honokiol exerts broad-range anticancer activity in vitro and in vivo by regulating numerous signalling pathways. These include induction of G0/G1 and G2/M cell cycle arrest (via the regulation of cyclin-dependent kinase (CDK) and cyclin proteins), epithelial–mesenchymal transition inhibition via the downregulation of mesenchymal markers and upregulation of epithelial markers. Additionally, honokiol possesses the capability to supress cell migration and invasion via the downregulation of several matrix-metalloproteinases (activation of 5′ AMP-activated protein kinase (AMPK) and KISS1/KISS1R signalling), inhibiting cell migration, invasion, and metastasis, as well as inducing anti-angiogenesis activity (via the down-regulation of vascular endothelial growth factor (VEGFR) and vascular endothelial growth factor (VEGF)). Combining these studies provides significant insights for the potential of honokiol to be a promising candidate natural compound for chemoprevention and treatment.

Keywords: honokiol; anticancer; mechanism; signalling pathway

---

1. Introduction

Cancer is the outcome of rampant cell division which is associated with cell cycle disorganisation [1], leading to uncontrolled cell proliferation. In addition, it also involves the dysregulation of apoptosis, immune evasion, inflammatory responses, and ultimately, metastatic spread [2]. Over the last few decades, our progressive understanding of the aetiology of cancer together with advancement of cancer treatment, detection, and prevention, have contributed towards receding cancer mortality around the world [3]. However, more than half of cancer cases were diagnosed at a later stage of cancer progression [4]. According to a study by Bray et al. [5], the worldwide estimated number of new cancer cases for the year 2018 was 18.1 million in both sexes and across all ages. Amongst all the cancer types, lung, breast, and colorectum have topped the charts with approximately 2.1 million, 2.1 million, and 1.8 million cases, respectively. On the other hand, the estimated number of deaths was approximately 9.6 million. Asia accounted for more than half of the cancer deaths (57.3%), followed by Europe (20.3%), and America (14.4%). Lung cancer has caused the highest number of deaths due to substandard prognoses. Attempts to develop the effective prevention of cancer may diminish the incidence rate for some cancers, for instance lung cancer in North America and Northern Europe. These western countries have implemented tobacco control in order to avert involuntary exposure to tobacco and minimise active smoking within the community. Unfortunately, a majority of the population are still facing an upsurge of cancer diagnosis, demanding treatment and care [5].

The common treatment regimens for cancer patients include surgery, chemotherapy, and radiotherapy [6]. Although some of these regimens represent the first-in-line options for cancer treatment, the lack of selectivity towards neoplastic cells and the development of drug toxicity has caused these therapeutic effects to recede slowly, rendering it ineffective over the years [7]. Additionally, multidrug resistance tumours pose a severe threat and have been responsible for numerous cancer-related deaths [8]. A modern approach to target multiple cell regulating pathways is mandatory in order to provide highly efficient and targeted cancer therapy. For instance, combination therapy that targets different pathways exhibit significantly lower toxicity towards normal cells compared to mono-therapy [9]. Currently, the development of anticancer drugs possessing the capability to overcome common mechanisms of chemoresistance with minimal toxicity effects would be considered a breakthrough in cancer research [2].

Approximately 70–95% of the world population continues to use traditional medicinal herbs, plants, and fruits which contain valuable bioactive compounds with therapeutic effects to maintain health, as well as to prevent or treat physical and mental illnesses [10]. These biologically active compounds provide extensive opportunities in uncovering competent anticancer agents [2,11]. A majority of the anticancer drugs that are currently in use originate from plants, marine organisms, and microorganisms, such as the well-known plant-derived anti-cancer drugs Paclitaxel (Taxol®) and Camptothecin (CPT) [12].

The *Magnolia* genus is widely distributed throughout the world, especially in East and South-East Asia [13]. Among the *Magnolia* species, *Magnolia officinalis* and *Magnolia obovata* are commonly used in traditional Chinese (known as "Houpu") and Japanese herbal medicine [13,14]. The traditional prescriptions named Hange-koboku-to and Sai-boku-to, which contain the *Magnolia* bark, are still used in modern clinical practice in Japan [15]. There are several potent bioactive compounds in the *Magnolia* species have been identified including honokiol, magnolol, obovatol, 4-*O*-methylhonokiol, and several other neolignan compounds [13,15,16]. This paper highlights the potential anticancer effect of a simple biphenyl neolignan found in this *Magnolia* family, namely honokiol.

Honokiol was traditionally used for anxiety and stroke treatment, as well as the alleviation of flu symptoms [14]. In recent studies, this natural product displayed diverse biological activities, including anti-arrhythmic, anti-inflammatory, anti-oxidative, anti-depressant, anti-thrombocytic, and anxiolytic activities [13,14,16]. Furthermore, it was also shown to exert potent broad-spectrum anti-fungal, antimicrobial, and anti-human immunodeficiency virus (HIV) activities [13]. Due to its ability to cross the blood–brain barrier, honokiol has been deemed beneficial towards neuronal protection through various mechanism, such as the preservation of Na^+/K^+ ATPase, phosphorylation of pro-survival factors, preservation of mitochondria, prevention of glucose, reactive oxgen species (ROS), and inflammatory mediated damage [17]. Hence, honokiol was described as a promiscuous rather than selective agent due to its known pharmacologic effects. Recent studies have been focused on the anti-cancer properties of honokiol, emphasising its tremendous potential as an anticancer agent. In this review, we summarise the anti-cancer properties of honokiol, together with its mechanism of action, based on in vitro and in vivo experimental evidence. In addition, we also summarize the current data on its pharmacological relevance and potential delivery routes for future applications in cancer prevention and treatment.

2. Research Methodology

A systematic search was performed to identify all relevant research papers published on the use of honokiol as a potent anticancer treatment using PubMed (1994–present) and Web of

Sciences (1994–present). The search strategy was performed using several keywords to track down the relevant research articles including 'honokiol', 'cancer', 'cancer statistics', 'structural', 'metabolites', 'mechanism', 'cell death', 'apoptosis', 'anti-inflammatory', 'anti-tumour', 'antioxidant', 'cell proliferation', 'cytotoxicity', 'cell cycle arrest', 'metastasis', 'tumour', 'angiogenesis', 'absorption', 'metabolism', 'toxicity', 'distribution', 'elimination', 'solubility', 'nanoparticles', and 'delivery'.

3. Structure Activity Relationship and Its Derivatives

Honokiol bioactive compounds are easily found in the root and stem bark of the *Magnolia* species, although some studies have also found them in seed cones [13,18]. Due to the structural resemblance of both honokiol and magnolol in the *Magnolia* bark, the extraction of pure honokiol and magnolol cannot be achieved using conventional column chromatography nor thin-layer chromatography. Eventually, their purification process requires a costly alternative like electromigration [16]. The only difference between honokiol and magnolol in terms of structure is only in the position of the hydroxyl group, as shown in Figure 1. In 2007, Chen et al. developed a rapid separation technique using high-capacity high-speed counter-current chromatography (HSCCC) to isolate and purify honokiol and magnolol from crude extracts of *Magnolia* plants. Within 20 min, the resulting fraction has a purity of 98.6% honokiol, indicating that this method exhibited substantial efficiency in honokiol extraction [19]. Two years later, another team of researchers formulated a time-effective synthetic method while providing higher yielding honokiol using Suzuki-Miyaura coupling and Claisen rearrangement as key steps of the synthetic pathway of honokiol. The five steps of the honokiol synthesis pathway includes bromination, Suzuki coupling, allylation, one-pot Claisen's rearrangement, and demethylation, eventually resulting in a 32% overall yield [20]. The emergence of the synthetic method for honokiol has alleviated the risk of extinction of the *Magnolia* species.

Natural bioactive compounds often serve as lead templates and are subjected to structural modification to improve pharmacological activity, physiochemical properties, along with pharmacokinetics, to generate clinically useful structures [21]. According to Anand et al. [22], a comprehensive study of the natural and synthetic analogues of a drug molecule is crucial to determining its fundamental pharmacophores. As seen in Figure 1, honokiol contains two phenyl rings substituted with hydroxyl and allyl groups. In a study conducted by Bohmdorfer et al. [23], it was found that the predominant metabolic pathways of honokiol in the human liver was through sulfation and glucuronidation (Phase II metabolism) of the free hydroxyl groups, inducing rapid excretion and shortening its half-life [23]. Moreover, Lin et al. [24] have hypothesised that the hydroxyl groups on the biphenyl skeleton of honokiol could be subjected to metabolic oxidation by Phase I enzymes, thus diminishing its efficacy.

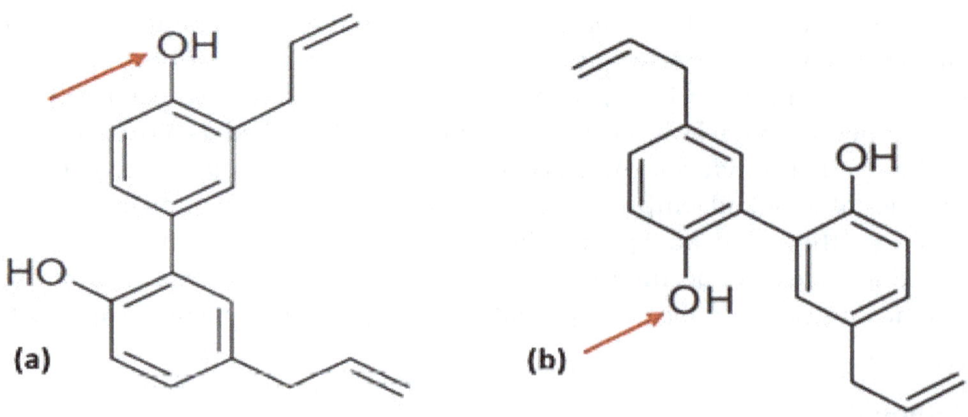

Figure 1. (**a**): The structure of honokiol [24]; (**b**): The structure of magnolol [25]. Arrow indicates the difference in the position of hydroxyl group between honokiol and magnolol.

Through the alteration of the top and bottom rings by changing the substitution pattern at its bottom ring and replacing the hydroxyl group in the top ring with a methoxy group, six different analogues were produced, as shown in Figure 2. A structure–activity relationship (SAR) study was conducted and it was found that replacing the hydroxyl group in the top ring of honokiol with a methoxy group greatly improved its cytotoxicity against lung, melanoma, and colon cancer cells. The two hydroxyl group substituted analogues (3′-Bromo-3,5′-dy-allyl-2′hydroxyl-4-methoxy-1,1′-biphenyl and 3,3′-Diallyl-4-methoxy-4′-hydroxy-1,1′-biphenyl) have induced G0/G1 phase cell cycle arrest and a swift decrement in Cdk1 and cyclin B1 protein levels, similarly to the parental honokiol compound [24]. Overall, obstruction of the potential oxidation of the phenolic hydroxyl group in the biphenyl group skeleton of honokiol improved its anti-cancer effect.

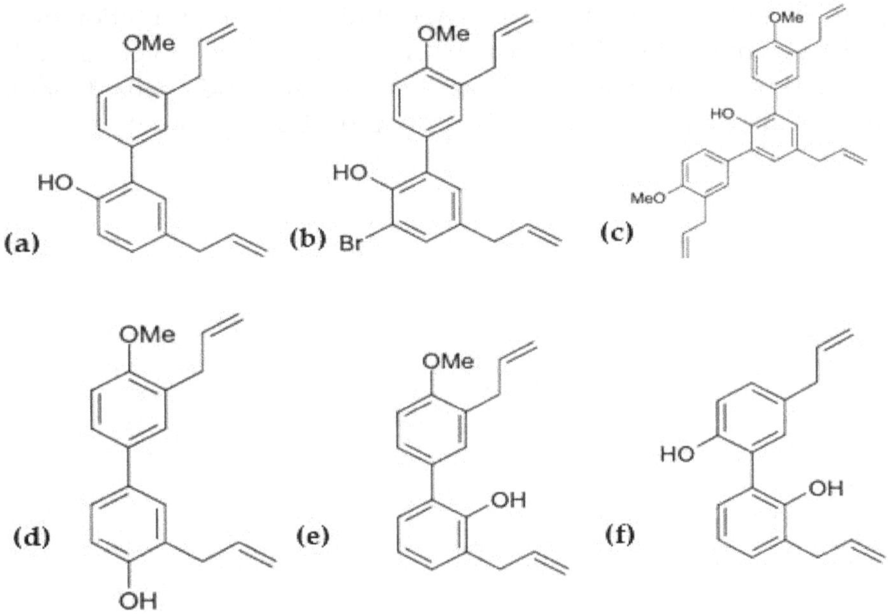

Figure 2. The structure of honokiol analogues. (**a**): 3,5′-Diallyl-2′-hydroxyl-4-methoxy-1,1′-biphenyl; (**b**): 3′-Bromo-3,5′-di-allyl-2′-hydroxyl-4-methoxy-1,1′-biphenyl; (**c**): 2,6-Di-(4′-methoxy-3′-allylphenyl)-1-phenol; (**d**): 3,3′-Diallyl-4-methoxy-4′-hydroxy-1,1′-biphenyl; (**e**): 3,3′Diallyl-2′-hydroxyl-4-methoxy-1,1′-biphenyl; (**f**): 3′,5-Diallyl-2,2′-di-hydroxy-1,1′-biphenyl [24].

4. Anticancer Properties of Honokiol

4.1. *In Vitro Studies*

Honokiol has been shown to exhibit antiproliferation effects against numerous cancer cells, including bone, bladder, brain, breast, blood, and colon, as shown in Table 1. Generally, the concentrations used for the in vitro studies are between 0–150 μM, which majority of these concentration ranges have been shown to significantly inhibit cell proliferation or cell viability of various cancer cell lines. The trend for the IC_{50} values of numerous cancer cell lines were time-dependent, whereby the IC_{50} values decreases as duration of the experiment increases. As seen in Table 1, human blood cancer Raji cells were highly susceptible to honokiol treatment (IC_{50} = 0.092) compared to highly resistant human nasopharyngeal cancer HNE-1 cells (IC_{50} = 144.71 μM). Interestingly, honokiol has been shown to exhibit minimal cytotoxicity against on normal cell lines, including human fibroblast FB-1, FB-2, Hs68, and NIH-3T3 cells [25–28]. The low cytotoxicity of honokiol treatment against normal cell lines should be emphasised as current chemotherapeutic regimens have a considerable amount of side effects that harm cancer patients.

Many chemotherapeutic agents have been shown to induce severe systemic toxicity and several side effects due to their deficient pharmacokinetic profiles and non-specific distribution in the body [29]. In Yang et al.'s study [30], they have encapsulated honokiol into nanopolymers to enhance its permeability and specificity against cancer cells. They utilised the active targeting nanoparticles-loaded honokiol (ANTH) in their in vitro studies against human nasopharyngeal cancer HNE-1 cells, and this incorporation exhibited significantly lower IC_{50} values compared to free honokiol treatment. As a result, the incorporation or encapsulation of honokiol in transporting vehicles can improve the anticancer effects and concurrently overcome the water solubility issue of honokiol itself. This has shown to be a promising regimen for anticancer treatment in the future.

Furthermore, it is worthy to note that honokiol can enhance the antineoplastic effects of several chemotherapeutic agents when cells are treated in combination treatment of both honokiol and the chemotherapeutic agent. In Wang et al.'s study [31], they have shown that honokiol has enhanced the in vitro cytotoxicity of paclitaxel against human cervix cancer cell lines. The combination treatment has resulted in approximately 10–60% increase of apoptotic cells and inhibition of cell viability when compared to honokiol treatment alone [31]. In another study, honokiol potentiated the apoptotic effect of both doxorubicin and paclitaxel against human liver cancer HepG2 cells. Honokiol enhanced the apoptotic effects of paclitaxel and doxorubicin by 22% and 24% respectively [32].

Table 1. The anticancer effects of honokiol against cancer cells in in vitro experiments.

	Cell Lines	Mechanism of Action	Concentration Used	Efficacy/IC_{50} (Exposure Time)	References
Colorectal cancer	RKO	Inhibit cell proliferation Induce G1 phase cell cycle arrest Induce apoptosis ↓ Bcl-xL; ↑ Caspase-3 & caspase-9	0–150 µM	46.76 µM (68 h)	[33]
	HCT116, HCT116-CH2, HCT116-CH3	Inhibit cell proliferation Induce G0/G1 & G2/M phase cell cycle arrest: ↓ cyclin D1 & A1; ↑ p53 phosphorylation Induce apoptosis: ↓ Caspase-3; ↓ Bcl-2; ↑ Bax protein	25 µM Honokiol with 2.5 or 5.0 Gy IR	N/A	[34]
	HT-29	Inhibit cell growth & proliferation Induce G1 phase cell cycle arrest: ↓ Cdk1 & cyclin B1	0–50 µM followed by 0–5 Gy IR	23.05 µM (24 h) 13.24 µM (72 h)	[24]
	HCT116 & SW480	Inhibit cell proliferation via Inhibition of Notch signalling: ↓ Notch1 & Jagged-1; ↓ Hey-1 & Hes1; ↓ γ-secretase complex; ↓ Skip1 Induce apoptosis: ↑ caspase-3/-7 activity; ↓ Bcl-2 & Bcl-xL; ↑ Bax protein; ↓ cyclin D1 & c-Myc; ↑ $p21^{WAF1}$ protein Inhibit primary and secondary colonosphere formation	0–50 µM	N/A	[35]
	RKO & HCT116	Inhibit cell viability Induce apoptosis: ↑ caspase-3, caspase-8 & caspase-9 activation; ↑ DR5 & cleaved PARP proteins; ↑ survivin protein; ↑ phosphorylated p53 & p53 proteins; ↓ PUMA protein	0–60 µM	RKO: 38.25 µM (24 h) HCT116: 39.64 µM (24 h)	[36]
Blood cancer	B-CLL	Inhibit cell viability Induce apoptosis: ↑ caspase-3 activity; ↑ caspase-8 & caspase-9 activation; ↓ caspase-9; ↑ Bax protein; ↓ Mcl-1 protein	0–100 µM	49 µM (6 h) 38 µM (24 h)	[37]
	Raji, Molt-4	Inhibit cell growth ↓ p65; ↓ NF-κB Induce apoptosis: ↑ JNK activation Increase ROS activity: ↑ Nrf2 & c-Jun protein activation	0–2.5 µM	Raji: 3.500 µM (24 h) 0.092 µM (72 h) Molt-4: 0.521 µM (24 h)	[38]
Breast cancer	MCF-7, MDA-MB-231, SKBR-3, ZR-75-1, BT-474	Inhibit cell viability and growth: ↓ EGFR; ↓ MAPK/PI3K pathway activity Induce apoptosis: ↑ PARP protein degradation; ↓ caspase-8; ↑ Bax proteins Induce G1 phase cell cycle arrest: ↓ cyclin D1; ↑ p21 & p27	0–100 µM	MCF-7: 40 µM (24 h) MDA-MB-231: 33 µM (24 h) SKBR-3: 29 µM (24 h) ZR-75-1: 39 µM (24 h) BT-474: 50 µM (24 h)	[39]
	MCF-7, MDA-MB-231	Inhibit cell clonogenicity Inhibit cell anchorage-dependent colony formation Inhibit cell growth, migration & invasion: ↓ pS6K & 4EBP1 phosphorylation; ↑ AMPK activation; ↓ mTORC1 function; ↑ LKB1 & cytosolic localisation	1–25 µM	N/A	[40]
	MCF-7, MDA-MB-231, SUM149, SUM159	Inhibit cell migration & invasion: ↑ AMPK phosphorylation; ↑ LKB1 Inhibit stem-like characteristics: ↓ Oct4, Nanog & Sox4 protein; ↓ STAT3; ↓ iPSC inducer mRNA	5 µM	N/A	[41]

Table 1. *Cont.*

Cell Lines	Mechanism of Action	Concentration Used	Efficacy/IC_{50} (Exposure Time)	References
MCF-7, MDA-MB-231, T47D, SKBR-3, Zr-75, BT-474	Inhibit cell growth: ↓ PI3K/Akt/mTOR signalling Inhibit cell invasion Induce G0/G1 phase cell cycle arrest: ↓ cyclin D1 & cyclin E; ↓ Cdk2 & c-myc; ↑ PTEN Induce apoptosis: ↑ caspase-3, caspase-6 & caspase-9 activation	0–40 μM	MCF7: 34.9 μM (24 h) 13.7 μM (48 h) 13.5 μM (72 h) 10.5 μM (96 h) MDA-MB-231: 56.9 μM (24 h) 44.4 μM (48 h) 16.0 μM (72 h) 12.0 μM (96 h) T47D: 47.7 μM (24 h) 41.6 μM (48 h) 17.6 μM (72 h) 7.1 μM (96 h) SKBR-3: 76.1 μM (24 h) 68.1 μM (48 h) 62.7 μM (72 h) 15.7 μM (96 h) ZR-75: 71.1 μM (24 h) 58.1 μM (48 h) 28.7 μM (72 h) 14.5 μM (96 h) BT-474: 80.2 μM (24 h) 65.6 μM (48 h) 39.5 μM (72 h) 15.1 μM (96 h)	[42]
MDA-MB-231	Inhibit cell proliferation: ↓ c-Src/EGFR-mediated signalling pathway; ↓ c-Myc protein Induce G0/G1 phase cell cycle arrest: ↓ cyclin A, cyclin D1 & cyclin E; ↓ Cdk2, Cdk4 & p-pRb^{Ser780}; ↑ p27^{Kip-1} Induce apoptosis: ↑ caspase-3, caspase-8 & caspase-9 cascade; ↓ Bcl-2 & Bid protein; ↑ PARP cleavage	0–100 μM	59.5 μM (72 h)	[43]

Table 1. *Cont.*

	Cell Lines	Mechanism of Action	Concentration Used	Efficacy/IC_{50} (Exposure Time)	References
Lung cancer	A549	Inhibit cell growth & proliferation Induce G0/G1 phase cell cycle arrest: ↓ Cdk1 & cyclin B1	0–50 µM	12.51 µM (24 h) 7.75 µM (72 h)	[24]
	A549, H460, H226, H1299	Reduce invasive potential Inhibit PGE_2-induced cell migration: ↓ PGE_2 production ↓ COX-2 ↑ β-catenin degradation ↓ NF-κB/p65 activity ↓ IKKα	0–20 µM	N/A	[44]
	A549, H1299	Inhibit cell viability and growth: ↓ class I HDAC proteins; ↓ HDAC activity; ↑ histone acetyltransferase (HAT) activity; ↑ histone H3 & H4 Induce G1 phase cell cycle arrest: ↓ cyclin D1 & cyclin D2; ↓ Cdk2, Cdk4 & Cdk6	0–60 µM	N/A	[45]
	H460 & A549	Inhibit cell proliferation Induce apoptosis: ↑ cathepsin D; ↑ cleaved PARP; ↑ caspase-3 Inhibit autophagy: ↑ p62; ↑ LC3-II	0–60 µM	H460: ~30 µM (48 h) A549: ~40 µM (48 h)	[46]
	Pc9-BrM3 & H2030-BrM3 (brain metastatic)	Inhibit cell proliferation and cell invasion: ↓ STAT3 protein phosphorylation; ↓ STAT-3 mediated mitochondrial respiratory function	0–50 µM	PC9-BrM3: 28.4 µM (48 h) H2030-BrM3: 25.7 µM (48 h)	[47]
	H23, A549 & HCC827	Inhibit cell growth Induce G1 phase cell cycle arrest: ↓EGFR; ↓ class I HDAC; ↓ class IIb HDAC6 activity; ↑ Hsp90 acetylation & EGFR degradation	0–40 µM	A549: 23.55 µM (24h)	[48]
	H460, A549, H358	Inhibit cell growth: ↓ c-RAF, ERK & AKT phosphorylation Inhibit colony formation capacity Induce apoptosis: ↑ Bax protein; ↓ Bcl-2 protein; ↑ PARP cleavage Induce G1 phase cell cycle arrest: ↓ cyclin D1; ↑ p21 & p27; ↓ P70S6k kinase activity Induce autophagy: ↑ LC3-I conversion to LC3-II; ↑ Sirt3 mRNA & protein; ↓ Hif-1α protein	0–80 µM	H460: 30.42 µM (72 h) A549: 50.58 µM (72 h) H358: 59.38 µM (72 h)	[49]
	A549 & 95-D	Inhibit cell viability Induce apoptosis: ↑ ER stress signalling pathway activation; ↑ GRP78, phosphorylation PERK & phosphorylated IRE1α; ↑ cleaved caspase-9 & CHOP; ↓ Bcl-2 protein; ↑ Bax, caspase-3 & caspase-9 Inhibit cell migration	0–60 µM	N/A	[50]
	CH27, H460 & H1299	Inhibit cell growth Induce apoptosis: ↓ Bcl-XL; ↑ mitochondrial cytochrome c release; ↑ BAD protein; ↑ caspase-1, caspase-2, caspase-3, caspase-6, caspase-8 & caspase-9 activity; ↑ PARP cleavage	0–100 µM	CH27: 40.9 µM (24 h) H460: 41.4 µM (24 h) H1299: 34.7 µM (24 h)	[25]
	MSTO-211H	Inhibit cell viability Induce apoptosis: ↑ PARP cleavage; ↑ caspase-3 activation; ↓ Bid & Bcl-xL protein; ↑ Bax protein; ↓ Mcl-1 & survivin protein; ↓ Sp1 Induce G1 phase cell cycle arrest: ↓ cyclin D1	0–22.5 µM	N/A	[51]

Table 1. *Cont.*

Cell Lines		Mechanism of Action	Concentration Used	Efficacy/IC_{50} (Exposure Time)	References
Skin cancer	SK-MEL2 & MeWo	Inhibit cell growth & cell proliferation Induce apoptosis via DNA degradation Induce cell death via mitochondrial depolarization	0–100 µM	N/A	[52]
	A431	Inhibit cell viability & proliferation Induce G0/G1 phase cell cycle arrest: ↓ cyclin A, cyclin D1, cyclin D2 & cyclin E; ↓ Cdk2, Cdk4 & Cdk6; ↑ p21 & p27 Induce cell apoptosis: ↑ PARP	0–75 µM	N/A	[53]
	B16-F10	Inhibit cell proliferation Induce cell death: ↑ Autophagosome (vacuoles) formation; ↓ cyclin D1; ↓ AKT/mTOR & Notch signalling	0–50 µM	N/A	[54]
	B16/F-10 & SKMEL-28	Inhibit cell proliferation & viability: ↓ Notch signalling; ↓ TACE & γ-secretase complex proteins Inhibit clonogenicity Induce G0/G1 phase cell cycle arrest Induce autophagy: ↑ autophagosome formation; ↑ LC3B cleavage Inhibit cell stemness: ↓ CD271, CD166, Jarid1B & ABCB5	0–60 µM	N/A	[55]
	UACC903	Inhibit cell growth & proliferation	0–50 µM	7.45 µM (24 h) 5.10 µM (72 h)	[24]
	SKMEL-2	Inhibit cell proliferation & viability Induce apoptotic death: ↑ caspase-3, caspase-6, caspase-8 & caspase-9; ↑ PARP cleavage; ↓ procaspase-3, procaspase-8 & procaspase-9 Induce G2/M phase cell cycle arrest: ↓ cyclin B1, cyclin D1, cyclin D2 & PCNA; ↓ Cdk2 & Cdk4; ↑ p21 & p53	0–100 µM	N/A	[56]
	UACC-62	Inhibit cell proliferation & viability Induce apoptotic death: ↑ caspase-3, caspase-6, caspase-8 & caspase-9; ↑ cleaved PARP; ↓ procaspase-3, procaspase-8 & procaspase-9 Induce G0/G1 phase cell cycle arrest: ↓ cyclin B1, cyclin D1 & cyclin D2; ↓ Cdk2, Cdk4 & Cdc2p34; ↓ p21 & p27	0–100 µM	N/A	[56]
Renal cancer	A498	Inhibit cell proliferation Inhibit colony formation capability Inhibit cell migration and invasion: ↓ Epithelial-mesenchymal transition (EMT); ↓ cancer stem cells (CSC) properties; ↑ miR-141; ↓ ZEB2 Inhibit tumoursphere formation	0–80 µM	~12 µM (72 h)	[57]
Cervix cancer	KB-3-1, KB-8-5, KB-C1, KB-V1	Inhibit cell viability: ↓ EGFR-STAT3 signalling Induce mitochondria-dependent & death receptor-dependent apoptosis: ↓ Bcl-2, Mcl-1 & survivin; ↑ PARP & caspase-3 cleavage; ↑ mitochondrial release of cytochrome c; ↑ DR5 Enhances in vitro cytotoxicity of Paclitaxel	0–75 µM	KB-3-1: 12.56 µM (72 h) KB-8-5: 12.08 µM (72 h) KB-C1: 11.40 µM (72 h) KB-V1: 10.39 µM (72 h)	[31]

Table 1. *Cont.*

Cell Lines		Mechanism of Action	Concentration Used	Efficacy/IC_{50} (Exposure Time)	References
Pancreatic cancer	MiaPaCa & Colo-357	Suppress plating efficiency of cells Reduce anchorage-independent clonogenicity growth Suppress migration and invasion ability	0–5 µM	N/A	[58]
	MiaPaCa & Panc1	Inhibit cell growth Induce G1 phase cell cycle arrest: ↓ cyclin D1 & cyclin E; ↓ Cdk2 & Cdk4; ↑ p21 & p27 Induce apoptosis: ↓ Bcl-2 & Bcl-xL proteins; ↑ Bax protein; ↓ IKB-α phosphorylation; ↓ NF-κB constitutive activation	0–60 µM	MiaPaCa: 43.25 µM (24 h) 31.08 µM (48 h) 18.54 µM (72 h) Panc1: 47.44 µM (24 h) 34.17 µM (48 h) 21.86 µM (72 h)	[59]
Thyroid cancer	ARO, WRO	Inhibit cell growth & proliferation: ↓ ERK, JNK & p37 activation and expression; ↓ mTOR & p70S6K Inhibit colony formation Induce apoptosis: ↑ PARP cleavage; ↑ caspase-3, caspase-8 & PARP activation; ↓ PI3K/AKT & MAPK pathways Induce G0/G1 cell cycle arrest: ↓ cyclin D1; ↓ Cdk2 & Cdk4; ↑ p21 & p27 Induce autophagy & autophagy flux: ↑ LC3-II	ARO & WRO: 0–60 µM SW579: 0–40 µM	ARO: 36.3 µM (24 h) 40.1 µM (48 h) 44.8 µM (72 h) WRO: 37.7 µM (24 h) 31.8 µM (48 h) 30.7 µM (72 h) SW579: 19.9 µM (24 h) 10.5 µM (48 h) 8.8 µM (72 h)	[60]
Nasopharyngeal cancer	HNE-1	Inhibit cell growth Induce apoptosis Induce G1 phase cell cycle arrest	0–150 µM (Honokiol & ATNH—Active targeting nanoparticles-loaded honokiol)	Honokiol: 144.71 µM (24 h) ATNH: 69.04 µM (24 h)	[30]
Brain cancer	U251	Inhibit cell growth Inhibit cell proliferation Induce apoptosis	0–120 µM	61.43 µM (24 h)	[61]
	T98G	Inhibit cell viability Inhibit cell invasion Induce cell apoptosis: ↑ Bax protein; ↓ Bcl-2; ↑ Bax/Bcl-2 ratio	0–50 µM	N/A	[62]
	GBM8401 (Parental) & GBM8401 SP	Inhibit cell proliferation & viability Induce sub-G1 phase cell cycle arrest Induce apoptosis: ↓ Notch3/Hes1 pathway	0–20 µM	GBM8401 (Parental): 5.30 µM (48 h) GBM8401 SP: 11.20 µM (48 h)	[36]
	U251 & U-87 MG	Inhibit cell viability & proliferation: ↓ PI3K/Akt & MAPK/Erk signalling pathways Inhibit cell invasion & migration: ↓ MMP2 & MMP9; ↓ NF-κB-mediated E-cadherin pathway Inhibit colony formation Induce apoptosis: ↓ Bcl-2, p-AKT & p-ERK; ↑ Bax protein; ↑ caspase-3 cleavage; ↓ EGFR-STAT3 signalling Reduce spheroid formation: ↓ CD133 & Nestin protein	0–60 µM	U251: 54.00 µM (24 h) U-87 MG: 62.50 µM (24 h)	[63]

Table 1. *Cont.*

	Cell Lines	Mechanism of Action	Concentration Used	Efficacy/IC_{50} (Exposure Time)	References
	DBTRG-05MG	Inhibit cell growth Induce apoptosis: ↓ Rb protein; ↑ PARP & Bcl-x(S/L) cleavage Induce autophagy: ↑ Beclin-1 & LC3-II	0–50 μM	~30 μM	[64]
	U87 MG (Human) BMEC (Mouse)	Inhibit cell viability Inhibit epithelial-mesenchymal transition (EMT): ↓ Snail, β-catenin & N-cadherin; ↑ E-cadherin Inhibit cell adhesion & invasion: ↓ VCAM-1; ↓ phosphor-VE-cadherin-mediated BMEC permeability	0–20 μM	U87MG: 22.66 μM (24 h) BMEC: 13.09 μM (24 h)	[65]
	U87 MG	Inhibit cell viability Induce G1 phase cell cycle arrest: ↑ p21 & p53; ↓ cyclin D1; ↓ Cdk4 & Cdk6; ↓ p-Rb protein; ↓ E2F1 Induce apoptosis: ↓ procaspase-3; ↑ caspase-8 & caspase-9 activity	0–100 μM	52.70 μM	[66]
Bone cancer	HOS & U20S	Inhibit cell proliferation Inhibit colony formation Induce G0/G1 phase cell cycle arrest: ↓ cyclin D1 & cyclin E; ↓ Cdk4 Induce mitochondria-mediated apoptosis: ↑ caspase-3 & caspase-9 activation; ↑ PARP cleavage; ↓ Bcl-2, Bcl-xL & survivin; ↑ ERK activation; ↓ proteasome activity; ↑ ER stress and subsequent ROS overgeneration; ↑ GRP78 Induce autophagy: ↑ Atg7 protein activation; ↑ Atg5; ↑ LC3B-II	0–30 μM	HOS: 17.70 μM (24 h) U20S: 21.50 μM (24 h)	[67]
	SAOS-2, HOS, 143B, MG-63 M8, HU09, HU09 M132 Dunn, LM5, LM8 & LM8-LacZ (Mouse)	Inhibit cell metabolic activity Inhibit cell proliferation Inhibit cell migration Induce rapid cell death via Honokiol-provoked vacuolation	0–150 μM	(72 h) SAOS-2: 48.38 μM HOS: 51.38 μM 143B: 41.63 μM MG-63M8: 34.88 μM HU09: 59.25 μM HU09M132: 31.88 μM (72 h) Dunn: 36.00 μM LM5: 30.00 μM LM8: 31.13 μM	[68]
	Saos-2 & MG-63	Inhibit cell viability Induce apoptosis: ↑ caspase-3 & PARP cleavage; ↑ Bax protein; ↓ Bcl-2; ↓ PI3K/AKT signalling pathway; ↓ miR-21	0–100 μM	Saos-2: 37.85 μM (24 h) MG-63: 38.24 μM (24h)	[69]

Table 1. *Cont.*

	Cell Lines	Mechanism of Action	Concentration Used	Efficacy/IC_{50} (Exposure Time)	References
Oral cancer	OC2 & OCSL	Inhibit cell growth Induce G0/G1 phase cell cycle arrest: ↑ cyclin E accumulation; ↑ p21 & p27; ↓ cyclin D1, ↓ Cdk2 & Cdk4 Induce apoptosis: ↓ caspase-8 & caspase-9; ↑ caspase-3 cleavage; ↓ Bid protein Induce autophagy and autophagic flux: ↑ LC3-II; ↓ Akt/mTORC1 pathway; ↑ AMPK signalling pathway; ↑ p62	0–60 μM	OC2: 35.00 μM (24 h) 22.00 μM (48 h) OCSL: 33 μM (24 h) 13 μM (48 h)	[26]
	HN-22 & HSC-4	Inhibit cell viability Induce apoptosis: ↓ Sp1 protein; ↑ p21 & p27; ↑ PARP & caspase-3 activation; ↓ Mcl-1 & survivin protein Induce G1 phase cell cycle arrest: ↓ cyclin D1	0–37.5 μM	HN-22: 26.63 μM (48 h) HSC-4: 30.00 μM (48 h)	[70]
Liver cancer	HepG2	Inhibit cell growth & proliferation: ↓ β-catenin protein Induce apoptosis: ↑ BAD protein; ↓ Bcl-2 protein Upregulation of BAD protein expression Downregulation of Bcl-2 protein level	0–2 μM	N/A	[71]
	SMMC-7721	Inhibit cell growth Induce G0/G1 phase cell cycle arrest Induce apoptosis: ↓ mitochondrial potential; ↑ ROS production; ↓ Bcl-2 protein; ↑ Bax protein	0–37.5 μM	N/A	[72]
	HepG2, HUH7, PLC/PRF5, Hep3B	Inhibit cell proliferation: ↓ STAT3 activation; ↓ IL-induced Akt phosphorylation; ↓ c-Src activation; ↓ JAK1 & JAK2; ↑ SHP-1 protein Induce sub-G1 phase cell cycle arrest: ↓ cyclin D1 Downregulation of cyclin D1 level Induce apoptosis: ↓ Bcl-2 & Bcl-xL; ↓ survivin & Mcl-1 protein; ↑ caspase-3 activation; ↑ PARP cleavage Enhance apoptotic effect of doxorubicin & paclitaxel	0–100 μM	N/A	[32]
Ovarian cancer	A2780s & A2780cp	Inhibit cell growth Induce apoptosis	0–100 μM	A2780s: 36.00 μM (48 h) A2780cp: 34.70 μM (48 h)	[73]
	SKOV3 & Caov-3	Inhibit cell proliferation and growth Inhibit colony formation Induce apoptosis: ↑ AMPK pathway activation; ↑ caspase-3, caspase-7 & caspase-9 activation; ↑ PARP cleavage Induce G0/G1 phase cell cycle arrest Inhibit cell migration and invasion	0–100 μM	SKOV: 48.71 μM (24 h) Caov-3: 46.42 μM (24 h)	[28]
	SKOV3, COC1, Angelen & A2780	Inhibit cell proliferation Induce cell apoptosis: ↓ Bcl-xL; ↑ BAD protein; ↑ caspase-3 activation Induce G1 phase cell cycle arrest	0–93.75 μM	SKOV3: 62.63 μM (24 h) COC1: 73.50 μM (24 h) Angelen: 61.50 μM (24 h) A2780: 55.85 μM (24 h)	[74]

Table 1. *Cont.*

Cell Lines		Mechanism of Action	Concentration Used	Efficacy/IC_{50} (Exposure Time)	References
Prostate cancer	PC-3 & LNCaP	Inhibit cell viability Induce G0/G1 phase cell cycle arrest: ↓ cyclin D1 & cyclin E; ↓ Cdk2, Cdk4 & Cdk6; ↑ p21 & p53; ↓ Rb & E2F1 proteins; ↓ Rb phosphorylation at $Ser^{807/811}$; ↑ ROS generation	0–60 µM	N/A	[75]
	PC-3, LNCaP & C4-2	Inhibit cell growth Induce apoptosis: ↑ caspase-3, caspase-8 & caspase-9 activation; ↑ PARP cleavage Induce apoptosis via DNA fragmentation: ↑ Bax & Bak proteins; ↓ Mcl-1 protein	0–75 µM	18.75–37.50 µM (24 h)	[76]
	PC-3, LNCaP	Inhibit cell viability Induce autophagy: ↑ LC3-BII protein; ↓ mTOR pathway Induce apoptosis via DNA fragmentation: ↑ ROS generation	0–40 µM	N/A	[77]
Head & neck squamous cancer	Cal-33 & MD-1483	Inhibit cell growth Induce cell apoptosis and cell cycle arrest: ↓ EGFR signalling pathway; ↓ STAT3 signalling pathway; ↓ Bcl-xL & cyclin D1; ↓ phosphorylation p42/p44 MAPK & phosphorylated Akt	0–100 µM	Cal-33: 3.80 µM (72 h) 1483: 7.44 µM (72 h)	[78]
Neuroblastoma	Neuro-2a	Induce apoptosis via DNA fragmentation: ↑ caspase-3, caspase-6 & caspase-9 activation; ↑ Bax protein; ↓ mitochondrial membrane potential; ↑ cytochrome c releaseInduce sub-G1 phase cell cycle arrest	0–100 µM	63.3 µM (72 h)	[79]
	Neuro-2a & NB41A3	Inhibit cell viability Induce autophagy: ↑ LC3-II; ↑ PI3K/Akt/mTOR signalling pathway; ↑ Grp78; ↑ ROS generation; ↑ ERK1/2; ↑ p-ERK1Induce apoptosis via DNA fragmentation Inhibit cell migration	0–100 µM	Neuro-2a: ~50 µM (72 h)	[80]
Bladder cancer	T24 & 5637	Inhibit cell viability and induce apoptosis: ↑ Bax protein; ↑ PARP cleavage; ↓ Bcl-2 protein Inhibit clonogenicity Induce G1 phase cell cycle arrest: ↓ cyclin D1; ↑ p21 & p27 Inhibit sphere formation capacity Inhibit cell migration & invasion: ↓ EZH2 gene expression; ↓ MMP9 Inhibit cell stemness: ↓ EZH2 gene expression; ↓ CD44 & Sox2; ↑ miR-143 overexpression	0–72 µM	N/A	[81]

4.2. *In Vivo Studies*

Based on the in vivo studies, honokiol possessed the capability to inhibit tumour growth, metastasis, and angiogenesis using different animal models, as shown in Table 2. The degree of tumour inhibition was shown to be significantly effective against each distinct cancer cell line, ranging from 0–150 mg/kg via various delivery methods of honokiol between oral gavage or injection (intraperitoneal, caudal vein, or intravenous). Honokiol was shown to downregulate the expression of Oct4, Nanog, and Sox2 which were known to be expressed in osteosarcoma, breast carcinoma and germ cell tumours [41]. According to Wang et al.'s study, they have found that the average tumour size was significantly lower than the control group without affecting their body weight, suggesting inconsequential toxicity under tested conditions when treated with a combination of honokiol and paclitaxel [31]. Indisputably, honokiol was once again proven to exhibit minor to no toxicity against normal cells.

Over the years, the development of chemo-resistance in ovarian cancer cells has hindered the outcome of treatment regimen towards ovarian cancer [82]. Despite the effectiveness of honokiol to inhibit cancer cell proliferation, delivering effective concentration towards the tumour site was deemed challenging due to its water insolubility [73]. The encapsulation of honokiol in liposome, namely Lipo-HNK by Luo and his team has displayed substantial efficacy against cisplatin-resistance ovarian cancer cell line A2780cp. The tumour volume for Lipo-HNK treated mice was 408 ± 165 mm^3 compared to liposome-treated mice and control mice were 2575 ± 701 mm^3 and 2828 ± 796 mm^3 respectively after 21 days [73]. In addition, Lipo-HNK was also shown to prolong survival and induce intra-tumoral apoptosis in vivo. The promising in vivo properties of honokiol should consolidate its importance as a potential anticancer agent for future researches.

Zebrafish (*Danio rerio*) model has emerged as a newly important cancer model that complements against traditional cell culture assays and mice model due to its small size, heavy brood, and rapid maturation time. Importantly, its transparent body wall enables visibility of tumour progression and the ease of experimentation [83,84]. It was known that juvenile zebrafish (*Danio rerio*) or zebrafish embryos have the competency to study cancer cell invasion, metastasis, tumour-induced angiogenesis. Honokiol reduced U-87 MG human glioma/glioblastoma cell proliferation and migration in zebrafish yolk sac and in vivo xenograft nude mouse model [63]. These observations are associated with a reduction in EGFR, phosphorylated STAT3, CD133 and Nestin levels, thus highlighting the regulation of honokiol in EGFR-mediated STAT3/JAK signalling pathway to induce anti-tumour and anti-metastasis.

The subsections below will further discuss the mechanism of anticancer actions of honokiol including the induction of cancer cell death, inhibition of cell cycle progression, induction of autophagy, prevention of epithelial–mesenchymal transition (EMT), as well as the suppression of migration, invasion, and angiogenesis of cancer cells.

Table 2. The antitumour effect of honokiol in in vivo tumour bearing animal models.

Cancer Cell Line	Animal Model & Site of Tumour Xenograft	Dose, Duration & Route of Administration	Observation & Mechanism of Action	Efficacy on Tumour Inhibition	References
		Breast cancer			
MDA-MB-231 cells	Both flanks of athymic nude mice	100 mg/kg/day 28 days IP	Induce tumour growth arrest	Complete arrest of tumour growth from week 2 onwards	[39]
MDA-MB-231 cells	Right gluteal region of athymic nude mice	3 mg/mouse/day Three times a week 28 days IP	Inhibit tumour progression: ↓ Ki-67; ↑ LKB1 & pAMPK; ↑ ACC phosphorylation, ↓ pS6K & 4EBP1 phosphorylation	Tumour weight of honokiol-treated group was 0.22 g compared to control group which was 1.58 g	[40]
MDA-MB-231-pLKO.1 & MDA-MB-231-LKB1^{shRNA} cells	Right gluteal region of athymic nude mice	3 mg/mouse/day Three times a week 42 days Oral gavage	Inhibit cell stemness: ↓ Oct4, Nanog & Sox2; ↓ pSTAT3 & Ki-67 Inhibit mammosphere formation	Decreased expression of Oct4, Nanog, Sox2 Reduce number of tumour cells showing Ki-67 & pStat3 expression	[41]
		Colorectal cancer			
RKO cells	Axilla of BALB/c nude mice	80 mg/kg/day Treatment on days 8–11, 14–17, 21–24, 28–31 51 days IP	Inhibit tumour growth Prolong survival of mice	709.9% increase in tumour growth rate in honokiol-treated group compared to 1627.6% and 1408.2% in control and vehicle groups respectively	[33]
HCT116 cells	Flank of athymic nude mice	200 µg/kg/day + 5 Gy irradiation Once a week 21 days IP	Inhibit tumour growth: ↓ CSC proteins → ↓ DCLK1, Sox-9, CD133 & CD44	Significantly lower tumour weight (<800 mg) in honokiol-IR combination, (~1500 mg) in honokiol treatment group compared to (~3300 mg) in control group	[35]
		Cervical cancer			
KB-8-5 cells	Athymic nu/nu nude mice (site of xenograft not stated)	50 mg/kg Honokiol Three times a week + 20 mg/kg Paclitaxel Once a week 28 days IP (honokiol) Tail vein injection (paclitaxel)	Suppress tumour growth: ↓ Ki-67 tissue level Induce apoptosis	Significantly lower average tumour volume for honokiol-paclitaxel combination treatment (573.9 mm^3) compared to control (2585.4 mm^3)	[31]
		Lung cancer			
H2030-BrM3 cells	Left ventricle of NOD/SCID mice	2 or 10 mg/kg/day 28 days Oral gavage	Prevent metastasis of lung cancer cells to brain	10 mg/kg: Decrease brain metastasis for >70%	[47]
H2030-BrM3 cells	Left lung via left ribcage of athymic nude mice	2 or 10 mg/kg/day Five days a week 28 days Oral gavage	Decrease lung tumour growth Inhibit metastasis to lymph node	10 mg/kg: Significantly reduce incidence of mediastinal adenopathy, decrement of weight of mediastinal lymph node for >80%, only 2/6 mice have lymphatic metastasis	[47]

Table 2. *Cont.*

Cancer Cell Line	Animal Model & Site of Tumour Xenograft	Dose, Duration & Route of Administration	Observation & Mechanism of Action	Efficacy on Tumour Inhibition	References
Blood cancer					
Raji cells	Back of BALB/c nude mice	5 mg/20 g & 10 mg/20 g Treatment on days 8–12 & 15–19 20 days (Route of administration not specified)	Inhibit cell proliferation Inhibit tumour growth	Tumour growth of honokiol-treated mice was significantly lower (~90 cm^3) compared to control mice (~270 cm^3)	[38]
HL60 cells	Inoculated intraperitoneally into SCID mice	100 mg/kg/day Treatment on Day 1–6 17 days IP	Prolong survival of mice	Median survival time of honokiol-treated mice are longer (37.5 days) compared to vehicle-treated mice (24.5 days)	[85]
Pancreatic cancer					
MiaPaCa cells	Pancreas of immunocompromised mice	150 mg/kg/day 28 days IP	Suppress tumour growth Inhibit metastasis: ↓ CXCR & SHH; ↓ NF-κB & downstream pathway Inhibit desmoplastic reaction: ↓ ECM protein; ↓ collagen I	Significant decrease in tumour growth for honokiol-treated mice (99.6 mm^3) compared to vehicle-treated mice (1361.0 mm^3)	[58]
Skin cancer					
SKMEL-2 or UACC-62 cells	Right flank of athymic nude mice	30 mg/kg Three times a week 14–54 days IP	Decrease tumour growth	SKMEL-2: 40% reduction in tumour volume UACC-62: 50% reduction in tumour volume	[56]
Thyroid cancer					
ARO cells	BALB/cAnN.Cg-Foxn1nu/CrlNarl mice (site of xenograft not stated)	5 or 15 mg/kg/mouse Every three days 21 days Oral gavage	Decrease tumour volume & tumour weight Induce apoptosis & autophagy	Control: ~1000 mm^3; 700 mg 5 mg/kg Honokiol: ~600 mm^3; 400 mg 15 mg/kg Honokiol: ~400 mm^3; 200 mg	[60]
Nasopharyngeal cancer					
HNE-1 cells	Right dorsal aspect of right foot of BALB/c athymic nude mice	Active-targeting nanoparticles-loaded HK (ATNH), Non-active-targeting nanoparticles-loaded HK (NATNH), Free Honokiol (HK) 3 mg/mouse/day Every three days Euthanise 50% mice after 12 days, rest are left to observe tumour growth & survival time up to 60 days; IV	Inhibit tumour progression, Induce apoptosis Potential inhibitor of angiogenesis & proliferation	Efficiency in tumour delay: ATNH > NATNH > Free HK Median survival time: Control: 28.5 days Free HK: 34 days NATNH: 42.5 days ATNH: 57.5 days	[30]

Table 2. *Cont.*

Cancer Cell Line	Animal Model & Site of Tumour Xenograft	Dose, Duration & Route of Administration	Observation & Mechanism of Action	Efficacy on Tumour Inhibition	References
Brain cancer					
U21 cells	Right flank of athymic nude mice	20 mg/kg Twice a week 27 days Caudal vein injection	Inhibit tumour growth Inhibit angiogenesis	Honokiol-treated mice have significant inhibition of tumour volume by 50.21% compared to vehicle Significantly lower microvessel present in honokiol-treated cells	[61]
U-87 MG cell suspension pre-treated with honokiol or vehicle for 48h	Yolk sac of Zebrafish larvae	(Concentration N/A) 3 days Injection of cells into zebrafish	Inhibit cell proliferation Inhibit cell migration	Reduced number of cell mass compared to vehicle-treated cells	[63]
U-87 MG cells	Right flank near upper extremity of nude mice	100 mg/kg/day Treatment at days 1–7 21 days IP	Reduce tumour growth: ↓ EGFR, pSTAT3, CD133 & Nestin	Increased number of apoptotic cells in honokiol-treated tissue, Significantly lower tumour volume & tumour weight in honokiol-treated mice	[63]
Bone cancer					
HOS cells	Dorsal area of BALB/c-nu mice	40 mg/kg/day 7 days IP	Reduce tumour growth Induce apoptosis & autophagy: ↑ cleaved caspase-3; ↑ LC3B-II & phosphor-ERK (ROS/ERK1/2 signalling pathway)	Significant decrease in tumour volume & weight of honokiol-treated mice (200 mm^3; 0.2 g) compared to control group (~500 mm^3; 0.5 g) Increased number of TUNEL-positive cells	[26]
LM8-LacZ cells	Left flank of C3H/HeNCrl mice	150 mg/kg/day 25 days; IP	Inhibit metastasis	Mean number of micrometastases decreased significantly by 41.4% in honokiol-treated mice compared to control mice	[68]
Oral cancer					
SAS cells	Right flank of BALB/cAnN.Cg-Foxn1nu.CrlNarl nude mice	5 mg/kg or 15 mg/kg Treatment on day 1, 4, 7, 10, 13, 16, 19, 22 35 days Oral	Reduce tumour growth & volume	Significantly reduction in tumour growth in honokiol-treated mice 29% reduction (5 mg/kg; 21 days), 40% reduction (15 mg/kg; 21 days) 41% reduction (5 mg/kg; 35 days), 56% reduction (15 mg/kg; 35 days)	[26]

Table 2. *Cont.*

Cancer Cell Line	Animal Model & Site of Tumour Xenograft	Dose, Duration & Route of Administration	Observation & Mechanism of Action	Efficacy on Tumour Inhibition	References
		Prostate cancer			
C4-2 cells	Bilateral tibia of BALB/c nu/nu athymic nude mice	100 mg/kg/day 12 days IP	Inhibit cell proliferation: ↑ Ki-67 Induce apoptosis: ↑ M-31 Inhibit angiogenesis: ↑ CD-31	Lower PSA value in honokiol-treated mice compared to control group	[76]
PC-3 cells	Left & right flanks above hind limb of nude mice	1 or 2 mg/mice Monday, Wednesday & Friday two weeks before tumour implantation and duration of experiment after implantation 77 days Oral gavage	Inhibit tumour growth Inhibit cell proliferation Inhibit neovascularisation Induce apoptosis	Tumour volume of honokiol-treated mice are significantly lower (~330 mm^3; 1 mg), (~50 mm^3; 2 mg) compared to control (~400 mm^3)	[18]
		Gastric cancer			
MKN45 cells	Dorsal side of BALB/c nude mice (nu/nu)	0.5 mg/kg/day & 1.5 mg/kg/day 10 days Injection (route not stated)	Inhibit tumour growth: ↓ GRP94 overexpression	30% reduction in tumour volume (0.5 mg/kg) 60% reduction in tumour volume (1.5 mg/kg) Decreased accumulation of GRP94	[86]
MKN45 & SCM-1 cells	Peritoneal cavity of BALB/c nude mice	5 mg/kg Twice a week 28 days IP	Inhibit metastasis Inhibit angiogenesis	Honokiol inhibited STAT-3 signalling and VEGF signalling induced by calpain/SHP-1	[87]
		Ovarian cancer			
SKOV3 cells	Right axilla of BALB/c nude mice	1 mg liposome-encapsulated honokiol/day 48 days IP	Inhibit tumour growth Inhibit angiogenesis	Reduction in tumour growth rate in liposome-encapsulated honokiol-treated mice by 67–70% compared to control	[73,88]
A2780s cells	Right flank of athymic BALB/c nude mice	10 mg/kg Lipo-Honokiol Twice a week 21 days IV	Inhibit cancer growth Prolong survival of mice Increase intra-tumoural apoptosis Inhibit intra-tumoural angiogenesis	Lipo-HNK treated mice have significantly smaller tumour volume (222 ± 71 mm^3) compared to liposome-treated mice (1823 ± 606 mm^3) and control mice (3921 ± 235 mm^3)	[73]
A2780cp cells	Right flank of athymic BALB/c nude mice	10 mg/kg Lipo-Honokiol Twice a week 21 days IV	Inhibit cancer growth Prolong survival Increase intra-tumoural apoptosis Inhibit intra-tumoural angiogenesis	Lipo-HNK treated mice have significantly smaller tumour volume (408 ± 165 mm^3) compared to liposome-treated mice (2575 ± 701 mm^3) and control mice (2828 ± 796 mm^3)	[73]

5. Mechanism of Action of Honokiol

5.1. Dual Induction of Apoptotic and Necrotic Cell Death

Apoptosis is a normal physiological process that maintains the homeostatic cellular balance in multicellular organisms [89]. Generally, apoptosis can be classified into two central pathways, namely the intrinsic pathway (mitochondrial-mediated pathway) and extrinsic pathway (death receptor-mediated pathway) [90]. The intrinsic pathway is associated with changes in mitochondrial membrane permeability that lead to imbalance in Bax/Bak ratio and release of cytochrome *c* and other mitochondrial proteins into cytosol [89,90]. The released cytochrome *c* interacts with apoptosis protease-activating factor 1 (Apaf1) and forms an apoptosome complex [91], which promotes the activation of caspase-9 and later caspase-3, initiating the caspase cascade, which executes cell death in a coordinated way [91]. For the extrinsic pathway, the binding of ligands such as tumour necrosis factor (TNF), Fas ligand (Fas-L), and TNF-related apoptosis-inducing ligand (TRAIL) to their respective death receptors (type 1 TNF receptor (TNFR1), Fas (also called CD95/Apo-1) and TRAIL receptors will turn procaspase-8 into active caspase-8 to induce apoptosis [91–93].

Honokiol has been shown tp initiate caspase-dependent apoptotic pathways in different types of cancer (Table 1). Chen et al. [14] found that JJ012 human chondrosarcoma cells lose their mitochondrial membrane potential when treated at 10 μM of honokiol, thus leading to apoptosis. Other studies have also shown that honokiol markedly disrupted the balance of Bax/Bcl-2 ratio [13,18,34,63,94–97]. The increasing ratio of proapoptotic to antiapoptotic Bcl-2 family proteins (Bax/Bcl-2) will induce the release of cytochrome *c* and other apoptogenic proteins through the mitochondrial membrane to the cytosol, subsequently leading to the activation of caspase cascade and apoptosis [34]. Furthermore, honokiol downregulated the expression of several other anti-apoptosis mRNA and proteins such as Bcl-xL [13,18,25,64], survivin [67,98], and MCL-1 [18], as well as upregulated other pro-apoptotic proteins such as BAD, BAX, and BAK proteins [18,25].

Moreover, honokiol has been shown to effectively induce apoptosis in p53-deficient cancer cells, such as MDA-MD-231 breast cancer cells, as well as lung and bladder cancer cell lines by inhibiting the activation of ras-phospholipase D [39,99,100]. Besides p53, other tumour suppressor genes that will be activated in honokiol treatment include p21 [53], p21/waf1 [101], p27 [53], p38 MAPK [102,103], and p62 [26,46].

Besides the intrinsic pathway, honokiol is capable of targeting death receptors TNF-related apoptosis-inducing ligand (TRAIL) receptors and tumour necrosis factor receptors (TNFR) resulting in a sequential activation of caspase-8 and -3, which cleaves target proteins and then leads to apoptosis [104–106]. Activation of the death receptor mediated apoptotic pathway is primarily inhibited by cellular-caspase-8/FADD-like IL-1β-converting enzyme (FLICE) inhibitory protein (c-FLIP), which inhibits caspase-8 activation by preventing the recruitment of caspase-8 to the death inducing signalling complex [106]. However, honokiol was able to downregulate c-FLIP through the ubiquitin/proteasome-mediated mechanism, resulting in the sensitisation of non-small cell lung cancer cells to TRAIL-mediated apoptosis [107,108].

Other than intrinsic and extrinsic pathways, honokiol can also induce apoptosis by the endoplasmic reticulum (ER) stress-induced mechanism. A variety of ER stresses result in unfolded protein accumulation responses [109,110]. For survival, the cells induce ER chaperone proteins to increase protein aggregation, temporarily halt translation, and activate the proteasome machinery to degrade misfolded proteins. However, under severe and prolonged ER stress, an unfolded protein response activates unique pathways that lead to cell death through apoptosis [111]. According to a study by Zhu et al. [50], honokiol can upregulate the expressions of ER stress-induced apoptotic signalling molecules such as GRP78, phosphorylated PERK, phosphorylated eIF2α, CHOP, Bcl-2, Bax, and cleaved caspase-9 in human lung cancer cells. Chiu et al. [112] found that honokiol also led to an increase in ER stress activity in melanoma cell lines B16F10 (mouse), human malignant melanoma, and human metastatic melanoma. Honokiol activated ER stress and down-regulated peroxisome proliferator-activated receptor-γ (PPARγ) activity resulting in PPARγ and CRT degradation through calpain-II activity in human gastric cancer cell lines [86,113,114] and human chondrosarcoma cells [14]. This was due to the ability of honokiol to upregulate and bind effectively to the glucose regulated protein 78 (GRP78) to activate apoptosis [14,115]. However, this was opposed by another study where treatment of various human gastric cancer cells with honokiol led to the induction of GRP94 cleavage but did not affect GRP78 [86].

Necrosis is known as unprogrammed cell death whereby cell swelling and destabilisation of the cell membrane results in the leakage of cellular cytoplasmic contents into the extracellular space, thus causing inflammation [116]. Besides apoptosis, honokiol has also been found to induce necrotic cell death in MCF-7 (40 μg/mL honokiol) [117], human oesophageal adenocarcinoma cells CP-A and CP-C [118], and primary human acute myelogenous leukemia HL60 [85] via p16ink4a pathway by targeting cyclophilin D to affect several downstream mechanisms. This phenomenon was also observed in transformed Barrett's and oesophageal adenocarcinoma cells when treated with honokiol (<40 μM) by targeting their STAT3 signalling pathway, thus resulting in a decrease of Ras activity and phosphorylated ERK1/2 expression [119]. The phosphorylation of Ser727 STAT3 induces translocation towards the mitochondria followed by ROS production, ultimately leading to the induction of necrosis [120]. Taken together, honokiol demonstrates the dual induction of apoptotic and necrotic cell death.

5.2. Cell Cycle Arrest

Cancer is attributed to uncontrolled proliferation resulting from abnormal activity of different cell cycle proteins. Therefore, cell cycle regulators are becoming attractive targets in cancer therapy. Honokiol can induce cell cycle arrest in several types of cancer cells, such as in lung squamous cell carcinoma [121], prostate cancer cells [75,122], oral squamous cancer [70], UVB-induced skin cancer [123], and more as listed in Table 1, by generally inducing G0/G1 and G2/M arrest. This arrest is associated with the suppression of cyclin-B1, CDC2, and cdc25C in honokiol-treated human gastric carcinoma and human neuroglioma cells [97,124,125], downregulation of cyclin dependent kinase (CDK)-2 and CDK-4, and the upregulation of cell cycle suppressors p21 and p27 in human oral squamous cell carcinoma (OSCC) cells [26,97]. In addition, the downregulation of c-Myc and class I histone deacetylases was also identified as other contributors to cell cycle arrest at the G0/G1 phase in prostate cancer cells [97,122] and acute myeloid leukemia respectively [11,101,108].

5.3. Autophagy

Autophagy is an evolutionary conserved catabolic process that involves the delivery of dysfunctional cytoplasmic components for lysosomal degradation [126,127]. The activation of autophagy promotes cell survival and regulates cell growth during harsh and stressful conditions via a reduction of cellular energy requirements by breaking down unnecessary components [82,127]. In cancer cells, autophagy facilitates both tumour suppression and tumourigenesis by the induction of cell death and tumour growth promotion, respectively [128,129]. The regulation of mTORC complexes mTORC1 and mTORC2 is involved in controlling the autophagic process. The activation of mTORC1 plays an important role in phosphorylation of autophagy-related protein (ATG) and subsequently inhibiting autophagy, whereas the inhibition of mTORC1 complements the autophagic process [130,131]. The inhibition of mTORC1 complex will concurrently activate Unc-51-like autophagy-activating kinase (ULK) complex, inducing localisation to the phagophore and followed by class III PI3K activation [132,133]. Beclin-1 was known to play a role in tumour suppression by recruiting several proteins associated with autophagosome elongation and maturation [134]. ATGs regulate the autophagosome elongation. For instance, ATG5-ATG12/ATG16L complexes recruit microtubule-associated protein 1 light chain 3 (LC3), followed by conversion of pro-LC3 to active cytosolic isoform LC3 I by ATG4B [135,136]. Thereafter, the interaction with ATG3, ATG7, and phosphatidylethanolamine (PE) converts LC3 I to LC3 II. The LC3 II enables the autophagosome to bind to degraded substrates and mature autophagosomes are capable of fusing with lysosomes to selectively remove damaged organelles via autophagy [137].

Generally, there are two modes of autophagy known as conventional and alternative autophagy. Conventional autophagy (also known as Atg5/Atg7-dependent pathway) involves the activation of Atg5 and Atg7 which are core regulators of autophagy, and then leads to microtubule-associated protein 1A/1B light chain 3 (LC3) modification and translocation from cytosol to the isolation membrane. This LC3 translocation was considered as a reliable hallmark of autophagy. Contradictorily, alternative autophagy occurs independently without involving Atg5 and Atg7, as well as LC3 modification [128,129,137].

The regulation of autophagy in cancer remains controversial as it plays dual roles in tumour suppression and promotion. Autophagy is believed to contribute to the properties of cancer cells stemness, induction of recurrence, and the development of anticancer drugs. However, the actual mechanism of autophagy in cancer remains unclear. Several studies have highlighted the potential of honokiol to induce cell death via autophagy in human prostate cancer cells [77], human glioma cells [138], NSCLC cells [30], and human thyroid cancer cells [60].

The activation of Atg5/Atg7-dependent pathways through the upregulation of LC3B-II, Atg5, and Atg7 levels was observed in honokiol-treated osteosarcoma HOS and U2OS cells and leads to the accumulation of autophagic vacuoles [26]. According to a study by Chang et al. [64], the expression of two critical autophagic proteins, Beclin-1 and LC3, were found to have increased in the honokiol-treated glioblastoma multiforme cells (DBTRG-05MG cell line). Similarly, the expression of autophagosomal marker LC3-II was also increased in Kirsten rat sarcoma viral oncogene homolog (KRAS) mutated cell lines of non-small cell lung cancer (NSCLC).

Other signalling pathways are also found to be involved in honokiol-induced autophagy including the involvement of AMPK-mTOR signalling pathway which leads to autophagocytosis through the coordinated phosphorylation of Ulk1 in Kirsten rat sarcoma viral oncogene homolog (KRAS) mutant lung cancer and melanoma cells [55,60,66,97]. Besides this, the ROS/ERK1/2 signalling pathway is also believed to play a certain role in honokiol-induced autophagy though ERK activation and the generation of ROS in treated osteosarcoma cells [67,77,97]. All these recent studies have further supported the potential of honokiol in the induction of autophagy in cancer cells.

5.4. Epithelial-Mesenchymal Transition (EMT)

Migratory mesenchymal-like cells are involved in embryonic development, tissue repair, and regeneration, as well as several pathological processes like tissue fibrosis, tumour invasiveness, and metastasis [139,140]. These migratory mesenchymal cells originate from the conversion of the epithelial cells, and this process is known as epithelial-mesenchymal transition (EMT). This plasticity of cellular phenotypes provides a new insight into possible therapeutic interventions in cancer [140].

EMT is characterised by the loss of epithelial markers such as cytokeratins and E-cadherin, followed by an increase in mesenchymal markers such as N-cadherin and vimentin [141]. The cellular processes of EMT are composed of several key transcription factors (such as TWIST, SNAI1, SNAI2, ZEB1/2) that act in concert with epigenetic mechanisms and post-translational protein modifications to coordinate cellular alterations [139,142]. The application of gene expression signatures combining multiple EMT-linked genes has proven useful to evaluate EMT as a contributing factor in tumour development in human cancers. However, the EMT process was shown to be incomplete in tumours, venturing in between multiple translational states and expressing a mixture of both epithelial and mesenchymal genes. This hybrid in partial EMT can be more aggressive than tumour cells with a complete EMT phenotype [141]. In addition, EMT contributes to tumour metastatic progression and resistance towards cancer treatment, resulting in poor clinical outcomes [140,141].

Honokiol has been shown to block and inhibit EMT in many cancer cells such as breast cancer, melanoma, bladder cancer, human non-small cell lung cancer, and gastric cancer (Table 1). Honokiol reduced steroid receptor coactivator-3 (SRC-3), matrix metalloproteinase (MMP)-2, and Twist1, preventing the invasion of urinary bladder cancer cells [108,143]. In addition, honokiol was also capable of inducing E-cadherin and repressing N-cadherin expression, thus inhibiting the EMT process in J82 bladder cancer cells [108,143]. In breast cancer cells, honokiol inhibits the recruitment of Stat3 on mesenchymal transcription factor Zeb1 promoter, resulting in decreased Zeb1 expression and nuclear translocation [144]. In addition, honokiol increases E-cadherin expression via the Stat3-mediated release of Zeb1 from E-cadherin promoter [144]. Collectively, many studies have reported that honokiol effectively inhibits EMT in breast cancer cells, evidence has been found to support a cross-talk between honokiol and Stat3/Zeb1/E-cadherin axis [144]. On the other hand, EMT is inhibited by modulating the miR-141/ZEB2 signalling in renal cell carcinoma (A-498) [57].

Honokiol inhibited the EMT-driven migration of human NSCLC cells in vitro by targeting c-FLIP through N-cadherin/snail signalling as N-cadherin and snail are downstream targets of c-FLIP [145]. Twist1, a basic helix-loop-helix domain-containing transcription factor, promotes tumour metastasis by inducing EMT, and can be upregulated by multiple factors, including SRC-1, STAT3, MSX2, HIF-1α, integrin-linked kinase, and NF-κB. The capability of honokiol in targeting Twist1 can be regarded as a promising therapy for metastatic cancer [108,146].

Honokiol was found to inhibit breast cancer cell metastasis and eliminate human oral squamous cell carcinoma cell by blocking EMT through the modulation of Snail/Slug protein translation [147,148]. Honokiol markedly downregulated endogenous Snail, Slug, and vimentin expression and upregulated E-cadherin expression in MDA-MB-231, MCF7, and 4T1 breast cancer cells [148]. As primary EMT inducers, Snail and Slug dictate the induction of EMT by targeting E-cadherin and vimentin [144,148]. Furthermore, when cells were treated with honokiol, Snail and Slug expression levels were decreased from 12 h to 24 h in a time-dependent manner, suggesting that honokiol can reverse the EMT process via the downregulation of Snail and Slug in breast cancer cell lines [148]. Besides that, EMT was inhibited in human oral squamous cell carcinoma cell via the disruption of Wnt/β-catenin signalling pathway [147]. It was reported that the protein levels of mesenchymal markers such as Slug and Snail were markedly suppressed, while β-catenin and its downstream Cyclin D1 were inhibited [147]. It is known that β-catenin could mediate EMT [147,149], which plays a crucial role in cancer invasion and metastasis. The EMT markers such as Snail and Slug are also the target genes of β-catenin [150]. Therefore, the suppression of Snail and Slug in honokiol treated human oral squamous cell carcinoma cells was believed to be due to the inhibition of Wnt/β-catenin signalling pathway [147]. Similarly, in U87MG human glioblastoma cell and melanoma cells, Snail, N-cadherin and β-catenin expression levels were decreased, whereas E-cadherin expression was increased after honokiol treatment [65,112].

5.5. *Suppression of Migration, Invasion and Angiogenesis of Cancer Cells*

Metastasis is known to be the major cause of death in cancer patients [151]. It involves the migration and invasion of tumour cells into neighbouring tissues and distant organs via intravasation into blood or lymphatic system [152,153]. The formation of invadopodium was stimulated by epidermal growth factor (EGF) and is crucial for the degradation of the extracellular matrix and remodelling membrane proteins, promoting metastasis [151]. Therefore, one of the important steps in cancer management is to control tumour cell metastasis, especially for early-stage cancer patients [153]. Various studies have reported that honokiol has the capability to suppress tumour metastasis in different types of cancer including breast cancer [40,148,154], non-small cell lung cancer [44,155] ovarian carcinoma cells [28], lung cancer [50], U251 human glioma, as well as U-87MG and T98G human glioblastoma cell [63,65,94], oral squamous cell carcinoma (OSCC) [26], bladder cancer cell [143], pancreatic cancer [58], renal cell carcinoma [156,157], and gastric cancer cells [113]. For instance, the percentage of invading urinary bladder cancer (UBC) cells was significantly reduced by 67% and 92% upon 2.4 μg/mL and 4.8 μg/mL of honokiol treatment, respectively [143]. Similarly, tumour cell migration was inhibited by 38–66% in A549 cells, by 37–62% in H1299 cells, 12% to 58% in H460 cells and 32% to 69% in H226 cells, in a concentration-dependent manner after treatment with honokiol [44].

Furthermore, honokiol also demonstrated an inhibitory effect on the expression of matrix metalloproteinases (MMPs) such as MMP-2 and MMP-9 proteins, which play an essential role in the metastatic process of tumour cells, as well as the regulation of angiogenesis in the maintenance of tumour cell survivability [44,63,143]. MMPs are a group of extracellular matrix degrading enzymes that control various normal cellular processes, such as cell growth, differentiation, apoptosis, and migration [153]. However, MMP activity was increased in many tumour cells. The overexpression of MMP-2 and MMP-9 are associated with pro-oncogenic events such as neovascularisation, tumour cell proliferation, and metastasis because it can degrade the extracellular matrix, basement membranes, and adhesion molecules (intercellular adhesion molecule, ICAM, and vascular cell adhesion molecule) and become invasive [58,153,158].

The transition from an epithelial-to-mesenchymal (EMT) phenotype facilitates the breakdown of extracellular matrix followed by the subsequent invasion of the surrounding tissues in order to enter the bloodstream and/or lymph nodes, and travel to distant organ sites. Once cells have reached the distant organ sites, they undergo mesenchymal-to-epithelial transition and begin the establishment of distal metastasis by the surviving cancer cells followed by the outgrowth of secondary tumours [58,159]. Honokiol has been shown to inhibit the invasion of HT-1080 human fibrosarcoma cells and U937 leukemic cells by inhibiting MMP-9 [160]. In addition, honokiol also reduced the protein levels of MMP2 and MMP9 in U251 human glioma and U-87 MG human glioblastoma cell lines in a dose-dependent manner [63]. The expression of MMP-2 and MMP-9 were also found to be decreased in both honokiol-treated A549 and H1299 cells (NSCLC cell lines), consistent with the decreased nuclear accumulation of β-catenin as both MMP-2 and MMP-9 are the downstream targets of β-catenin [44,161,162]. In the J82 bladder cancer cell, honokiol repressed the expression of SRC-3, MMP-2, and Twist1 genes which were involved in cancer cell invasion [143].

Another proposed mechanism for the inhibitory effects of honokiol on invasion and metastasis is through the liver kinase B1 (LKB1)/adenine monophosphate-activated protein kinase (AMPK) axis. Honokiol treatment increased the expression and cytoplasmic translocation of tumour-suppressor LKB1 in breast cancer cells, which led to the phosphorylation and functional activation of AMPK and resulted in the inhibition of cell invasion and metastasis [40,58]. The activation of AMPK suppresses mTOR signalling, decreasing the phosphorylation of p70 kDA ribosomal protein S6 kinase 1 (p70S6K1) and eukaryotic translation initiation factor 4E (eIF4E)-binding protein (4EBP1). This will ultimately inhibit the reorganisation of the actin cytoskeleton in cells, subsequently inhibiting cell migration [40].

In human renal carcinoma cell (RCC) 786-0, honokiol significantly upregulated the expression of metastasis suppressor gene (KISS-1), genes encoding TIMP metalloproteinase inhibitor 4 (TIMP4), and KISS-1 receptor (KISS-1R). In addition, honokiol markedly suppressed the expression of genes encoding chemokine (C-X-C motif) ligand 12 (CXCL12), chemokine (C-C motif) ligand 7 (CCL7), interleukin-18 (IL18) and matrix metalloproteinase 7 (MMP7). It was proven that honokiol significantly upregulated KISS1 and KISS1R in the 786-0 cells when treated with honokiol since recent studies showed that the activation of KISS1/KISS1R signalling by kisspeptin treatment decreases the motility and invasive capacity of conventional RCC, and overexpression of KISS1 inhibits the invasion of RCC cells Caki-1 [14,163]. In short, the activation of KISS1/KISS1R signalling by honokiol suppresses the multistep process of metastasis, including invasion and colony formation, in RCC cells 786-0 [163].

Angiogenesis is the formation of new blood vessels for supplying nutrients and oxygen to tissues and cells. In tumourigenesis, angiogenesis is important for the development and progression of malignant tumours [164]. The endothelial cells in growing cancer are active due to the release of cell growth and motility promoting proteins, creating a network of blood vessels to overcome its oxygen tension [165]. Vascular endothelial growth factor (VEGF) and fibroblast growth factor-2 (FGF2) are among the factors that play an important role in tumour angiogenesis [153]. In human renal cancer cell lines (786-0 and Caki-1), honokiol induced down-regulation of the expression of VEGF and heme oxygenase-1 (HO-1) via the Ras signalling pathway thus inhibit angiogenesis [166,167].

In retinal pigment epithelial (RPE) cell lines, honokiol inhibited the binding of hypoxia-inducible-factor (HIF) to hypoxia-response elements present on the VEGF promoter, thereby inhibiting the secretion of VEGF protein [168,169]. This decrement of VEGF levels resulted in reduced proliferation of human retinal microvascular endothelial cells (hRMVECs) [168]. Therefore, honokiol is said to possess both anti-HIF and anti-angiogenic properties.

In the overexpression of VEGF-D Lewis lung carcinoma cell-induced tumours in C57BL/6 mice, honokiol was shown to significantly inhibit tumour-associated lymphangiogenesis and metastasis. Furthermore, a remarkable delay in tumour growth and prolonged life span in honokiol-treated mice were also observed [170]. In another study, honokiol inhibited VEGF-D-induced survival, proliferation, and microcapillary tube formation in both human umbilical vein endothelial cells (HUVECs) and lymphatic vascular endothelial cells (HLECs). These observations are believed to be due to the inhibition in Akt and MAPK phosphorylation and downregulation of VEGFR-2 expressions in HUVECs as well as VEGFR-3 of HLECs [101,160,171]. Collectively, honokiol has been shown to exert direct and indirect effects on tumour suppression via anti-metastasis, anti-angiogenesis, and anti-lymphangiogenesis by mainly affecting HIF- and VEGF/VEGFR- dependent pathways. However, an in-depth mechanism of honokiol on the inhibition of metastatic progression and spread should be further explored in the future.

6. Effect of Honokiol on Various Signalling Pathways

6.1. Nuclear Factor Kappa B (NF-κB)

The nuclear factor kappa B (NFκB) family comprises of five DNA-binding proteins (p50, p52, p65, cRel, and RelB) that differentially modulate the transcription of genes that are involved in various cellular processes such as inflammation, migration, invasion, angiogenesis, proliferation, and apoptosis [172,173]. The continuous activation of NFκB has been reported in different types of cancers. Honokiol affects the constitutive activation of NFκB and expression of NFκB-regulated gene products involved in apoptosis (survivin, Bcl-2, Bcl-xL, IAP1, IAP2, cFLIP and TRAF1), inflammation (cyclooxygenase-2, COX-2), proliferation (cyclin D1 and c-myc), invasion (ICAM-1 and MMP-9), and angiogenesis (VEGF), thereby enhancing apoptosis and suppressing cancer progression [58,174]. Several studies support the inhibitory activity of honokiol against NFκB in different types of cancer cells, including breast cancer [42,117,175], head and neck squamous cell carcinoma (HNSCC) [176], colon cancer cells [177], non-small cell lung cancer (NSCLC) cells [44], pancreatic cancer cells [13], human leukemic cell [104], embryonic kidney cells, T-cell leukemia, multiple myeloma, lung adenocarcinoma, and squamous cell carcinoma [174].

Honokiol was found to repress the transcriptional activity of NFκB in both pancreatic MiaPaCa and Panc1 cancer cells. It was found that honokiol treatment significantly reduced nuclear NFκB levels with an increase of cytoplasmic NFκB fraction in MiaPaCa and Panc1 cells, in a dose-dependent manner [13]. The cellular distribution of NFκB is controlled by the relative expression of its biological inhibitor IκB, which keeps NFκB sequestered in the cytoplasm in an inactive complex [172]. Upon honokiol treatment, IκB-α levels were increased due to the stabilisation of IκB-α post-treatment, concurrently inducing the downregulation of IκB-α phosphorylation [13]. Furthermore, honokiol has also been shown to inhibit the TNF-α-induced phosphorylation and degradation of the cytosolic NFκB inhibitor IκBa and suppression of IKK activation [104,174,178]. In addition, honokiol was also found to inhibit the nuclear translocation and phosphorylation of p65 subunit of NFκB [44,104]. Honokiol suppressed NF-κB-regulated gene products including MMP-9, TNF-α, IL-8, ICAM-1, and MCP-1 [66].

6.2. Signal Transducers and Activators of Transcription (STATs)

Signal transducers and activators of transcription (STATs) is a well-known oncogene that is regulated by receptor tyrosine kinases, G-protein-coupled receptors, and interleukin families [179,180]. STAT3 are a group of transcription factors that upon phosphorylation will undergo dimerization and translocation to either the nucleus or mitochondria to control cell survival, cell cycle, cellular growth, and angiogenesis. STATs are aberrantly activated in several types of malignancies due to functional loss of their negative regulators, or the overexpression of upstream tyrosine kinases [179].

STAT3 can also localise into the mitochondria and mediate mitochondrial biogenesis. Honokiol has been shown to target STAT3 to reduce its expression and phosphorylation in many cancer cells such as human glioblastoma [47,63,100], lung cancer [47,181], oral squamous cell carcinoma (OSCC) [95], breast cancer [41,144], human epidermoid carcinoma [31], colorectal cancers [182], gastric cancer [87], and esophageal adenocarcinoma [119].

Honokiol was found to inhibit EGFR expression and down-regulate STAT3 phosphorylation by reducing the CD133 and Nestin levels [63]. Similarly, honokiol also induces apoptosis through the suppression of JAK2/STAT3, Akt and Erk signalling pathways in human oral squamous cell carcinoma (SAS and OCEM-1) cell lines [95]. Similar effect was observed in oral cancer cells where honokiol suppressed JAK2/STAT3 activation and, inhibited IL-6-mediated cell migration [95,183]. Furthermore, another study indicated that honokiol induces apoptosis in human glioblastoma cell line U87 through suppressing the phosphorylation of STAT3 (Tyr705), down-regulating survivin, and upregulating cleaved caspase-3 expression [98].

Moreover, honokiol inhibited STAT3-phosphorylation/activation in an LKB1-dependent manner, preventing its recruitment to canonical binding-sites in the promoters of Nanog, Oct4, and Sox2 [41]. Thus, the inhibition of the coactivation function of STAT3 resulted in the suppression of expression of pluripotency factors in MCF7, MDA-MB-231, SUM149, and SUM159 breast cancer cells [41]. Furthermore, honokiol inhibited breast tumorigenesis in mice in an LKB1-dependent manner [41]. This showed that honokiol can support crosstalk between LKB1, STAT3, and pluripotency factors in breast cancer and effective anticancer modulation of this axis with honokiol treatment in both in vitro and in vivo [41]. Apart from that, honokiol suppressed metastasis and proliferation in both brain metastatic lung cancer cell lines PC9-BrM3 and H2030- BrM3 by inhibiting STAT3 phosphorylation [47].

In other studies, honokiol is proven to be an effective chemotherapeutic agent that exert its antitumour function by inhibiting the STAT3 signalling pathway. Honokiol can induce cell cycle arrest and apoptosis via the inhibition of survival signals in adult T-cell leukemia by suppressing the phosphorylation and DNA binding of different oncogene factors, such as NF-κB, activator protein 1, STAT3, and STAT5 [184]. Besides that, honokiol can induce necrosis and apoptosis in transformed Barrett's and oesophageal adenocarcinoma cells through the inhibition of the STAT3 signalling pathway [119]. Honokiol can inhibit the growth and peritoneal metastasis of gastric cancer in nude mice, which was correlated with the inhibition of STAT3 signalling via the upregulation of Src homology 2 (SH2)-containing tyrosine phosphatase 1 [87].

6.3. Epidermal Growth Factor Receptor (EGFR)

EGFR is a group of transmembrane receptor tyrosine kinases (RTKs) that are normally deregulated in various cancers [185,186]. The overexpression or activating mutations in EGFR results in increased cell proliferation, abnormal metabolism, and cell survival through the activation of the downstream mitogen-activated protein kinase (MAPK) and v-akt murine thymoma viral oncogene homolog 1 (AKT) signalling pathways, as well as phosphatidyl-inositol 3-kinase (PI3K)/Akt, and STAT3 signalling pathways [13,58]. EGFR activation occurs upon binding to its ligands, which then leads to its homo- or heterodimerization with other members of the ErbB family, and subsequent activation of downstream signalling cascades in many cancer cell types, including breast cancer and head and neck squamous cell carcinoma (HNSCC) [187,188].

Honokiol has been shown to inhibit EGFR signalling pathway through either inhibition of EGFR expression or inhibition of EGFR phosphorylation [78,189,190]. Honokiol (60 μM) was found to inhibit EGFR expression and down-regulate STAT3 phosphorylation in U251 and U-87 MG human glioma/glioblastoma cells via JAK-STAT3 signalling [63]. In another study, honokiol (2.5–7.5 μM) differentially suppressed proliferation (up to 93%) and induced the apoptosis (up to 61%) of EGFR overexpressing tumourigenic bronchial cells. These effects were observed in parallel with the downregulation of phospho-EGFR, phospho-Akt, phospho- STAT3, and cell cycle-related proteins [189]. Furthermore, in a mouse lung tumour bioassay, intranasal instillation of liposomal honokiol (5 mg/kg) for 14 weeks reduced the size and multiplicity (49%) of lung tumours and the level of total- and phospho-EGFR, phospho-Akt, and phospho-STAT3 [189]. Overall, honokiol has been proven to be a promising candidate to suppress the development and progression of lung tumours driven by EGFR deregulation. Moreover, honokiol induced mitochondria-dependent and death receptor-mediated apoptosis in multi-drug resistant (MDR) KB cells, which was associated with inhibition of EGFR-STAT3 signalling and downregulation of STAT3 target genes [31].

Furthermore, the downregulation of c-Src/EGFR-mediated signaling is involved in honokiol-induced cell cycle arrest and apoptosis in MDA-MB-231 human breast cancer cells. EGFR can also be activated in a ligand-independent manner by cellular Src (c-Src), a non-receptor tyrosine kinase. The tyrosine kinase c-Src is also upregulated in many human malignancies and promotes the activation of mitogenic signalling through EGFR [13,191]. In MDA-MB-231 human breast cancer cells, honokiol downregulated the expression and phosphorylation of c-Src, epidermal growth factor receptor (EGFR), and Akt, and consequently led to the inactivation of mTOR and its downstream signal molecules including 4E-binding protein (4E-BP) and p70 S6 kinase [43]. Besides that, inhibition of HER-2 signalling by specific human epidermal growth receptor 1/HER-2 (EGFR/HER-2) kinase inhibitor lapatinib synergistically enhanced the anti-cancer effects of honokiol in HER-2 over-expressed breast cancer cells [42].

The treatment of HNSCC cells with honokiol also decreased the expression of total EGFR as well as p-EGFR and its downstream target, mTOR. Since the activation of mTOR has been shown to contribute to tumour progression, it can be speculated that the honokiol-induced inhibition of cell proliferation in HNSCC cells is mediated through the downregulation of EGFR/mTOR signalling pathway [176,192]. These observations are consistent with the evidence that honokiol inhibits the growth of cancer cells by targeting EGFR and its downstream molecular targets and suggest that these mechanisms are in play in HNSCC.

6.4. Mammalian Target of Rapamycin (mTOR)

The mammalian target of rapamycin (mTOR) is a type of protein kinase which regulates cell metabolism, proliferation, and growth. The activation of PI3K/Akt pathway results in the aberrant activation of mTOR in most cancer cells [97,193,194]. It is known that mTOR controls the expression of many survival proteins via activating p70 S6 kinase (S6K) and inhibition of eIF4E inhibitor 4E-BP1 [193]. The mTOR signalling pathway is dysregulated in premalignant or early malignant human tissues and is highly implicated in the carcinogenic process. Honokiol suppresses the activation of mTOR and its signalling mediators (4E-BP1 and p70 S6 kinase) by inhibiting ERK and Akt pathways [43] or upregulating PTEN (Phosphatase and Tensin homolog) expression [42,157].

Honokiol was found to induce apoptosis and suppress migration and invasion in ovarian carcinoma cells (SKOV3 and Caov-3) via TSC1/TSC2 complex/AMPK/mTOR signalling pathway [28]. This is mediated via the regulation of the tumour suppressors p27, p53, and MMP-9 [28]. Furthermore, it was proven that honokiol was able to attenuate PI3K/Akt/mTOR signalling via the down-regulation of Akt phosphorylation and upregulation of PTEN expression in breast cancer cells (MCF-7, MCF-7/adr, and BT-474 cell lines) [42]. A combination of honokiol with the mTOR inhibitor rapamycin presented synergistic effects to induce apoptosis in breast cancer cells where the inhibition of PI3K/Akt/mTOR signalling by the mTOR inhibitor further sensitizes breast cancer cells to honokiol [42]. Other studies have also shown that honokiol induces autophagy in PC-3 and LNCaP prostate cancer cells via the suppression of mTOR and Akt phosphorylation [77]. Another study revealed that the treatment of neuroblastoma cells with honokiol caused significant downregulation of mTOR phosphorylation, which leads to the induction of autophagy of neuroblastoma cells (neuro-2a cells) through the PI3K/Akt/mTOR signalling pathways [96,195].

6.5. Hypoxia-Inducible-Factor (HIF) Pathway

The master regulator of neovascularisation, HIF, is a transcription factor that that plays an integral role in the body's response to low oxygen concentrations (i.e., hypoxia) [196,197]. Active HIF is composed of of two subunits: HIF-α and HIF-1/ARNT. Transcriptional regulation by oxygen is mediated by the HIF-α isoforms. In humans, three isoforms of α-subunit (HIF-1α, HIF-2α, and HIF-3α) have been identified. Recent studies suggest that transcriptional adaptation to hypoxia involves epigenetic changes in histone methylation. Strong evidence has established that the expression of pro-angiogenic factors (VEGF), which play a critical role in pathological neovascularisation in cancer, is elevated due to the activation of HIF pathway under hypoxia conditions [198].

An activation of the HIF pathway leading to hypoxia-induced neovascularisation is the central cause of pathogenesis in almost all solid tumours and ischemic retinal diseases [198,199]. There are studies reporting the capability of honokiol to inhibit HIF isoforms and the expression of hypoxic markers, as well as the binding of HIF to hypoxia-response elements present on VEGF promoter in D407 cells (human retinal pigment epithelial cells) [168]. In KRAS mutant lung cancer cells, it was discovered that Sirt3 was significantly up-regulated in honokiol-treated KRAS mutant lung cancer cells, leading to the destabilisation of its target gene Hif-1α and induction of G1 arrest and apoptosis. This suggests that the anticancer property of honokiol is regulated via a novel mechanism associated with the Sirt3/Hif-1α [49].

6.6. Notch Signalling Pathway

Notch signalling has been implicated in maintaining tissue homeostasis, including the regulation of self-renewal in adult stem cells, organ development, and embryonic development [200–202]. In mammals, the Notch receptor family comprises of four receptors (Notch-1, Notch-2, Notch-3, and Notch-4) and five ligands (Delta-like-1, Delta-like-3, Delta-like-4, Jagged-1, and Jagged-2). Each Notch receptor is activated through cell membrane-associated ligands. A series of proteolytic cleavage processes lead to the maturation and activation of Notch receptors. The first cleavage was catalysed by ADAM-family metalloprotease TACE, followed by the second cleavage mediated by γ-secretase, an enzyme complex that contains presenilin, nicastrin, presenilin enhancer 2 (PEN2), and anterior pharynx-defective 1 (APH1). The series of cleavages will lead to the release and translocation of Notch intracellular domain (NICD) into the nucleus [202]. Activated NICD is able to bind to activator proteins, including mastermind-like proteins (MAML) and recombination signalling binding protein-J (RBPJ) to form a nuclear transcriptional activator complex to regulate the transcription of downstream target genes, such as the hairy and enhancer of split (Hes) gene, Hey family genes, c-myc, cyclin D1, and p21/Waf1 [200]. The Notch pathway plays a complex role in the tumourigenesis of both hematologic and solid tissues. In fact, Notch signalling plays a vital role in regulating cellular differentiation, angiogenesis, proliferation, and apoptosis [201].

It has been shown that honokiol can eliminate cancer stem-like cells and potentiation of temozolomide (TMZ) sensitivity in glioblastoma multiforme (GBM) cells [36]. It was shown that honokiol enhanced the sensitization of GBM cells to MGMT inhibitor O6 benzylguanine (O6-BG) through the downregulation of Notch3 as well as the expression of its downstream target, Hes1 [36]. Furthermore, honokiol has been shown to inhibit B16/F-10, SKMEL-28 melanoma cell lines and SW480 colon cancer cells by targeting Notch signalling pathways [203,204]. Honokiol treatment resulted in reduced levels of cleaved Notch, particularly the Notch-2 receptor, along with a decrease in the expression of downstream target proteins, including Hes-1, cyclin D1, as well as TACE and γ-secretase complex proteins in melanoma cells [55].

Apart from that, honokiol in combination with radiation treatment reduced the number of DCLK1+ (cancer stem cell marker protein) colon cancer cells, which was accompanied by reduced levels of activated Notch-1, its ligand Jagged-1, and the downstream target gene Hes-1 [35,204]. Furthermore, the expression of components of the Notch-1 activating γ-secretase complex, presenilin 1, nicastrin, Pen2, and APH-1 were also suppressed [35]. To determine the effect of a honokiol–IR combination on tumour growth in vivo, nude mice tumour xenografts were administered honokiol intraperitoneally and exposed to IR. The honokiol–IR combination significantly inhibited tumour xenograft growth [35]. In addition, there were reduced levels of DCLK1 and the Notch signalling–related proteins in the xenograft tissues. Together, these data suggest that honokiol is a potent inhibitor of colon cancer growth that targets the stem cells by inhibiting the γ-secretase complex and the Notch signalling pathway [35,204].

6.7. *Downregulation of P-Glycoprotein*

The principal mechanism of multidrug resistance is due to the active transport of drugs out of cells [205]. Among the efflux transporters, P-glycoprotein (P-gp, gene symbol ABCB1) plays an important role in the resistance of cancer cells to a variety of chemotherapeutic treatments [205,206]. Furthermore, P-gp is distributed throughout the body where it interacts with various drugs of different structures to limit their bioavailability [207]. Therefore, the development of effective inhibitors of P-gp expression and/or functional activity should reverse drug resistance and enhance the bioavailability of P-gp substrates. One of the effective ways to overcome P-gp mediated drug resistance is either to block its drug-pump function or to inhibit its expression. To date, there are a total of three generations of P-gp inhibitors that have been discovered [207,208]. However, these compounds were not used widely due to toxicity at the doses required for attenuating P-gp activity, poor specificity, or unpredictable pharmacokinetic interactions. Honokiol was shown to downregulate the expression of P-gp at mRNA and protein levels in MCF-7/ADR, a human breast MDR cancer cell line [209,210]. The downregulation of P-gp was accompanied by a partial recovery of intracellular drug accumulation [210]. In MDR ovarian cancer cells (NCI/ADR-RES), honokiol has also been shown to downregulate the expression of P-gp in a concentration- and time-dependent manner [208].

7. Metabolism, Bioavailability, and Pharmacological Relevance of Honokiol

Pharmacokinetics involves the study of drug movement within the body, which includes the time course of absorption, distribution, metabolism, and excretion (ADME). Honokiol is mainly metabolized in the liver and undergoes in vivo biotransformation, whereby glucuronidation and sulfation are the main metabolic pathways to convert honokiol into mono-glucuronide honokiol and sulphated mono-hydroxyhonokiol before elimination [23]. This extensive biotransformation of honokiol may contribute to its low bioavailability. Currently, studies are being conducted to determine whether the metabolites of honokiol possess any biological activities that can extend the half-life of honokiol while maintaining its biological properties.

Most of the studies have reported that honokiol undergoes a rapid distribution and absorption, but slow elimination after intravenous (i.v.) administration [13,58,211,212]. For i.v. administration, it has been found that there was a rapid rate of distribution followed by a slower rate of elimination (elimination half-life $t_{1/2}$ = 49.22 min and 56.2 min for 5 mg or 10 mg of honokiol, respectively) observed in Sprague Dawley rats [213]. In another study, Liang et al. [214] investigated the pharmacokinetic properties of honokiol in beagle dogs after intravenous guttae, whereby the blood plasma of both male and female dogs was assessed. The elimination half-life ($t_{1/2}$ in hours) was found to be 20.13 (female), 9.27 (female), 7.06 (male), 4.70 (male), and 1.89 (male) after administration of doses of 8.8, 19.8, 3.9, 44.4, and 66.7 mg/kg, respectively. The $t_{1/2}$ decreases with an increase in the dose and length of infusion [214]. In another study, Wang et al. [61] discovered for the first time that honokiol is able to cross the blood–brain barrier (BBB) and blood–cerebrospinal fluid barrier (BCSFB) after i.v. administration when tested on intracerebral gliosarcoma model in Fisher 344 rats and human U251 xenograft glioma model in nude mice. It was also reported that the honokiol was distributed in the order of: lungs > plasma > liver > brain > kidney > heart > spleen after i.v. administration [61].

Furthermore, honokiol has been studied via an intraperitoneal route of administration. Chen et al. [33] reported a maximum plasma concentration of honokiol at 27.179 ± 6.252 min, with the $t_{1/2}$ of 312.08 ± 51.66 min after intraperitoneal injection of 250 mg/kg in BALB/c mice. On another note, studies have also shown that the presence of rhubarb and immature orange fruit extract in the decoction influenced the pharmacokinetics of honokiol, where a single oral dose of honokiol in Houpu decoction (a compound prescription of honokiol; 5 g/kg body weight) in Wistar rats demonstrated an elimination $t_{1/2}$ of 526.6 min [215]. Honokiol has a rapid absorption (Tmax = 20 min) and slow elimination ($t_{1/2}z$ = 290 min) after a single dose of oral gavage at 40 mg/kg in healthy rats [216]. In another study, honokiol showed a peak plasma concentration at 72 min, and $t_{1/2}$ of 186 min, and the absolute bioavailability for honokiol was found to be 5.3% when rats underwent oral administration of Magnolol/Honokiol emulsion (4:1) at 50 mg/kg [217]. After the rats were administered with honokiol orally, the honokiol was distributed rapidly to all parts of organs with the highest concentration being accumulated in the liver, followed by the brain and kidneys [216]. This was opposed to their discovery in tumour-bearing mice, where the highest concentration was found in the liver, followed by the kidneys and lungs [218]. This may be due to the different types of species being used as well as the tumor-burdened mice possibly affecting drug distribution [47]. With the rectal administration of Houpo extract at a dose of 245 mg/kg (equivalent to 13.5 mg/kg of honokiol) in Wistar rats, the maximal plasma concentration of honokiol found was approximately six times to that administered orally at an identical dose, indicating that rectal dosing avoids first-pass metabolism to some extent [219].

Meanwhile, the topical application of honokiol on UVB-induced contact hypersensitivity (CHS) as a model in C3H/HeN mice was also evaluated [68,220]. The topical application of honokiol (0.5 and 1.0 mg/cm^2 skin area) had a significant preventive effect on the UVB-induced suppression of the CHS response. The inflammatory mediators COX-2 and PGE_2 played a key role in this effect, as indicated by the honokiol-mediated inhibition of cyclooxygenase-2 (COX-2) expression and PGE_2 production in the UVB-exposed skin. Besides that, both topical application and oral administration of honokiol significantly inhibited (38% to 46%, $p < 0.001$) UVB-induced suppression of CHS in mice compared with the mice that were not treated with honokiol but exposed to UVB radiation. Prominently, the level of inhibition of CHS was not significantly different between the two modes of administration of honokiol [220].

Apart from that, Gao et al. [221] investigated the enhancement in the transdermal and localised delivery of honokiol through breast tissue. It was reported that microneedle-porated dermatome significantly increased the delivery of honokiol by nearly three-fold (97.81 ± 18.96 $\mu g/cm^2$) compared with passive delivery (32.56 ± 5.67 $\mu g/cm^2$). Oleic acid was found to be the best chemical penetration enhancer, increasing the delivery almost 27-fold (868.06 ± 100.91 $\mu g/cm^2$). The addition of oleic acid also resulted in a better retention of drugs in porcine mammary papilla (965.41 ± 80.26 $\mu g/cm^2$) compared with breast skin (294.16 ± 8.49 $\mu g/cm^2$) [221]. In summary, both microneedles and chemical enhancers can improve the absorption of honokiol through the skin. Directly applying honokiol on mammary papilla is a potential administration route which can increase localized delivery into breast tissue [183].

On another note, some studies have addressed the poor solubility of honokiol in hydrophilic environment. Wang et al. [222] developed polyethylene glycol-coated (PEGylated) liposomal honokiol to improve its solubility compared to free honokiol. PEGylated (polyethylene glycol coated) liposomal honokiol was shown to enhance the serum honokiol concentration and decrease clearance. The pharmacokinetic analysis of PEGylated liposomal honokiol showed a two-fold increase in elimination $t_{1/2}$ value as compared to that of free honokiol when being injected through the i.v. route (20 mg/kg body weight) in Balb/c mice (from 26 min in PEGylated liposomal honokiol to 13 min in free honokiol) [222]. Moreover, the $AUC_{0\rightarrow\infty}$ (mean concentration of drug in plasma) of PEGylated liposomal honokiol was about 1.85-fold higher than free honokiol. The protein-binding ability of honokiol in plasma was reported to be between 60% and 65% as revealed by equilibrium dialysis [222]. In another study, plasma honokiol concentrations were maintained above 30 and 10 μg/mL for 24 and 48 h, respectively, in liposomal honokiol-treated mice. However, it was reduced rapidly (<5 μg/mL) by 12 h in free honokiol-treated mice bearing A549 xenograft tumors, suggesting that liposomal honokiol extended blood circulation times in tumor-bearing mice compared to free honokiol [223].

8. Potential Drug Delivery of Honokiol

Due to the low water solubility and bioavailability of honokiol, multiple studies have been performed to develop proper honokiol delivery systems to improve its pharmacological effectiveness. A few studies have been performed to develop efficient drug carriers to deliver honokiol to its respective target, including the development of nanoparticles [224–226], micelles [227–229], and liposomes [73,171,223].

For honokiol delivery in the form of nanoparticles, Zheng et al. [230] developed monomethoxy poly(ethylene glycol)–poly(lactic acid) (MPEG–PLA) via ring opening polymerisation and then processed into nanoparticle for honokiol delivery. The honokiol-loaded MPEG–PLA nanoparticles were mono-dispersed and stable in the aqueous solution [230]. It was found that only 53% of honokiol was released from the nanoparticles within 24 h, while 100% of free honokiol was released into the outside media, suggesting that the honokiol loaded MPEG–PLA nanoparticle is a novel honokiol formulation which could meet the requirement of intravenous injection. In comparison, honokiol loaded MPEG-PLA nanoparticles significantly decreased the viability of A2780s cells (human ovarian cancer cells) than free honokiol, indicating that honokiol loaded MPEG–PLA nanoparticles might possess great potential applications for anticancer effect on cisplatin-sensitive A2780s cells in vitro [230]. In addition, the incorporation of both honokiol and doxorubicin in MPEG-PLA nanoparticles exhibited stronger anticancer activity than its individual form against A2780s cells [231].

In another study, emulsion solvent evaporation was used to develop the active targeting nanoparticle-loaded honokiol (ATNH) using copolymerpoly (ε-caprolactone)-poly (ethylene glycol)-poly (ε-caprolactone) (PCEC), which was modified with folate (FA) by introducing polyethylenimine (PEI) [30]. It was reported that ATNH showed a suitable size distribution, high encapsulation efficiency, gradual release, and targeting uptake by human nasopharynx carcinoma cells (HNE-1). Moreover, ATNH significantly inhibited tumour growth, metabolism, proliferation, micro-vessel generation, and caused cell-cycle arrest at the G1 phase [30]. Apart from that, epigallocatechin-3-gallate functionalized chitin loaded with honokiol nanoparticles (CE-HK NP), developed by Tang et al. [224], inhibit HepG2 cell growth and induce apoptosis through the suppression of mitochondrial membrane potential. Furthermore, CE-HK NPs (40 mg/kg) inhibited tumour growth by 83.55% ($p < 0.05$), which was far higher than the 30.15% inhibition of free honokiol (40 mg/kg). The proposed delivery system exhibits better tumour selectivity and growth reduction in both in vitro and in vivo models (male BALB/c nude mice treated with honokiol administrated by intertumoral injection) and did not induce any side effects [224]. Therefore, the CE-HK NPs may act as an effective delivery system for liver cancer. Recently, Yu et al. [232] further improved the design of nanoparticles for targeted delivery in breast cancer by surface modifying the honokiol nanoparticles through conjugation with folic acid to the surface of honokiol nanoparticles coated with polydopamine (HK-PDA-FA-NPs) as a pH-sensitive targeting anchor for nanoparticles. The targeted nanoparticles (HK-PDA-FA-NPs) can be stably present in various physiological media and exhibit pH sensitivity during drug release in vitro. HK-PDA-FA-NPs have better targeting ability to 4T1 cells than normal HK-NPs. Targeted nanoparticles have a tumour inhibition rate of greater than 80% in vivo (female Balb/c mice injected intraperitoneally with 40 mg/kg HK-PDA-FA-NPs), which is significantly higher than conventional HK-NPs [232].

For honokiol delivery in the form of micelles, researchers developed poly(ethylene glycol)-poly(ε-caprolactone)-poly(ethylene glycol) (PECE) micelle loaded with honokiol [229]. The cytotoxicity results showed that the composite drug delivery system is a safe carrier and the encapsulated honokiol retained its potent antitumor effect when tested against murine melanoma cell line B16 [233]. The IC_{50} values of free honokiol, honokiol nanoparticles, and honokiol micelles were 5.357, 6.274, and 6.746 μg/mL, respectively. The result indicated that the cytotoxicity of the honokiol micelles was lower than that of free honokiol, which was attributed to the sustained release behaviour of honokiol from honokiol micelles [233]. Further, comparing with honokiol nanoparticles, the cytotoxicity of honokiol micelles was a little lower, which might be due to the absence of organic solvent and surfactant in the honokiol micelles [233]. To increase the hydrophilicity of honokiol, Qiu et al. [234] developed an amphiphilic polymer–drug conjugate via the condensation of low molecular weight monomethoxy-poly(ethylene glycol) (MPEG)-2000 with honokiol through an ester linkage. The MPEG–honokiol (MPEG–HK) conjugate prepared formed nano-sized micelles, with a mean particle size of less than 20 nm (MPEG–HK, 360 $\mu g{\cdot}mL^{-1}$) in water, in which they could be well dispersed, and the results showed that only 20% of the conjugated honokiol was released in 2 h in beagle dog plasma, while in phosphate-buffered saline, the time required to reach 20% of honokiol release was >200 h [234]. Meanwhile, the inhibitory activity of the honokiol conjugate was found to be retained in vitro against LL/2 cell lines with an IC_{50} value of 10.7 μg/mL [234]. These results suggest that the polymer–drug conjugate provides a potential new approach to hydrophobic drugs, such as honokiol, in formulation design. In another study, nanomicellar honokiol (HNK-NM) with the size range of 20–40 nm was developed and compared against honokiol free drug (HNK-FD) [212]. Compared to HNK-FD, HNK-NM resulted in a significant increase in oral bioavailability. Cmax (4.06 and 3.60-fold) and AUC (6.26 and 5.83-fold) were significantly increased in comparison to oral 40 and 80 mg/kg HNK-FD, respectively, when tested in triple negative breast cancer cell lines (MDA-MB-231, MDA-MB-453, and MDA-MB-468). The anticancer effects of these formulations were also studied in BALB/c nude mice transplanted with orthotopic MDA-MB-231 cell induced xenografts [212]. After four weeks of daily oral administration of HNK-NM formulation, a significant reduction in the tumour volumes and weights compared to free drug ($p < 0.001$) treated groups was observed. Furthermore, in 25% of the mice, the treatment resulted in a complete eradication of tumours. Increased apoptosis and antiangiogenic effects were observed in HNK-NM groups compared to HNK-FD and untreated control mice [212].

Wang et al. [228] prepared paclitaxel (PTX) and honokiol (HK) combination methoxy poly(ethylene glycol) poly(caprolactone) micelles (P–H/M) via the solid dispersion method against breast cancer (4T1). The particle size of P–H/M was 28.7 ± 2.5 nm and spherical in shape. Both the cytotoxicity and the cellular uptake of P–H/M were increased in 4T1 cells, and P–H/M induced more apoptosis than PTX-loaded micelles or HK-loaded micelles. Furthermore, the antitumor effect of P–H/M was significantly improved compared with PTX-loaded micelles or HK-loaded micelles in vivo (Female Balb/c mice and female Balb/c nude mice treated with intravenous injection) [31,228]. P–H/M were more effective in inhibiting tumour proliferation, inducing tumour apoptosis, and decreasing the density of microvasculature accumulated more in tumour tissues compared to the free drug. After that, Wang et al. [235] developed paclitaxel (PTX) and honokiol (HNK) which are co-encapsulated into pH-sensitive polymeric micelles based on poly(2-ethyl-2-oxazoline)-poly(D,L-lactide) (PEOz-PLA). Results showed efficient inhibition of tumour metastasis by dual drug-loaded PEOz-PLA micelles in vitro anti-invasion and anti-migration assessment in MDA-MB-231 cells and in vivo in nude mice [235]. The suppression of MDR and metastasis by the micelles was assigned to the synergistic effects of pH-triggered drug release and HNK/PEOz-PLA-aroused P-gp inhibition, and pH-triggered drug release and PTX/HNK-aroused MMPs inhibition, respectively. After that, Wang et al. [236] proceeded to modify the paclitaxel plus honokiol micelles with dequalinium and tested it in non-small-cell lung cancer. When tested on Lewis lung tumour (LLT) cells, the polymeric micelles show powerful cytotoxicity, effective suppression on vasculogenic mimicry (VM) channels and tumour metastasis, as well as the activation of apoptotic enzymes caspase-3 and caspase-9, and down-regulation of FAK, PI3K, MMP-2, and MMP-9 [236]. In vivo assays (C57BL/6 mice treated through intravenous injection) indicated that polymeric micelles could increase the selective accumulation of chemotherapeutic drugs at tumour sites and showed a conspicuous anti-tumour efficacy [236].

For liposomes loaded with honokiol, Luo et al. [73] created liposomal honokiol and tested it on cisplatin-sensitive (A2780s) and -resistant (A2780cp) human ovarian cancer models. The administration of liposomal honokiol resulted in significant inhibition (84–88% maximum inhibition relative to controls) in the growth of A2780s and A2780cp tumour xenografts and prolonged the survival of the treated mice (treated twice weekly with intravenous administration) [73]. These anti-tumour responses were associated with marked increases in tumour apoptosis, and reductions in intratumoural microvessel density. Jiang et al. [223] incorporated honokiol in combination with cisplatin in the liposomes and tested it in A549 lung cancer xenograft nude mice model through intraperitoneal administration. This combination effectively suppressed tumour growth and significantly increased life span of treated mice compared to liposomal honokiol alone [223]. A similar result was observed in murine CT26 colon cancer models, where the systemic administration of liposomal honokiol with cisplatin resulted in the inhibition of subcutaneous tumour growth beyond the effects observed with either liposomal honokiol or cisplatin alone due to elevated levels of apoptosis and reduced endothelial cell density significantly [237]. In a recent study, hyaluronic acid (HA) modified daunorubicin plus honokiol cationic liposomes were prepared and characterised for the treatment of breast cancer by eliminating vasculogenic mimicry (VM) [238]. Studies found that the HA modified daunorubicin plus honokiol cationic liposomes enhanced the cellular uptake and destroyed VM channels. In addition, these liposomes prolonged their circulation time in the blood, and significantly accumulated at the tumour site to maximise its anticancer efficacy.

9. Future Perspective

Up to date, many in vitro and in vivo studies have identified the protective effects of honokiol in various types of cancers. However, the exact anticancer mechanism of honokiol is still insufficiently elucidated, especially its application in treating human cancer clinically. Since honokiol is being extensively metabolised in the body into different metabolites, it is vital to recognise the different types of metabolites circulating in the body in order to gain a better insight into the fate of honokiol after administration. The characterisation of honokiol metabolites would enable a better understanding of the overall bioactivity of honokiol as well as to determine the relationship between the bioactivity of the core molecule and its metabolites circulating within the target tissue. Moreover, future studies could focus on improving the methods used for in vitro studies to mimic more favourable in vivo conditions by considering the actual metabolites detected and concentrations found in the respective cancer tissues in order to better understand the mode of action of honokiol in cancer. Apart from that, it is essential to study the anticancer properties of the derivatives of honokiol as very few studies have been performed on the derivatives. It is important to study its derivatives as they might have improved and enhanced anticancer properties due to the change in structures and functional groups.

In short, more research can be done to confirm the anticancer properties of honokiol in more detail in order to come up with a safe and effective dosage to be used in chemoprevention and chemotherapy. Furthermore, more research can be done on the metabolism of honokiol via different routes of administration to find out the most effective route of administration for different types of cancer. The pre-formulation as well as formulation of honokiol can also be developed to prepare the transition of honokiol from pre-clinical to clinical studies in the future.

10. Conclusions

For centuries, researchers have been searching for strategies to control cancer progression through different approaches. Honokiol is a potential natural compound that exerts multiple effects on different cellular processes in various cancer models. Honokiol has been shown to regulate cell cycle arrest, induction of apoptosis, necrosis, and autophagy, as well as the inhibition of metastasis and angiogenesis through various signalling pathways. In addition, its effects are also validated in several in vivo studies with promising results where it can inhibit tumour growth and prolong survival in mouse cancer models. Current efforts are focusing on developing numerous drug delivery systems to improve the pharmacological, pharmacokinetics, and pharmacodynamic properties of honokiol. This review concludes that honokiol may be considered as a potential candidate for anticancer drug development.

Author Contributions: The literature searches and data collection were performed by W.L.L., C.P.O. and Y.Q.T. The manuscript was written by W.L.L., C.P.O., Y.Q.T. and W.H.Y. The manuscript was critically reviewed and edited by Y.Q.T. and W.H.Y. The project was conceptualized by W.H.Y. All authors have read and agreed to the published version of the manuscript.

References

1. Foster, I. Cancer: A cell cycle defect. *Radiography* **2008**, *14*, 144–149. [CrossRef]
2. Cabral, C.; Efferth, T.; Pires, I.M.; Severino, P.; Lemos, M.F.L. Natural Products as a Source for New Leads in Cancer Research and Treatment. *Evid.-Based Complement. Altern. Med.* **2018**, *2018*, 8243680. [CrossRef] [PubMed]
3. Wu, S.; Zhu, W.; Thompson, P.; Hannun, Y.A. Evaluating intrinsic and non-intrinsic cancer risk factors. *Nat. Commun.* **2018**, *9*, 3490. [CrossRef] [PubMed]
4. Siegel, R.L.; Miller, K.D.; Jemal, A. Cancer statistics, 2019. *CA Cancer J. Clin.* **2019**, *69*, 7–34. [CrossRef]
5. Bray, F.; Ferlay, J.; Soerjomataram, I.; Siegel, R.L.; Torre, L.A.; Jemal, A. Global cancer statistics 2018: GLOBOCAN estimates of incidence and mortality worldwide for 36 cancers in 185 countries. *CA Cancer J. Clin.* **2018**, *68*, 394–424. [CrossRef]
6. DeVita, V.T.; Canellos, G.P. New therapies and standard of care in oncology. *Nat. Rev. Clin. Oncol.* **2011**, *8*, 67–68. [CrossRef]
7. Marqus, S.; Pirogova, E.; Piva, T.J. Evaluation of the use of therapeutic peptides for cancer treatment. *J. Biomed. Sci.* **2017**, *24*, 21. [CrossRef]
8. Mitra, S.; Dash, R. Natural Products for the Management and Prevention of Breast Cancer. *Evid.-Based Complement. Altern. Med.* **2018**, *2018*, 8324696. [CrossRef]
9. Bayat Mokhtari, R.; Homayouni, T.S.; Baluch, N.; Morgatskaya, E.; Kumar, S.; Das, B.; Yeger, H. Combination therapy in combating cancer. *Oncotarget* **2017**, *8*, 38022–38043. [CrossRef]
10. Robinson, M.M.Z.; Zhang, X. *The World Medicines Situation 2011. Traditional Medicines: Global Situation, Issues and Challenges*; World Health Organization: Geneva, Switzerland, 2011.
11. Seelinger, M.; Popescu, R.; Giessrigl, B.; Jarukamjorn, K.; Unger, C.; Wallnöfer, B.; Fritzer-Szekeres, M.; Szekeres, T.; Diaz, R.; Jäger, W.; et al. Methanol extract of the ethnopharmaceutical remedy Smilax spinosa exhibits anti-neoplastic activity. *Int. J. Oncol.* **2012**, *41*, 1164–1172. [CrossRef]
12. Amaral, R.G.; dos Santos, S.A.; Andrade, L.N.; Severino, P.; Carvalho, A.A. Natural Products as Treatment against Cancer: A Historical and Current Vision. *Clin. Oncol.* **2019**, *4*, 1562.
13. Arora, S.; Singh, S.; Piazza, G.A.; Contreras, C.M.; Panyam, J.; Singh, A.P. Honokiol: A novel natural agent for cancer prevention and therapy. *Curr. Mol. Med.* **2012**, *12*, 1244–1252. [CrossRef] [PubMed]
14. Chen, Y.J.; Wu, C.L.; Liu, J.F.; Fong, Y.C.; Hsu, S.F.; Li, T.M.; Su, Y.C.; Liu, S.H.; Tang, C.H. Honokiol induces cell apoptosis in human chondrosarcoma cells through mitochondrial dysfunction and endoplasmic reticulum stress. *Cancer Lett.* **2010**, *291*, 20–30. [CrossRef] [PubMed]
15. Lee, J.D.; Lee, J.Y.; Baek, B.J.; Lee, B.D.; Koh, Y.W.; Lee, W.-S.; Lee, Y.-J.; Kwon, B.-M. The inhibitory effect of honokiol, a natural plant product, on vestibular schwannoma cells. *Laryngoscope* **2012**, *122*, 162–166. [CrossRef]
16. Amblard, F.; Delinsky, D.; Arbiser, J.L.; Schinazi, R.F. Facile purification of honokiol and its antiviral and cytotoxic properties. *J. Med. Chem.* **2006**, *49*, 3426–3427. [CrossRef]
17. Woodbury, A.; Yu, S.P.; Wei, L.; García, P. Neuro-modulating effects of honokiol: A review. *Front. Neurol.* **2013**, *4*, 130. [CrossRef]
18. Hahm, E.R.; Arlotti, J.A.; Marynowski, S.W.; Singh, S.V. Honokiol, a constituent of oriental medicinal herb magnolia officinalis, inhibits growth of PC-3 xenografts in vivo in association with apoptosis induction. *Clin. Cancer Res.* **2008**, *14*, 1248–1257. [CrossRef]
19. Chen, L. Rapid purification and scale-up of honokiol and magnolol using high-capacity high-speed counter-current chromatography A. *J. Chromatogr.* **2007**, *1142*, 115–122. [CrossRef]

20. Chen, C.-M.; Liu, Y.-C. ChemInform Abstract: A Concise Synthesis of Honokiol. *Tetrahedron Lett.* **2009**, *50*, 1151–1152. [CrossRef]
21. Gupta, M. Pharmacological Properties and Traditional Therapeutic Uses of Important Indian Spices: A Review. *Int. J. Food Prop.* **2010**, *13*, 1092–1116. [CrossRef]
22. Anand, K.W.; Wakode, S. Development of drugs based on Benzimidazole Heterocycle: Recent advancement and insights. *Int. J. Chem. Stud.* **2017**, *5*, 350–362.
23. Bohmdorfer, M.; Maier-Salamon, A.; Taferner, B.; Reznicek, G.; Thalhammer, T.; Hering, S.; Hufner, A.; Schuhly, W.; Jager, W. In vitro metabolism and disposition of honokiol in rat and human livers. *J. Pharm. Sci.* **2011**, *100*, 3506–3516. [CrossRef] [PubMed]
24. Lin, J.M.; Prakasha Gowda, A.S.; Sharma, A.K.; Amin, S. In vitro growth inhibition of human cancer cells by novel honokiol analogs. *Bioorg. Med. Chem.* **2012**, *20*, 3202–3211. [CrossRef] [PubMed]
25. Yang, S.E.; Hsieh, M.T.; Tsai, T.H.; Hsu, S.L. Down-modulation of Bcl-XL, release of cytochrome c and sequential activation of caspases during honokiol-induced apoptosis in human squamous lung cancer CH27 cells. *Biochem. Pharmacol.* **2002**, *63*, 1641–1651. [CrossRef]
26. Huang, K.J.; Kuo, C.H.; Chen, S.H.; Lin, C.Y.; Lee, Y.R. Honokiol inhibits in vitro and in vivo growth of oral squamous cell carcinoma through induction of apoptosis, cell cycle arrest and autophagy. *J. Cell. Mol. Med.* **2018**, *22*, 1894–1908. [CrossRef] [PubMed]
27. Huang, L.; Zhang, K.; Guo, Y.; Huang, F.; Yang, K.; Chen, L.; Huang, K.; Zhang, F.; Long, Q. Honokiol protects against doxorubicin cardiotoxicity via improving mitochondrial function in mouse hearts. *Sci. Rep.* **2017**, *7*, 11989. [CrossRef] [PubMed]
28. Lee, J.S.; Sul, J.Y.; Park, J.B.; Lee, M.S.; Cha, E.Y.; Ko, Y.B. Honokiol induces apoptosis and suppresses migration and invasion of ovarian carcinoma cells via AMPK/mTOR signaling pathway. *Int. J. Mol. Med.* **2019**, *43*, 1969–1978. [CrossRef]
29. Olusanya, T.O.B.; Haj Ahmad, R.R.; Ibegbu, D.M.; Smith, J.R.; Elkordy, A.A. Liposomal Drug Delivery Systems and Anticancer Drugs. *Molecules* **2018**, *23*, 907. [CrossRef]
30. Yang, B.; Ni, X.; Chen, L.; Zhang, H.; Ren, P.; Feng, Y.; Chen, Y.; Fu, S.; Wu, J. Honokiol-loaded polymeric nanoparticles: An active targeting drug delivery system for the treatment of nasopharyngeal carcinoma. *Drug Deliv.* **2017**, *24*, 660–669. [CrossRef]
31. Wang, X.; Beitler, J.J.; Wang, H.; Lee, M.J.; Huang, W.; Koenig, L.; Nannapaneni, S.; Amin, A.R.M.R.; Bonner, M.; Shin, H.J.C.; et al. Honokiol Enhances Paclitaxel Efficacy in Multi-Drug Resistant Human Cancer Model through the Induction of Apoptosis. *PLoS ONE* **2014**, *9*, e86369. [CrossRef]
32. Rajendran, P.; Li, F.; Shanmugam, M.K.; Vali, S.; Abbasi, T.; Kapoor, S.; Ahn, K.S.; Kumar, A.P.; Sethi, G. Honokiol inhibits signal transducer and activator of transcription-3 signaling, proliferation, and survival of hepatocellular carcinoma cells via the protein tyrosine phosphatase SHP-1. *J. Cell. Physiol.* **2012**, *227*, 2184–2195. [CrossRef] [PubMed]
33. Chen, F.; Wang, T.; Wu, Y.-F.; Gu, Y.; Xu, X.-L.; Zheng, S.; Hu, X. Honokiol: A potent chemotherapy candidate for human colorectal carcinoma. *World J. Gastroenterol.* **2004**, *10*, 3459–3463. [CrossRef] [PubMed]
34. He, Z.; Subramaniam, D.; Ramalingam, S.; Dhar, A.; Postier, R.G.; Umar, S.; Zhang, Y.; Anant, S. Honokiol radiosensitizes colorectal cancer cells: Enhanced activity in cells with mismatch repair defects. *Am. J. Physiol.-Gastrointest. Liver Physiol.* **2011**, *301*, G929–G937. [CrossRef] [PubMed]
35. Ponnurangam, S.; Mammen, J.M.; Ramalingam, S.; He, Z.; Zhang, Y.; Umar, S.; Subramaniam, D.; Anant, S. Honokiol in combination with radiation targets notch signaling to inhibit colon cancer stem cells. *Mol. Cancer Ther.* **2012**, *11*, 963–972. [CrossRef] [PubMed]
36. Lai, I.C.; Shih, P.-H.; Yao, C.-J.; Yeh, C.-T.; Wang-Peng, J.; Lui, T.-N.; Chuang, S.-E.; Hu, T.-S.; Lai, T.-Y.; Lai, G.-M. Elimination of Cancer Stem-Like Cells and Potentiation of Temozolomide Sensitivity by Honokiol in Glioblastoma Multiforme Cells. *PLoS ONE* **2015**, *10*, e0114830. [CrossRef] [PubMed]
37. Battle, T.E.; Arbiser, J.; Frank, D.A. The natural product honokiol induces caspase-dependent apoptosis in B-cell chronic lymphocytic leukemia (B-CLL) cells. *Blood* **2005**, *106*, 690–697. [CrossRef]
38. Gao, D.Q.; Qian, S.; Ju, T. Anticancer activity of Honokiol against lymphoid malignant cells via activation of ROS-JNK and attenuation of Nrf2 and NF-kappaB. *J. BUON* **2016**, *21*, 673–679.
39. Wolf, I.; O'Kelly, J.; Wakimoto, N.; Nguyen, A.; Amblard, F.; Karlan, B.Y.; Arbiser, J.L.; Koeffler, H.P. Honokiol, a natural biphenyl, inhibits in vitro and in vivo growth of breast cancer through induction of apoptosis and cell cycle arrest. *Int. J. Oncol.* **2007**, *30*, 1529–1537. [CrossRef]

40. Nagalingam, A.; Arbiser, J.L.; Bonner, M.Y.; Saxena, N.K.; Sharma, D. Honokiol activates AMP-activated protein kinase in breast cancer cells via an LKB1-dependent pathway and inhibits breast carcinogenesis. *Breast Cancer Res.* **2012**, *14*, R35. [CrossRef]
41. Sengupta, S.; Nagalingam, A.; Muniraj, N.; Bonner, M.Y.; Mistriotis, P.; Afthinos, A.; Kuppusamy, P.; Lanoue, D.; Cho, S.; Korangath, P.; et al. Activation of tumor suppressor LKB1 by honokiol abrogates cancer stem-like phenotype in breast cancer via inhibition of oncogenic Stat3. *Oncogene* **2017**, *36*, 5709–5721. [CrossRef]
42. Liu, H.; Zang, C.; Emde, A.; Planas-Silva, M.D.; Rosche, M.; Kuhnl, A.; Schulz, C.O.; Elstner, E.; Possinger, K.; Eucker, J. Anti-tumor effect of honokiol alone and in combination with other anti-cancer agents in breast cancer. *Eur. J. Pharmacol.* **2008**, *591*, 43–51. [CrossRef] [PubMed]
43. Park, E.J.; Min, H.Y.; Chung, H.J.; Hong, J.Y.; Kang, Y.J.; Hung, T.M.; Youn, U.J.; Kim, Y.S.; Bae, K.; Kang, S.S.; et al. Down-regulation of c-Src/EGFR-mediated signaling activation is involved in the honokiol-induced cell cycle arrest and apoptosis in MDA-MB-231 human breast cancer cells. *Cancer Lett.* **2009**, *277*, 133–140. [CrossRef] [PubMed]
44. Singh, T.; Katiyar, S.K. Honokiol Inhibits Non-Small Cell Lung Cancer Cell Migration by Targeting PGE2-Mediated Activation of β-Catenin Signaling. *PLoS ONE* **2013**, *8*, e60749. [CrossRef] [PubMed]
45. Singh, T.; Prasad, R.; Katiyar, S.K. Inhibition of class I histone deacetylases in non-small cell lung cancer by honokiol leads to suppression of cancer cell growth and induction of cell death in vitro and in vivo. *Epigenetics* **2013**, *8*, 54–65. [CrossRef]
46. Lv, X.; Liu, F.; Shang, Y.; Chen, S.Z. Honokiol exhibits enhanced antitumor effects with chloroquine by inducing cell death and inhibiting autophagy in human non-small cell lung cancer cells. *Oncol. Rep.* **2015**, *34*, 1289–1300. [CrossRef]
47. Pan, J.; Lee, Y.; Zhang, Q.; Xiong, D.; Wan, T.C.; Wang, Y.; You, M. Honokiol Decreases Lung Cancer Metastasis through Inhibition of the STAT3 Signaling Pathway. *Cancer Prev. Res.* **2017**, *10*, 133–141. [CrossRef]
48. Liou, S.-F.; Hua, K.-T.; Hsu, C.-Y.; Weng, M.-S. Honokiol from Magnolia spp. induces G1 arrest via disruption of EGFR stability through repressing HDAC6 deacetylated Hsp90 function in lung cancer cells. *J. Funct. Foods* **2015**, *15*, 84–96. [CrossRef]
49. Luo, L.-X.; Li, Y.; Liu, Z.-Q.; Fan, X.-X.; Duan, F.-G.; Li, R.-Z.; Yao, X.-J.; Leung, E.L.-H.; Liu, L. Honokiol Induces Apoptosis, G1 Arrest, and Autophagy in KRAS Mutant Lung Cancer Cells. *Front. Pharmacol.* **2017**, *8*, 199. [CrossRef]
50. Zhu, J.; Xu, S.; Gao, W.; Feng, J.; Zhao, G. Honokiol induces endoplasmic reticulum stress-mediated apoptosis in human lung cancer cells. *Life Sci.* **2019**, *221*, 204–211. [CrossRef]
51. Chae, J.I.; Jeon, Y.J.; Shim, J.H. Downregulation of Sp1 is involved in honokiol-induced cell cycle arrest and apoptosis in human malignant pleural mesothelioma cells. *Oncol. Rep.* **2013**, *29*, 2318–2324. [CrossRef]
52. Mannal, P.W.; Schneider, J.; Tangada, A.; McDonald, D.; McFadden, D.W. Honokiol produces anti-neoplastic effects on melanoma cells in vitro. *J. Surg. Oncol.* **2011**, *104*, 260–264. [CrossRef] [PubMed]
53. Chilampalli, C.; Guillermo, R.; Kaushik, R.S.; Young, A.; Chandrasekher, G.; Fahmy, H.; Dwivedi, C. Honokiol, a chemopreventive agent against skin cancer, induces cell cycle arrest and apoptosis in human epidermoid A431 cells. *Exp. Biol. Med.* **2011**, *236*, 1351–1359. [CrossRef] [PubMed]
54. Kaushik, G.; Ramalingam, S.; Subramaniam, D.; Rangarajan, P.; Protti, P.; Rammamoorthy, P.; Anant, S.; Mammen, J.M. Honokiol induces cytotoxic and cytostatic effects in malignant melanoma cancer cells. *Am. J. Surg.* **2012**, *204*, 868–873. [CrossRef] [PubMed]
55. Kaushik, G.; Kwatra, D.; Subramaniam, D.; Jensen, R.A.; Anant, S.; Mammen, J.M.V. Honokiol affects melanoma cell growth by targeting the AMP-activated protein kinase signaling pathway. *Am. J. Surg.* **2014**, *208*, 995–1002. [CrossRef] [PubMed]
56. Guillermo-Lagae, R.; Santha, S.; Thomas, M.; Zoelle, E.; Stevens, J.; Kaushik, R.S. Antineoplastic Effects of Honokiol on Melanoma. *Biomed Res. Int.* **2017**, *2017*, 5496398. [CrossRef] [PubMed]
57. Li, W.; Wang, Q.; Su, Q.; Ma, D.; An, C.; Ma, L.; Liang, H. Honokiol suppresses renal cancer cells' metastasis via dual-blocking epithelial-mesenchymal transition and cancer stem cell properties through modulating miR-141/ZEB2 signaling. *Mol. Cells* **2014**, *37*, 383–388. [CrossRef] [PubMed]
58. Averett, C.; Bhardwaj, A.; Arora, S.; Srivastava, S.K.; Khan, M.A.; Ahmad, A.; Singh, S.; Carter, J.E.; Khushman, M.D.; Singh, A.P. Honokiol suppresses pancreatic tumor growth, metastasis and desmoplasia by interfering with tumor–stromal cross-talk. *Carcinogenesis* **2016**, *37*, 1052–1061. [CrossRef] [PubMed]

59. Arora, S.; Bhardwaj, A.; Srivastava, S.K.; Singh, S.; McClellan, S.; Wang, B.; Singh, A.P. Honokiol arrests cell cycle, induces apoptosis, and potentiates the cytotoxic effect of gemcitabine in human pancreatic cancer cells. *PLoS ONE* **2011**, *6*, e21573. [CrossRef] [PubMed]
60. Lu, C.H.; Chen, S.H.; Chang, Y.S.; Liu, Y.W.; Wu, J.Y.; Lim, Y.P.; Yu, H.I.; Lee, Y.R. Honokiol, a potential therapeutic agent, induces cell cycle arrest and program cell death in vitro and in vivo in human thyroid cancer cells. *Pharmacol. Res.* **2017**, *115*, 288–298. [CrossRef]
61. Wang, X.; Duan, X.; Yang, G.; Zhang, X.; Deng, L.; Zheng, H.; Deng, C.; Wen, J.; Wang, N.; Peng, C.; et al. Honokiol crosses BBB and BCSFB, and inhibits brain tumor growth in rat 9L intracerebral gliosarcoma model and human U251 xenograft glioma model. *PLoS ONE* **2011**, *6*, e18490. [CrossRef]
62. Jeong, J.J.; Lee, J.H.; Chang, K.C.; Kim, H.J. Honokiol exerts an anticancer effect in T98G human glioblastoma cells through the induction of apoptosis and the regulation of adhesion molecules. *Int. J. Oncol.* **2012**, *41*, 1358–1364. [CrossRef] [PubMed]
63. Fan, Y.; Xue, W.; Schachner, M.; Zhao, W. Honokiol Eliminates Glioma/Glioblastoma Stem Cell-Like Cells Via JAK-STAT3 Signaling and Inhibits Tumor Progression by Targeting Epidermal Growth Factor Receptor. *Cancers* **2018**, *11*, 22. [CrossRef] [PubMed]
64. Chang, K.H.; Yan, M.D.; Yao, C.J.; Lin, P.C.; Lai, G.M. Honokiol-induced apoptosis and autophagy in glioblastoma multiforme cells. *Oncol. Lett.* **2013**, *6*, 1435–1438. [CrossRef] [PubMed]
65. Joo, Y.N.; Eun, S.Y.; Park, S.W.; Lee, J.H.; Chang, K.C.; Kim, H.J. Honokiol inhibits U87MG human glioblastoma cell invasion through endothelial cells by regulating membrane permeability and the epithelial-mesenchymal transition. *Int. J. Oncol.* **2014**, *44*, 187–194. [CrossRef]
66. Lin, C.J.; Chen, T.L.; Tseng, Y.Y.; Wu, G.J.; Hsieh, M.H.; Lin, Y.W.; Chen, R.M. Honokiol induces autophagic cell death in malignant glioma through reactive oxygen species-mediated regulation of the p53/PI3K/Akt/mTOR signaling pathway. *Toxicol. Appl. Pharmacol.* **2016**, *304*, 59–69. [CrossRef]
67. Huang, K.; Chen, Y.; Zhang, R.; Wu, Y.; Ma, Y.; Fang, X.; Shen, S. Honokiol induces apoptosis and autophagy via the ROS/ERK1/2 signaling pathway in human osteosarcoma cells in vitro and in vivo. *Cell Death Dis.* **2018**, *9*, 157. [CrossRef]
68. Steinmann, P.; Walters, D.K.; Arlt, M.J.; Banke, I.J.; Ziegler, U.; Langsam, B.; Arbiser, J.; Muff, R.; Born, W.; Fuchs, B. Antimetastatic activity of honokiol in osteosarcoma. *Cancer* **2012**, *118*, 2117–2127. [CrossRef]
69. Yang, J.; Zou, Y.; Jiang, D. Honokiol suppresses proliferation and induces apoptosis via regulation of the miR21/PTEN/PI3K/AKT signaling pathway in human osteosarcoma cells. *Int. J. Mol. Med.* **2018**, *41*, 1845–1854. [CrossRef]
70. Kim, D.W.; Ko, S.M.; Jeon, Y.J.; Noh, Y.W.; Choi, N.J.; Cho, S.D.; Moon, H.S.; Cho, Y.S.; Shin, J.C.; Park, S.M.; et al. Anti-proliferative effect of honokiol in oral squamous cancer through the regulation of specificity protein 1. *Int. J. Oncol.* **2013**, *43*, 1103–1110. [CrossRef]
71. Xu, Q.; Tong, F.; He, C.; Song, P.; Xu, Q.; Chen, Z. The inhibition effect of Honokiol in liver cancer. *Int. J. Clin. Exp. Med.* **2018**, *11*, 10673–10678.
72. Han, L.L.; Xie, L.P.; Li, L.H.; Zhang, X.W.; Zhang, R.Q.; Wang, H.Z. Reactive oxygen species production and Bax/Bcl-2 regulation in honokiol-induced apoptosis in human hepatocellular carcinoma SMMC-7721 cells. *Environ. Toxicol. Pharmacol.* **2009**, *28*, 97–103. [CrossRef] [PubMed]
73. Luo, H.; Zhong, Q.; Chen, L.J.; Qi, X.R.; Fu, A.F.; Yang, H.S.; Yang, F.; Lin, H.G.; Wei, Y.Q.; Zhao, X. Liposomal honokiol, a promising agent for treatment of cisplatin-resistant human ovarian cancer. *J. Cancer Res. Clin. Oncol.* **2008**, *134*, 937–945. [CrossRef] [PubMed]
74. Li, Z.; Liu, Y.; Zhao, X.; Pan, X.; Yin, R.; Huang, C.; Chen, L.; Wei, Y. Honokiol, a natural therapeutic candidate, induces apoptosis and inhibits angiogenesis of ovarian tumor cells. *Eur. J. Obstet. Gynecol. Reprod. Biol.* **2008**, *140*, 95–102. [CrossRef] [PubMed]
75. Hahm, E.R.; Singh, S.V. Honokiol causes G0-G1 phase cell cycle arrest in human prostate cancer cells in association with suppression of retinoblastoma protein level/phosphorylation and inhibition of E2F1 transcriptional activity. *Mol. Cancer Ther.* **2007**, *6*, 2686–2695. [CrossRef] [PubMed]
76. Shigemura, K.; Arbiser, J.L.; Sun, S.Y.; Zayzafoon, M.; Johnstone, P.A.; Fujisawa, M.; Gotoh, A.; Weksler, B.; Zhau, H.E.; Chung, L.W. Honokiol, a natural plant product, inhibits the bone metastatic growth of human prostate cancer cells. *Cancer* **2007**, *109*, 1279–1289. [CrossRef] [PubMed]
77. Hahm, E.R.; Sakao, K.; Singh, S.V. Honokiol activates reactive oxygen species-mediated cytoprotective autophagy in human prostate cancer cells. *Prostate* **2014**, *74*, 1209–1221. [CrossRef]

78. Leeman-Neill, R.J.; Cai, Q.; Joyce, S.C.; Thomas, S.M.; Bhola, N.E.; Neill, D.B.; Arbiser, J.L.; Grandis, J.R. Honokiol inhibits epidermal growth factor receptor signaling and enhances the antitumor effects of epidermal growth factor receptor inhibitors. *Clin. Cancer Res.* **2010**, *16*, 2571–2579. [CrossRef]
79. Lin, J.W.; Chen, J.T.; Hong, C.Y.; Lin, Y.L.; Wang, K.T.; Yao, C.J.; Lai, G.M.; Chen, R.M. Honokiol traverses the blood-brain barrier and induces apoptosis of neuroblastoma cells via an intrinsic bax-mitochondrion-cytochrome c-caspase protease pathway. *Neuro-Oncology* **2012**, *14*, 302–314. [CrossRef]
80. Yeh, P.S.; Wang, W.; Chang, Y.A.; Lin, C.J.; Wang, J.J.; Chen, R.M. Honokiol induces autophagy of neuroblastoma cells through activating the PI3K/Akt/mTOR and endoplasmic reticular stress/ERK1/2 signaling pathways and suppressing cell migration. *Cancer Lett.* **2016**, *370*, 66–77. [CrossRef]
81. Zhang, Q.; Zhao, W.; Ye, C.; Zhuang, J.; Chang, C.; Li, Y.; Huang, X.; Shen, L.; Li, Y.; Cui, Y.; et al. Honokiol inhibits bladder tumor growth by suppressing EZH2/miR-143 axis. *Oncotarget* **2015**, *6*, 37335–37348. [CrossRef]
82. Bao, L.; Jaramillo, M.C.; Zhang, Z.; Zheng, Y.; Yao, M.; Zhang, D.D.; Yi, X. Induction of autophagy contributes to cisplatin resistance in human ovarian cancer cells. *Mol. Med. Rep.* **2015**, *11*, 91–98. [CrossRef] [PubMed]
83. Zhang, Q.; Cheng, J.; Xin, Q. Effects of tetracycline on developmental toxicity and molecular responses in zebrafish (*Danio rerio*) embryos. *Ecotoxicology* **2015**, *24*, 707–719. [CrossRef] [PubMed]
84. Hill, D.; Chen, L.; Snaar-Jagalska, E.; Chaudhry, B. Embryonic zebrafish xenograft assay of human cancer metastasis. *F1000Research* **2018**, *7*, 1682. [CrossRef] [PubMed]
85. Li, L.; Han, W.; Gu, Y.; Qiu, S.; Lu, Q.; Jin, J.; Luo, J.; Hu, X. Honokiol Induces a Necrotic Cell Death through the Mitochondrial Permeability Transition Pore. *Cancer Res.* **2007**, *67*, 4894. [CrossRef] [PubMed]
86. Sheu, M.L.; Liu, S.H.; Lan, K.H. Honokiol induces calpain-mediated glucose-regulated protein-94 cleavage and apoptosis in human gastric cancer cells and reduces tumor growth. *PLoS ONE* **2007**, *2*, e1096. [CrossRef]
87. Liu, S.H.; Wang, K.B.; Lan, K.H.; Lee, W.J.; Pan, H.C.; Wu, S.M.; Peng, Y.C.; Chen, Y.C.; Shen, C.C.; Cheng, H.C.; et al. Calpain/SHP-1 Interaction by Honokiol Dampening Peritoneal Dissemination of Gastric Cancer in nu/nu Mice. *PLoS ONE* **2012**, *7*, e43711. [CrossRef]
88. Liu, Y.; Chen, L.; He, X.; Fan, L.; Yang, G.; Chen, X.; Lin, X.; Du, L.; Li, Z.; Ye, H.; et al. Enhancement of therapeutic effectiveness by combining liposomal honokiol with cisplatin in ovarian carcinoma. *Int. J. Gynecol. Cancer* **2008**, *18*, 652–659. [CrossRef]
89. Goldar, S.; Khaniani, M.S.; Derakhshan, S.M.; Baradaran, B. Molecular mechanisms of apoptosis and roles in cancer development and treatment. *Asian Pac. J. Cancer Prev.* **2015**, *16*, 2129–2144. [CrossRef]
90. Hassan, M.; Watari, H.; AbuAlmaaty, A.; Ohba, Y.; Sakuragi, N. Apoptosis and molecular targeting therapy in cancer. *Biomed Res. Int.* **2014**, *2014*, 150845. [CrossRef]
91. Wong, R.S.Y. Apoptosis in cancer: From pathogenesis to treatment. *J. Exp. Clin. Cancer Res.* **2011**, *30*, 87. [CrossRef]
92. Gerl, R.; Vaux, D.L. Apoptosis in the development and treatment of cancer. *Carcinogenesis* **2005**, *26*, 263–270. [CrossRef] [PubMed]
93. Letai, A. Apoptosis and Cancer. *Annu. Rev. Cancer Biol.* **2017**, *1*, 275–294. [CrossRef]
94. Jeong, Y.-H.; Hur, J.H.; Jeon, E.-J.; Park, S.-J.; Hwang, T.J.; Lee, S.A.; Lee, W.K.; Sung, J.M. Honokiol Improves Liver Steatosis in Ovariectomized Mice. *Molecules* **2018**, *23*, 194. [CrossRef] [PubMed]
95. Huang, J.-S.; Yao, C.-J.; Chuang, S.-E.; Yeh, C.-T.; Lee, L.-M.; Chen, R.-M.; Chao, W.-J.; Whang-Peng, J.; Lai, G.-M. Honokiol inhibits sphere formation and xenograft growth of oral cancer side population cells accompanied with JAK/STAT signaling pathway suppression and apoptosis induction. *BMC Cancer* **2016**, *16*, 245. [CrossRef] [PubMed]
96. Prasad, R.; Katiyar, S.K. Honokiol, an Active Compound of Magnolia Plant, Inhibits Growth, and Progression of Cancers of Different Organs. *Adv. Exp. Med. Biol.* **2016**, *928*, 245–265. [CrossRef] [PubMed]
97. Banik, K.; Ranaware, A.M.; Deshpande, V.; Nalawade, S.P.; Padmavathi, G.; Bordoloi, D.; Sailo, B.L.; Shanmugam, M.K.; Fan, L.; Arfuso, F.; et al. Honokiol for cancer therapeutics: A traditional medicine that can modulate multiple oncogenic targets. *Pharmacol. Res.* **2019**, *144*, 192–209. [CrossRef] [PubMed]
98. Wang, X.; Beitler, J.J.; Huang, W.; Chen, G.; Qian, G.; Magliocca, K.; Patel, M.R.; Chen, A.Y.; Zhang, J.; Nannapaneni, S.; et al. Honokiol Radiosensitizes Squamous Cell Carcinoma of the Head and Neck by Downregulation of Survivin. *Clin. Cancer Res.* **2018**, *24*, 858–869. [CrossRef]

99. Garcia, A.; Zheng, Y.; Zhao, C.; Toschi, A.; Fan, J.; Shraibman, N.; Brown, H.A.; Bar-Sagi, D.; Foster, D.A.; Arbiser, J.L. Honokiol Suppresses Survival Signals Mediated by Ras-Dependent Phospholipase D Activity in Human Cancer Cells. *Clin. Cancer Res.* **2008**, *14*, 4267. [CrossRef]
100. Fried, L.E.; Arbiser, J.L. Honokiol, a multifunctional antiangiogenic and antitumor agent. *Antioxid. Redox Signal.* **2009**, *11*, 1139–1148. [CrossRef]
101. Li, H.Y.; Ye, H.G.; Chen, C.Q.; Yin, L.H.; Wu, J.B.; He, L.C.; Gao, S.M. Honokiol induces cell cycle arrest and apoptosis via inhibiting class I histone deacetylases in acute myeloid leukemia. *J. Cell. Biochem.* **2015**, *116*, 287–298. [CrossRef]
102. Deng, J.; Qian, Y.; Geng, L.; Chen, J.; Wang, X.; Xie, H.; Yan, S.; Jiang, G.; Zhou, L.; Zheng, S. Involvement of p38 mitogen-activated protein kinase pathway in honokiol-induced apoptosis in a human hepatoma cell line (hepG2). *Liver Int.* **2008**, *28*, 1458–1464. [CrossRef] [PubMed]
103. Hasegawa, S.; Yonezawa, T.; Ahn, J.Y.; Cha, B.Y.; Teruya, T.; Takami, M.; Yagasaki, K.; Nagai, K.; Woo, J.T. Honokiol inhibits osteoclast differentiation and function in vitro. *Biol. Pharm. Bull.* **2010**, *33*, 487–492. [CrossRef] [PubMed]
104. Tse, A.K.; Wan, C.K.; Shen, X.L.; Yang, M.; Fong, W.F. Honokiol inhibits TNF-alpha-stimulated NF-kappaB activation and NF-kappaB-regulated gene expression through suppression of IKK activation. *Biochem. Pharmacol.* **2005**, *70*, 1443–1457. [CrossRef] [PubMed]
105. Li, J.; Shao, X.; Wu, L.; Feng, T.; Jin, C.; Fang, M.; Wu, N.; Yao, H. Honokiol: An effective inhibitor of tumor necrosis factor-alpha-induced up-regulation of inflammatory cytokine and chemokine production in human synovial fibroblasts. *Acta Biochim. Biophys. Sin.* **2011**, *43*, 380–386. [CrossRef]
106. Xu, H.L.; Tang, W.; Du, G.H.; Kokudo, N. Targeting apoptosis pathways in cancer with magnolol and honokiol, bioactive constituents of the bark of *Magnolia officinalis*. *Drug Discov. Ther.* **2011**, *5*, 202–210. [CrossRef]
107. Raja, S.M.; Chen, S.; Yue, P.; Acker, T.M.; Lefkove, B.; Arbiser, J.L.; Khuri, F.R.; Sun, S.Y. The natural product honokiol preferentially inhibits cellular FLICE-inhibitory protein and augments death receptor-induced apoptosis. *Mol. Cancer Ther.* **2008**, *7*, 2212–2223. [CrossRef]
108. Rauf, A.; Patel, S.; Imran, M.; Maalik, A.; Arshad, M.U.; Saeed, F.; Mabkhot, Y.N.; Al-Showiman, S.S.; Ahmad, N.; Elsharkawy, E. Honokiol: An anticancer lignan. *Biomed. Pharmacother.* **2018**, *107*, 555–562. [CrossRef]
109. Schroder, M.; Kaufman, R.J. ER stress and the unfolded protein response. *Mutat. Res.* **2005**, *569*, 29–63. [CrossRef]
110. Cao, S.S.; Kaufman, R.J. Endoplasmic reticulum stress and oxidative stress in cell fate decision and human disease. *Antioxid. Redox Signal.* **2014**, *21*, 396–413. [CrossRef]
111. Ferri, K.F.; Kroemer, G. Organelle-specific initiation of cell death pathways. *Nat. Cell Biol.* **2001**, *3*, E255–E263. [CrossRef]
112. Chiu, C.-S.; Tsai, C.-H.; Hsieh, M.-S.; Tsai, S.-C.; Jan, Y.-J.; Lin, W.-Y.; Lai, D.-W.; Wu, S.-M.; Hsing, H.-Y.; Arbiser, J.L.; et al. Exploiting Honokiol-induced ER stress CHOP activation inhibits the growth and metastasis of melanoma by suppressing the MITF and β-catenin pathways. *Cancer Lett.* **2019**, *442*, 113–125. [CrossRef] [PubMed]
113. Liu, S.H.; Shen, C.C.; Yi, Y.C.; Tsai, J.J.; Wang, C.C.; Chueh, J.T.; Lin, K.L.; Lee, T.C.; Pan, H.C.; Sheu, M.L. Honokiol inhibits gastric tumourigenesis by activation of 15-lipoxygenase-1 and consequent inhibition of peroxisome proliferator-activated receptor-γ and COX-2-dependent signals. *Br. J. Pharmacol.* **2010**, *160*, 1963–1972. [CrossRef] [PubMed]
114. Liu, S.H.; Lee, W.J.; Lai, D.W.; Wu, S.M.; Liu, C.Y.; Tien, H.R.; Chiu, C.S.; Peng, Y.C.; Jan, Y.J.; Chao, T.H.; et al. Honokiol confers immunogenicity by dictating calreticulin exposure, activating ER stress and inhibiting epithelial-to-mesenchymal transition. *Mol. Oncol.* **2015**, *9*, 834–849. [CrossRef] [PubMed]
115. Martin, S.; Lamb, H.K.; Brady, C.; Lefkove, B.; Bonner, M.Y.; Thompson, P.; Lovat, P.E.; Arbiser, J.L.; Hawkins, A.R.; Redfern, C.P. Inducing apoptosis of cancer cells using small-molecule plant compounds that bind to GRP78. *Br. J. Cancer* **2013**, *109*, 433–443. [CrossRef] [PubMed]
116. Lee, S.Y.; Ju, M.K.; Jeon, H.M.; Jeong, E.K.; Lee, Y.J.; Kim, C.H.; Park, H.G.; Han, S.I.; Kang, H.S. Regulation of Tumor Progression by Programmed Necrosis. *Oxidative Med. Cell. Longev.* **2018**, *2018*, 3537471. [CrossRef]
117. Tian, W.; Xu, D.; Deng, Y.-C. Honokiol, a multifunctional tumor cell death inducer. *Die Pharm. Int. J. Pharm. Sci.* **2012**, *67*, 811–816. [CrossRef]

118. Chen, G.; Izzo, J.; Demizu, Y.; Wang, F.; Guha, S.; Wu, X.; Hung, M.-C.; Ajani, J.A.; Huang, P. Different redox states in malignant and nonmalignant esophageal epithelial cells and differential cytotoxic responses to bile acid and honokiol. *Antioxid. Redox Signal.* **2009**, *11*, 1083–1095. [CrossRef]
119. Yu, C.; Zhang, Q.; Zhang, H.Y.; Zhang, X.; Huo, X.; Cheng, E.; Wang, D.H.; Arbiser, J.L.; Spechler, S.J.; Souza, R.F. Targeting the intrinsic inflammatory pathway: Honokiol exerts proapoptotic effects through STAT3 inhibition in transformed Barrett's cells. *Am. J. Physiol. Gastrointest. Liver Physiol.* **2012**, *303*, G561–G569. [CrossRef]
120. Meier, J.A.; Hyun, M. Stress-induced dynamic regulation of mitochondrial STAT3 and its association with cyclophilin D reduce mitochondrial ROS production. *Sci. Signal.* **2017**, *10*. [CrossRef]
121. Cen, M.; Yao, Y.; Cui, L.; Yang, G.; Lu, G.; Fang, L.; Bao, Z.; Zhou, J. Honokiol induces apoptosis of lung squamous cell carcinoma by targeting FGF2-FGFR1 autocrine loop. *Cancer Med.* **2018**, *7*, 6205–6218. [CrossRef]
122. Hahm, E.R.; Singh, K.B.; Singh, S.V. c-Myc is a novel target of cell cycle arrest by honokiol in prostate cancer cells. *Cell Cycle* **2016**, *15*, 2309–2320. [CrossRef] [PubMed]
123. Vaid, M.; Sharma, S.D.; Katiyar, S.K. Honokiol, a phytochemical from the Magnolia plant, inhibits photocarcinogenesis by targeting UVB-induced inflammatory mediators and cell cycle regulators: Development of topical formulation. *Carcinogenesis* **2010**, *31*, 2004–2011. [CrossRef] [PubMed]
124. Guo, C.; Ma, L.; Zhao, Y.; Peng, A.; Cheng, B.; Zhou, Q.; Zheng, L.; Huang, K. Inhibitory effects of magnolol and honokiol on human calcitonin aggregation. *Sci. Rep.* **2015**, *5*, 13556. [CrossRef] [PubMed]
125. Yan, B.; Peng, Z.Y. Honokiol induces cell cycle arrest and apoptosis in human gastric carcinoma MGC-803 cell line. *Int. J. Clin. Exp. Med.* **2015**, *8*, 5454–5461. [PubMed]
126. Grimmel, M.; Backhaus, C.; Proikas-Cezanne, T. WIPI-Mediated Autophagy and Longevity. *Cells* **2015**, *4*, 202–217. [CrossRef] [PubMed]
127. Yun, C.W.; Lee, S.H. The Roles of Autophagy in Cancer. *Int. J. Mol. Sci.* **2018**, *19*, 3466. [CrossRef]
128. Galluzzi, L.; Pietrocola, F.; Bravo-San Pedro, J.M.; Amaravadi, R.K.; Baehrecke, E.H.; Cecconi, F.; Codogno, P.; Debnath, J.; Gewirtz, D.A.; Karantza, V.; et al. Autophagy in malignant transformation and cancer progression. *EMBO J.* **2015**, *34*, 856–880. [CrossRef]
129. Lin, L.; Baehrecke, E.H. Autophagy, cell death, and cancer. *Mol. Cell Oncol.* **2015**, *2*, e985913. [CrossRef]
130. Paquette, M.; El-Houjeiri, L.; Pause, A. mTOR Pathways in Cancer and Autophagy. *Cancers* **2018**, *10*, 18. [CrossRef]
131. Murray, J.T.; Tee, A.R. Mechanistic Target of Rapamycin (mTOR) in the Cancer Setting. *Cancers* **2018**, *10*, 168. [CrossRef]
132. Itakura, E.; Mizushima, N. Atg14 and UVRAG: Mutually exclusive subunits of mammalian Beclin 1-PI3K complexes. *Autophagy* **2009**, *5*, 534–536. [CrossRef] [PubMed]
133. Torii, S.; Yoshida, T.; Arakawa, S.; Honda, S.; Nakanishi, A.; Shimizu, S. Identification of PPM1D as an essential Ulk1 phosphatase for genotoxic stress-induced autophagy. *EMBO Rep.* **2016**, *17*, 1552–1564. [CrossRef] [PubMed]
134. Maiuri, M.C.; Criollo, A.; Kroemer, G. Crosstalk between apoptosis and autophagy within the Beclin 1 interactome. *EMBO J.* **2010**, *29*, 515–516. [CrossRef] [PubMed]
135. Carlsson, S.R.; Simonsen, A. Membrane dynamics in autophagosome biogenesis. *J. Cell Sci.* **2015**, *128*, 193. [CrossRef] [PubMed]
136. Mochida, K.; Oikawa, Y.; Kimura, Y.; Kirisako, H.; Hirano, H.; Ohsumi, Y.; Nakatogawa, H. Receptor-mediated selective autophagy degrades the endoplasmic reticulum and the nucleus. *Nature* **2015**, *522*, 359–362. [CrossRef]
137. Wrighton, K.H. Selecting ER for eating. *Nat. Rev. Mol. Cell Biol.* **2015**, *16*, 389. [CrossRef]
138. Chio, C.C.; Chen, K.Y.; Chang, C.K.; Chuang, J.Y.; Liu, C.C.; Liu, S.H.; Chen, R.M. Improved effects of honokiol on temozolomide-induced autophagy and apoptosis of drug-sensitive and -tolerant glioma cells. *BMC Cancer* **2018**, *18*, 379. [CrossRef]
139. Nieto, M.A.; Huang, R.Y.; Jackson, R.A.; Thiery, J.P. EMT: 2016. *Cell* **2016**, *166*, 21–45. [CrossRef]
140. Brabletz, T.; Kalluri, R.; Nieto, M.A.; Weinberg, R.A. EMT in cancer. *Nat. Rev. Cancer* **2018**, *18*, 128–134. [CrossRef]
141. Roche, J. The Epithelial-to-Mesenchymal Transition in Cancer. *Cancers* **2018**, *10*, 52. [CrossRef]

142. Røsland, G.V.; Dyrstad, S.E.; Tusubira, D.; Helwa, R.; Tan, T.Z.; Lotsberg, M.L.; Pettersen, I.K.N.; Berg, A.; Kindt, C.; Hoel, F.; et al. Epithelial to mesenchymal transition (EMT) is associated with attenuation of succinate dehydrogenase (SDH) in breast cancer through reduced expression of SDHC. *Cancer Metab.* **2019**, *7*, 6. [CrossRef] [PubMed]
143. Shen, L.; Zhang, F.; Huang, R.; Yan, J.; Shen, B. Honokiol inhibits bladder cancer cell invasion through repressing SRC-3 expression and epithelial-mesenchymal transition. *Oncol. Lett.* **2017**, *14*, 4294–4300. [CrossRef] [PubMed]
144. Avtanski, D.B.; Nagalingam, A.; Bonner, M.Y.; Arbiser, J.L.; Saxena, N.K.; Sharma, D. Honokiol inhibits epithelial-mesenchymal transition in breast cancer cells by targeting signal transducer and activator of transcription 3/Zeb1/E-cadherin axis. *Mol. Oncol.* **2014**, *8*, 565–580. [CrossRef] [PubMed]
145. Lv, X.-Q.; Qiao, X.-R.; Su, L.; Chen, S.-Z. Honokiol inhibits EMT-mediated motility and migration of human non-small cell lung cancer cells in vitro by targeting c-FLIP. *Acta Pharmacol. Sin.* **2016**, *37*, 1574–1586. [CrossRef]
146. Qin, L.; Liu, Z.; Chen, H.; Xu, J. The steroid receptor coactivator-1 regulates twist expression and promotes breast cancer metastasis. *Cancer Res.* **2009**, *69*, 3819–3827. [CrossRef]
147. Yao, C.-J.; Lai, G.-M.; Yeh, C.-T.; Lai, M.-T.; Shih, P.-H.; Chao, W.-J.; Whang-Peng, J.; Chuang, S.-E.; Lai, T.-Y. Honokiol Eliminates Human Oral Cancer Stem-Like Cells Accompanied with Suppression of Wnt/β-Catenin Signaling and Apoptosis Induction. *Evid.-Based Complement. Altern. Med.* **2013**, *2013*, 146136. [CrossRef]
148. Wang, W.D.; Shang, Y.; Li, Y.; Chen, S.Z. Honokiol inhibits breast cancer cell metastasis by blocking EMT through modulation of Snail/Slug protein translation. *Acta Pharm. Sin.* **2019**, *40*, 1219–1227. [CrossRef]
149. Galichon, P.; Hertig, A. Epithelial to mesenchymal transition as a biomarker in renal fibrosis: Are we ready for the bedside? *Fibrogenesis Tissue Repair* **2011**, *4*, 11. [CrossRef]
150. Conacci-Sorrell, M.; Ngouenet, C.; Anderson, S.; Brabletz, T.; Eisenman, R.N. Stress-induced cleavage of Myc promotes cancer cell survival. *Genes Dev.* **2014**, *28*, 689–707. [CrossRef]
151. Yamaguchi, H.; Wyckoff, J.; Condeelis, J. Cell migration in tumors. *Curr. Opin. Cell Biol.* **2005**, *17*, 559–564. [CrossRef]
152. Seyfried, T.N.; Huysentruyt, L.C. On the origin of cancer metastasis. *Crit. Rev. Oncog.* **2013**, *18*, 43–73. [CrossRef] [PubMed]
153. Tay, R.Y.; Fernández-Gutiérrez, F.; Foy, V.; Burns, K.; Pierce, J.; Morris, K.; Priest, L.; Tugwood, J.; Ashcroft, L.; Lindsay, C.R.; et al. Prognostic value of circulating tumour cells in limited-stage small-cell lung cancer: Analysis of the concurrent once-daily versus twice-daily radiotherapy (CONVERT) randomised controlled trial. *Ann. Oncol.* **2019**, *30*, 1114–1120. [CrossRef] [PubMed]
154. Singh, T.; Katiyar, S.K. Honokiol, a phytochemical from *Magnolia* spp., inhibits breast cancer cell migration by targeting nitric oxide and cyclooxygenase-2. *Int. J. Oncol.* **2011**, *38*, 769–776. [CrossRef]
155. Zhang, J.; Zhang, Y.; Shen, W.; Fu, R.; Ding, Z.; Zhen, Y.; Wan, Y. Cytological effects of honokiol treatment and its potential mechanism of action in non-small cell lung cancer. *Biomed. Pharmacother.* **2019**, *117*, 109058. [CrossRef] [PubMed]
156. Cheng, S.; Castillo, V.; Welty, M.; Eliaz, I.; Sliva, D. Honokiol inhibits migration of renal cell carcinoma through activation of RhoA/ROCK/MLC signaling pathway. *Int. J. Oncol.* **2016**, *49*, 1525–1530. [CrossRef]
157. Balan, M.; Chakraborty, S.; Flynn, E.; Zurakowski, D.; Pal, S. Honokiol inhibits c-Met-HO-1 tumor-promoting pathway and its cross-talk with calcineurin inhibitor-mediated renal cancer growth. *Sci. Rep.* **2017**, *7*, 5900. [CrossRef]
158. Alizadeh, A.M.; Shiri, S.; Farsinejad, S. Metastasis review: From bench to bedside. *Tumor Biol.* **2014**, *35*, 8483–8523. [CrossRef]
159. Klein, C.A. Cancer. The metastasis cascade. *Science* **2008**, *321*, 1785–1787. [CrossRef]
160. Bai, X.; Cerimele, F.; Ushio-Fukai, M.; Waqas, M.; Campbell, P.M.; Govindarajan, B.; Der, C.J.; Battle, T.; Frank, D.A.; Ye, K.; et al. Honokiol, a small molecular weight natural product, inhibits angiogenesis in vitro and tumor growth in vivo. *J. Biol. Chem.* **2003**, *278*, 35501–35507. [CrossRef]
161. Kolligs, F.T.; Bommer, G.; Goke, B. Wnt/beta-catenin/tcf signaling: A critical pathway in gastrointestinal tumorigenesis. *Digestion* **2002**, *66*, 131–144. [CrossRef]
162. Hlubek, F.; Spaderna, S.; Jung, A.; Kirchner, T.; Brabletz, T. Beta-catenin activates a coordinated expression of the proinvasive factors laminin-5 gamma2 chain and MT1-MMP in colorectal carcinomas. *Int. J. Cancer* **2004**, *108*, 321–326. [CrossRef] [PubMed]

163. Cheng, S.; Castillo, V.; Eliaz, I.; Sliva, D. Honokiol suppresses metastasis of renal cell carcinoma by targeting KISS1/KISS1R signaling. *Int. J. Oncol.* **2015**, *46*, 2293–2298. [CrossRef] [PubMed]
164. Nishida, N.; Yano, H.; Nishida, T.; Kamura, T.; Kojiro, M. Angiogenesis in cancer. *Vasc. Health Risk Manag.* **2006**, *2*, 213–219. [CrossRef] [PubMed]
165. Rajabi, M.; Mousa, S.A. The Role of Angiogenesis in Cancer Treatment. *Biomedicines* **2017**, *5*, 34. [CrossRef] [PubMed]
166. Tonini, T.; Rossi, F.; Claudio, P.P. Molecular basis of angiogenesis and cancer. *Oncogene* **2003**, *22*, 6549–6556. [CrossRef] [PubMed]
167. Banerjee, P.; Basu, A.; Arbiser, J.L.; Pal, S. The natural product honokiol inhibits calcineurin inhibitor-induced and Ras-mediated tumor promoting pathways. *Cancer Lett.* **2013**, *338*, 292–299. [CrossRef]
168. Vavilala, D.T.; Ponnaluri, V.K.C.; Kanjilal, D.; Mukherji, M. Evaluation of anti-HIF and anti-angiogenic properties of honokiol for the treatment of ocular neovascular diseases. *PLoS ONE* **2014**, *9*, e113717. [CrossRef]
169. Vavilala, D.T.; O'Bryhim, B.E.; Ponnaluri, V.K.; White, R.S.; Radel, J.; Symons, R.C.; Mukherji, M. Honokiol inhibits pathological retinal neovascularization in oxygen-induced retinopathy mouse model. *Biochem. Biophys. Res. Commun.* **2013**, *438*, 697–702. [CrossRef]
170. Wen, J.; Wang, X.; Pei, H.; Xie, C.; Qiu, N.; Li, S.; Wang, W.; Cheng, X.; Chen, L. Anti-psoriatic effects of Honokiol through the inhibition of NF-kappaB and VEGFR-2 in animal model of K14-VEGF transgenic mouse. *J. Pharmacol. Sci.* **2015**, *128*, 116–124. [CrossRef]
171. Hu, J.; Chen, L.J.; Liu, L.; Chen, X.; Chen, P.L.; Yang, G.; Hou, W.L.; Tang, M.H.; Zhang, F.; Wang, X.H.; et al. Liposomal honokiol, a potent anti-angiogenesis agent, in combination with radiotherapy produces a synergistic antitumor efficacy without increasing toxicity. *Exp. Mol. Med.* **2008**, *40*, 617–628. [CrossRef]
172. Xia, Y.; Shen, S.; Verma, I.M. NF-κB, an active player in human cancers. *Cancer Immunol. Res.* **2014**, *2*, 823–830. [CrossRef] [PubMed]
173. Xia, L.; Tan, S.; Zhou, Y.; Lin, J.; Wang, H.; Oyang, L.; Tian, Y.; Liu, L.; Su, M.; Wang, H.; et al. Role of the NFκB-signaling pathway in cancer. *Onco Targets Ther.* **2018**, *11*, 2063–2073. [CrossRef] [PubMed]
174. Ahn, K.S.; Sethi, G.; Shishodia, S.; Sung, B.; Arbiser, J.L.; Aggarwal, B.B. Honokiol Potentiates Apoptosis, Suppresses Osteoclastogenesis, and Inhibits Invasion through Modulation of Nuclear Factor-κB Activation Pathway. *Mol. Cancer Res.* **2006**, *4*, 621. [CrossRef] [PubMed]
175. Wang, Z.; Zhang, X. Chemopreventive Activity of Honokiol against 7, 12—Dimethylbenz[a]anthracene-Induced Mammary Cancer in Female Sprague Dawley Rats. *Front. Pharmacol.* **2017**, *8*, 320. [CrossRef]
176. Katiyar, S.K. Emerging Phytochemicals for the Prevention and Treatment of Head and Neck Cancer. *Molecules* **2016**, *21*, 1610. [CrossRef]
177. Hua, H.; Chen, W.; Shen, L.; Sheng, Q.; Teng, L. Honokiol augments the anti-cancer effects of oxaliplatin in colon cancer cells. *Acta Biochim. Biophys. Sin.* **2013**, *45*, 773–779. [CrossRef]
178. Nabekura, T.; Hiroi, T.; Kawasaki, T.; Uwai, Y. Effects of natural nuclear factor-kappa B inhibitors on anticancer drug efflux transporter human P-glycoprotein. *Biomed. Pharmacother.* **2015**, *70*, 140–145. [CrossRef]
179. Furqan, M.; Akinleye, A.; Mukhi, N.; Mittal, V.; Chen, Y.; Liu, D. STAT inhibitors for cancer therapy. *J. Hematol. Oncol.* **2013**, *6*, 90. [CrossRef]
180. Yu, H.; Pardoll, D.; Jove, R. STATs in cancer inflammation and immunity: A leading role for STAT3. *Nat. Rev. Cancer* **2009**, *9*, 798–809. [CrossRef]
181. Pan, J.; Lee, Y.; Cheng, G.; Zielonka, J.; Zhang, Q.; Bajzikova, M.; Xiong, D.; Tsaih, S.-W.; Hardy, M.; Flister, M.; et al. Mitochondria-Targeted Honokiol Confers a Striking Inhibitory Effect on Lung Cancer via Inhibiting Complex I Activity. *iScience* **2018**, *3*, 192–207. [CrossRef]
182. He, Z.; Subramaniam, D.; Zhang, Z.; Zhang, Y.; Anant, S. Honokiol as a Radiosensitizing Agent for Colorectal cancers. *Curr. Colorectal Cancer Rep.* **2013**, *9*, 358–364. [CrossRef] [PubMed]
183. Bi, L.; Yu, Z.; Wu, J.; Yu, K.; Hong, G.; Lu, Z.; Gao, S. Honokiol Inhibits Constitutive and Inducible STAT3 Signaling via PU.1-Induced SHP1 Expression in Acute Myeloid Leukemia Cells. *Tohoku J. Exp. Med.* **2015**, *237*, 163–172. [CrossRef] [PubMed]
184. Ishikawa, C.; Arbiser, J.L.; Mori, N. Honokiol induces cell cycle arrest and apoptosis via inhibition of survival signals in adult T-cell leukemia. *Biochim. Biophys. Acta* **2012**, *1820*, 879–887. [CrossRef] [PubMed]
185. Sasaki, T.; Hiroki, K.; Yamashita, Y. The role of epidermal growth factor receptor in cancer metastasis and microenvironment. *BioMed Res. Int.* **2013**, *2013*, 546318. [CrossRef] [PubMed]

186. Normanno, N.; De Luca, A.; Bianco, C.; Strizzi, L.; Mancino, M.; Maiello, M.R.; Carotenuto, A.; De Feo, G.; Caponigro, F.; Salomon, D.S. Epidermal growth factor receptor (EGFR) signaling in cancer. *Gene* **2006**, *366*, 2–16. [CrossRef] [PubMed]
187. Kari, C.; Chan, T.O.; Rocha de Quadros, M.; Rodeck, U. Targeting the Epidermal Growth Factor Receptor in Cancer. *Cancer Res.* **2003**, *63*, 1. [PubMed]
188. Yewale, C.; Baradia, D.; Vhora, I.; Patil, S.; Misra, A. Epidermal growth factor receptor targeting in cancer: A review of trends and strategies. *Biomaterials* **2013**, *34*, 8690–8707. [CrossRef]
189. Song, J.M.; Anandharaj, A.; Upadhyaya, P.; Kirtane, A.R.; Kim, J.-H.; Hong, K.H.; Panyam, J.; Kassie, F. Honokiol suppresses lung tumorigenesis by targeting EGFR and its downstream effectors. *Oncotarget* **2016**, *7*, 57752–57769. [CrossRef]
190. Dai, X.; Li, R.-Z.; Jiang, Z.-B.; Wei, C.-L.; Luo, L.-X.; Yao, X.-J.; Li, G.-P.; Leung, E.L.-H. Honokiol Inhibits Proliferation, Invasion and Induces Apoptosis Through Targeting Lyn Kinase in Human Lung Adenocarcinoma Cells. *Front. Pharmacol.* **2018**, 9. [CrossRef]
191. Biscardi, J.S.; Ishizawar, R.C.; Silva, C.M.; Parsons, S.J. Tyrosine kinase signalling in breast cancer: Epidermal growth factor receptor and c-Src interactions in breast cancer. *Breast Cancer Res.* **2000**, *2*, 203–210. [CrossRef]
192. Singh, T.; Gupta, N.A.; Xu, S.; Prasad, R.; Velu, S.E.; Katiyar, S.K. Honokiol inhibits the growth of head and neck squamous cell carcinoma by targeting epidermal growth factor receptor. *Oncotarget* **2015**, *6*, 21268–21282. [CrossRef] [PubMed]
193. Dufour, M.; Dormond-Meuwly, A.; Demartines, N.; Dormond, O. Targeting the Mammalian Target of Rapamycin (mTOR) in Cancer Therapy: Lessons from Past and Future Perspectives. *Cancers* **2011**, *3*, 2478–2500. [CrossRef] [PubMed]
194. Hua, H.; Kong, Q.; Zhang, H.; Wang, J.; Luo, T.; Jiang, Y. Targeting mTOR for cancer therapy. *J. Hematol. Oncol.* **2019**, *12*, 71. [CrossRef] [PubMed]
195. Li, Z.; Dong, H.; Li, M.; Wu, Y.; Liu, Y.; Zhao, Y.; Chen, X.; Ma, M. Honokiol induces autophagy and apoptosis of osteosarcoma through PI3K/Akt/mTOR signaling pathway. *Mol. Med. Rep.* **2018**, *17*, 2719–2723. [CrossRef]
196. Pezzuto, A.; Carico, E. Role of HIF-1 in Cancer Progression: Novel Insights. A Review. *Curr. Mol. Med.* **2018**, *18*, 343–351. [CrossRef]
197. Masoud, G.N.; Li, W. HIF-1α pathway: Role, regulation and intervention for cancer therapy. *Acta Pharm. Sin. B* **2015**, *5*, 378–389. [CrossRef]
198. Semenza, G.L. Targeting HIF-1 for cancer therapy. *Nat. Rev. Cancer* **2003**, *3*, 721–732. [CrossRef]
199. Soni, S.; Padwad, Y.S. HIF-1 in cancer therapy: Two decade long story of a transcription factor. *Acta Oncol.* **2017**, *56*, 503–515. [CrossRef]
200. Aster, J.C.; Pear, W.S.; Blacklow, S.C. The Varied Roles of Notch in Cancer. *Annu. Rev. Pathol.* **2017**, *12*, 245–275. [CrossRef]
201. Venkatesh, V.; Nataraj, R.; Thangaraj, G.S.; Karthikeyan, M.; Gnanasekaran, A.; Kaginelli, S.B.; Kuppanna, G.; Kallappa, C.G.; Basalingappa, K.M. Targeting Notch signalling pathway of cancer stem cells. *Stem Cell Investig.* **2018**, *5*, 5. [CrossRef]
202. Nowell, C.S.; Radtke, F. Notch as a tumour suppressor. *Nat. Rev. Cancer* **2017**, *17*, 145–159. [CrossRef] [PubMed]
203. Kaushik, G.; Venugopal, A.; Ramamoorthy, P.; Standing, D.; Subramaniam, D.; Umar, S.; Jensen, R.A.; Anant, S.; Mammen, J.M. Honokiol inhibits melanoma stem cells by targeting notch signaling. *Mol. Carcinog.* **2015**, *54*, 1710–1721. [CrossRef] [PubMed]
204. Wynn, M.L.; Consul, N.; Merajver, S.D.; Schnell, S. Inferring the Effects of Honokiol on the Notch Signaling Pathway in SW480 Colon Cancer Cells. *Cancer Inform.* **2014**, *13*, 1–12. [CrossRef] [PubMed]
205. Callaghan, R.; Luk, F.; Bebawy, M. Inhibition of the multidrug resistance P-glycoprotein: Time for a change of strategy? *Drug Metab. Dispos.* **2014**, *42*, 623–631. [CrossRef]
206. Waghray, D.; Zhang, Q. Inhibit or Evade Multidrug Resistance P-Glycoprotein in Cancer Treatment. *J. Med. Chem.* **2018**, *61*, 5108–5121. [CrossRef]
207. Nanayakkara, A.K.; Follit, C.A.; Chen, G.; Williams, N.S.; Vogel, P.D.; Wise, J.G. Targeted inhibitors of P-glycoprotein increase chemotherapeutic-induced mortality of multidrug resistant tumor cells. *Sci. Rep.* **2018**, *8*, 967. [CrossRef]
208. Han, H.K.; Van Anh, L.T. Modulation of P-glycoprotein expression by honokiol, magnolol and 4-O-methylhonokiol, the bioactive components of Magnolia officinalis. *Anticancer Res.* **2012**, *32*, 4445–4452.

209. Wang, X.; Cho, K.; Chen, Z.; Arbiser, J.; Shin, D. Honokiol reduces drug resistance by inhibition of P-glycoprotein expression in multidrug resistant (MDR) squamous cell carcinoma of the head and neck (SCCHN). *Cancer Res.* **2007**, *67*, 2776.
210. Xu, D.; Lu, Q.; Hu, X. Down-regulation of P-glycoprotein expression in MDR breast cancer cell MCF-7/ADR by honokiol. *Cancer Lett.* **2006**, *243*, 274–280. [CrossRef]
211. Wang, H.; Liao, Z.; Sun, X.; Shi, Q.; Huo, G.; Xie, Y.; Tang, X.; Zhi, X.; Tang, Z. Intravenous administration of Honokiol provides neuroprotection and improves functional recovery after traumatic brain injury through cell cycle inhibition. *Neuropharmacology* **2014**, *86*, 9–21. [CrossRef]
212. Godugu, C.; Doddapaneni, R.; Singh, M. Honokiol nanomicellar formulation produced increased oral bioavailability and anticancer effects in triple negative breast cancer (TNBC). *Colloids Surf. B* **2017**, *153*, 208–219. [CrossRef] [PubMed]
213. Tsai, T.H.; Chou, C.J.; Cheng, F.C.; Chen, C.F. Pharmacokinetics of honokiol after intravenous administration in rats assessed using high-performance liquid chromatography. *J. Chromatogr. B* **1994**, *655*, 41–45. [CrossRef]
214. Liang, Y.; Cui, G.; Wang, X.; Zhang, W.; An, Q.; Lin, Z.; Wang, H.; Chen, S. Pharmacokinetics of honokiol after intravenous guttae in beagle dogs assessed using ultra-performance liquid chromatography-tandem mass spectrometry. *Biomed. Chromatogr.* **2014**, *28*, 1378–1383. [CrossRef] [PubMed]
215. Su, W.J.; Huang, X.; Qin, E.; Jiang, L.; Ren, P. Pharmacokinetics of honokiol in rat after oral administration of Cortex of Magnolia officinalis and its compound preparation Houpu Sanwu Decoction. *J. Chin. Med. Mater.* **2008**, *31*, 255–258.
216. Wang, J.; Miao, X.L.; Chen, J.Y.; Chen, Y. The Pharmacokinetics and Tissue Distribution of Honokiol and its Metabolites in Rats. *Eur. J. Drug Metab. Pharmacokinet.* **2016**, *41*, 587–594. [CrossRef]
217. Sheng, Y.L.; Xu, J.H.; Shi, C.H.; Li, W.; Xu, H.Y.; Li, N.; Zhao, Y.Q.; Zhang, X.R. UPLC-MS/MS-ESI assay for simultaneous determination of magnolol and honokiol in rat plasma: Application to pharmacokinetic study after administration emulsion of the isomer. *J. Ethnopharmacol.* **2014**, *155*, 1568–1574. [CrossRef]
218. Han, M.; Yu, X.; Guo, Y.; Wang, Y.; Kuang, H.; Wang, X. Honokiol nanosuspensions: Preparation, increased oral bioavailability and dramatically enhanced biodistribution in the cardio-cerebro-vascular system. *Colloids Surf. B* **2014**, *116*, 114–120. [CrossRef]
219. Wu, X.; Chen, X.; Hu, Z. High-performance liquid chromatographic method for simultaneous determination of honokiol and magnolol in rat plasma. *Talanta* **2003**, *59*, 115–121. [CrossRef]
220. Prasad, R.; Singh, T.; Katiyar, S.K. Honokiol inhibits ultraviolet radiation-induced immunosuppression through inhibition of ultraviolet-induced inflammation and DNA hypermethylation in mouse skin. *Sci. Rep.* **2017**, *7*, 1657. [CrossRef]
221. Gao, X.; Patel, M.G.; Bakshi, P.; Sharma, D.; Banga, A.K. Enhancement in the Transdermal and Localized Delivery of Honokiol Through Breast Tissue. *AAPS PharmSciTech* **2018**, *19*, 3501–3511. [CrossRef]
222. Wang, X.H.; Cai, L.L.; Zhang, X.Y.; Deng, L.Y.; Zheng, H.; Deng, C.Y.; Wen, J.L.; Zhao, X.; Wei, Y.Q.; Chen, L.J. Improved solubility and pharmacokinetics of PEGylated liposomal honokiol and human plasma protein binding ability of honokiol. *Int. J. Pharm.* **2011**, *410*, 169–174. [CrossRef] [PubMed]
223. Jiang, Q.Q.; Fan, L.Y.; Yang, G.L.; Guo, W.H.; Hou, W.L.; Chen, L.J.; Wei, Y.Q. Improved therapeutic effectiveness by combining liposomal honokiol with cisplatin in lung cancer model. *BMC Cancer* **2008**, *8*, 242. [CrossRef] [PubMed]
224. Tang, P.; Sun, Q.; Yang, H.; Tang, B.; Pu, H.; Li, H. Honokiol nanoparticles based on epigallocatechin gallate functionalized chitin to enhance therapeutic effects against liver cancer. *Int. J. Pharm.* **2018**, *545*, 74–83. [CrossRef] [PubMed]
225. Wu, W.; Wang, L.; Wang, L.; Zu, Y.; Wang, S.; Liu, P.; Zhao, X. Preparation of honokiol nanoparticles by liquid antisolvent precipitation technique, characterization, pharmacokinetics, and evaluation of inhibitory effect on HepG2 cells. *Int. J. Nanomed.* **2018**, *13*, 5469–5483. [CrossRef] [PubMed]
226. Guo, Y.; Zhao, Y.; Wang, T.; Zhao, S.; Qiu, H.; Han, M.; Wang, X. Honokiol nanoparticles stabilized by oligoethylene glycols codendrimer: In vitro and in vivo investigations. *J. Mater. Chem. B* **2017**, *5*, 697–706. [CrossRef]
227. Li, X.; Hou, X.; Ding, W.; Cong, S.; Zhang, Y.; Chen, M.; Meng, Y.; Lei, J.; Liu, Y.; Li, G. Sirolimus-loaded polymeric micelles with honokiol for oral delivery. *J. Pharm. Pharmacol.* **2015**, *67*, 1663–1672. [CrossRef] [PubMed]

228. Wang, N.; Wang, Z.; Nie, S.; Song, L.; He, T.; Yang, S.; Yang, X.; Yi, C.; Wu, Q.; Gong, C. Biodegradable polymeric micelles coencapsulating paclitaxel and honokiol: A strategy for breast cancer therapy in vitro and in vivo. *Int. J. Nanomed.* **2017**, *12*, 1499–1514. [CrossRef]
229. Gong, C.; Wei, X.; Wang, X.; Wang, Y.; Guo, G.; Mao, Y.; Luo, F.; Qian, Z. Biodegradable self-assembled PEG–PCL–PEG micelles for hydrophobic honokiol delivery: I. Preparation and characterization. *Nanotechnology* **2010**, *21*, 215103. [CrossRef]
230. Zheng, X.; Kan, B.; Gou, M.; Fu, S.; Zhang, J.; Men, K.; Chen, L.; Luo, F.; Zhao, Y.; Zhao, X.; et al. Preparation of MPEG–PLA nanoparticle for honokiol delivery in vitro. *Int. J. Pharm.* **2010**, *386*, 262–267. [CrossRef]
231. Wang, B.; Gou, M.; Zheng, X.; Wei, X.; Gong, C.; Wang, X.; Zhao, Y.; Luo, F.; Chen, L.; Qian, Z.; et al. Co-delivery honokiol and doxorubicin in MPEG-PLA nanoparticles. *J. Nanosci. Nanotechnol.* **2010**, *10*, 4166–4172. [CrossRef]
232. Yu, R.; Zou, Y.; Liu, B.; Guo, Y.; Wang, X.; Han, M. Surface modification of pH-sensitive honokiol nanoparticles based on dopamine coating for targeted therapy of breast cancer. *Colloids Surf. B* **2019**, *177*, 1–10. [CrossRef] [PubMed]
233. Gong, C.; Shi, S.; Wang, X.; Wang, Y.; Fu, S.; Dong, P.; Chen, L.; Zhao, X.; Wei, Y.; Qian, Z. Novel composite drug delivery system for honokiol delivery: Self-assembled poly(ethylene glycol)-poly(epsilon-caprolactone)-poly(ethylene glycol) micelles in thermosensitive poly(ethylene glycol)-poly(epsilon-caprolactone)-poly(ethylene glycol) hydrogel. *J. Phys. Chem. B* **2009**, *113*, 10183–10188. [CrossRef] [PubMed]
234. Qiu, N.; Cai, L.L.; Xie, D.; Wang, G.; Wu, W.; Zhang, Y.; Song, H.; Yin, H.; Chen, L. Synthesis, structural and in vitro studies of well-dispersed monomethoxy-poly(ethylene glycol)-honokiol conjugate micelles. *Biomed. Mater.* **2010**, *5*, 065006. [CrossRef] [PubMed]
235. Wang, Z.; Li, X.; Wang, D.; Zou, Y.; Qu, X.; He, C.; Deng, Y.; Jin, Y.; Zhou, Y.; Zhou, Y.; et al. Concurrently suppressing multidrug resistance and metastasis of breast cancer by co-delivery of paclitaxel and honokiol with pH-sensitive polymeric micelles. *Acta Biomater.* **2017**, *62*, 144–156. [CrossRef] [PubMed]
236. Wang, X.; Cheng, L.; Xie, H.-J.; Ju, R.-J.; Xiao, Y.; Fu, M.; Liu, J.-J.; Li, X.-T. Functional paclitaxel plus honokiol micelles destroying tumour metastasis in treatment of non-small-cell lung cancer. *Artif. Cells Nanomed. Biotechnol.* **2018**, *46*, 1154–1169. [CrossRef] [PubMed]
237. Cheng, N.; Xia, T.; Han, Y.; He, Q.J.; Zhao, R.; Ma, J.R. Synergistic antitumor effects of liposomal honokiol combined with cisplatin in colon cancer models. *Oncol. Lett.* **2011**, *2*, 957–962. [CrossRef] [PubMed]
238. Ju, R.J.; Cheng, L.; Qiu, X.; Liu, S.; Song, X.L.; Peng, X.M.; Wang, T.; Li, C.Q.; Li, X.T. Hyaluronic acid modified daunorubicin plus honokiol cationic liposomes for the treatment of breast cancer along with the elimination vasculogenic mimicry channels. *J. Drug Target.* **2018**, *26*, 793–805. [CrossRef]

5

Molecular Mechanisms Underlying Yatein-Induced Cell-Cycle Arrest and Microtubule Destabilization in Human Lung Adenocarcinoma Cells

Shang-Tse Ho [1,2], Chi-Chen Lin [3], Yu-Tang Tung [4,5,6,*] and Jyh-Horng Wu [1,*]

1 Department of Forestry, National Chung Hsing University, Taichung 402, Taiwan; s741129@hotmail.com
2 Agricultural Biotechnology Research Center, Academia Sinica, Taipei 115, Taiwan
3 Institute of Biomedical Science, National Chung Hsing University, Taichung 402, Taiwan; lincc@nchu.edu.tw
4 Graduate Institute of Metabolism and Obesity Sciences, Taipei Medical University, Taipei 110, Taiwan
5 Nutrition Research Center, Taipei Medical University Hospital, Taipei 110, Taiwan
6 Cell Physiology and Molecular Image Research Center, Wan Fang Hospital, Taipei Medical University, Taipei 116, Taiwan
* Correspondence: f91625059@tmu.edu.tw (Y.-T.T.); eric@nchu.edu.tw (J.-H.W.);

Abstract: Yatein is an antitumor agent isolated from *Calocedrus formosana* Florin leaves extract. In our previous study, we found that yatein inhibited the growth of human lung adenocarcinoma A549 and CL1-5 cells by inducing intrinsic and extrinsic apoptotic pathways. To further uncover the effects and mechanisms of yatein-induced inhibition on A549 and CL1-5 cell growth, we evaluated yatein-mediated antitumor activity in vivo and the regulatory effects of yatein on cell-cycle progression and microtubule dynamics. Flow cytometry and western blotting revealed that yatein induces G_2/M arrest in A549 and CL1-5 cells. Yatein also destabilized microtubules and interfered with microtubule dynamics in the two cell lines. Furthermore, we evaluated the antitumor activity of yatein in vivo using a xenograft mouse model and found that yatein treatment altered cyclin B/Cdc2 complex expression and significantly inhibited tumor growth. Taken together, our results suggested that yatein effectively inhibited the growth of A549 and CL1-5 cells possibly by disrupting cell-cycle progression and microtubule dynamics.

Keywords: *Calocedrus formosana*; lung cancer; yatein; cell-cycle arrest; xenograft

---

1. Introduction

Natural products have been used for treating disease for thousands of years. More recently, natural products are being continuously developed for pharmaceutical applications, particularly for anticancer, antibacterial, and antiviral applications [1]. To date, explorative and mechanistic studies on new bioactive compounds are still ongoing.

Cells routinely come in contact with endogenous and exogenous stress stimuli, such as toxic chemicals, UV radiation, and reactive oxygen species. These stress stimuli damage chromosomes, affecting DNA replication and chromosome segregation [2]. Each phase of the cell cycle, including G_0, G_1, S, G_2, and M phase, functions to maintain genetic material duplication and cell division. Abnormal expression of cell-cycle proteins disrupts the cell cycle and is thus closely associated with tumorigenesis [3]. Many natural products exhibit anticancer properties by interacting with cell-cycle proteins [4]. Thus, the identification of a new cell-cycle–targeting natural substance may provide new alternatives in cancer chemotherapy.

Calocedrus formosana is a valuable softwood species in Taiwan, which not only has high industrial economic value but also exhibits multiple bioactivities [5–14]. We previously found that the *C. formosana*

extract and its active phytocompound, yatein, inhibited the growth of human lung adenocarcinoma A549 and CL1-5 cells by inducing caspase-related apoptosis [15]. However, whether yatein regulates the cell cycle in human lung adenocarcinoma remains unclear. To uncover the mechanisms of yatein-mediated human lung adenocarcinoma growth inhibition, we examined the effects of yatein on cell-cycle progression, tubulin dynamics, and in vivo tumor growth.

2. Results

2.1. Yatein Induces Cell-Cycle Arrest at G_2/M Phase and Enhances G_2/M Phase-Related Protein Expression in Human A549 and CL1-5 Cells

To elucidate the mechanism underlying the anti-lung adenocarcinoma effects of yatein, cell-cycle distribution was analyzed in the yatein-treated A549 and CL1-5 cells. We found that 5 μM yatein treatment induced cell-cycle arrest at G_2/M phase in both cell lines (Figure 1). We further analyzed the kinetics of the effects of yatein on A549 and CL1-5 cells through flow cytometry (Figure 2). Compared with untreated cells, we found that more cells entered the G_2/M phase at 6 and 12 h after yatein treatment in both cell types. Next, we evaluated the effects of yatein on G_2/M arrest-related protein expression using western blot analysis (Figure 3). To this end, A549 and CL1-5 cells were treated with 5 μM yatein for 6 and 12 h, and the expression of Cdc2, Cdc25c, and cyclin B1 was analyzed (Figure 3). Cdc2, Cdc25c, and cyclin B1 are key regulators of the cell cycle (particularly in the G_2/M phase). Our results revealed that 6 and 12 h of yatein treatment upregulated cyclin B1, but not Cdc2 and Cdc25c, expression in A549 and CL1-5 cells. However, yatein treatment showed an increasing trend of Cdc2 phosphorylation in both cell types. Notably, yatein-induced Cdc2 phosphorylation was higher at 6 h than at 12 h in both the cell types, indicating that Cdc2 was involved in G_2/M phase regulation in A549 and CL1-5 cells at an early stage.

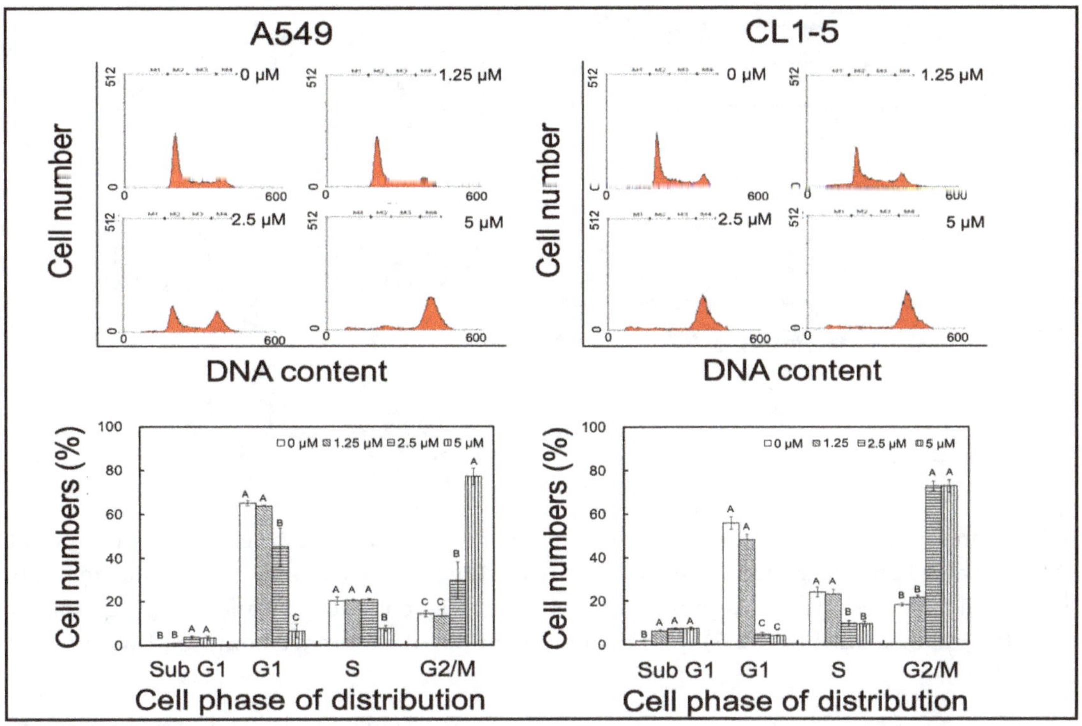

Figure 1. Effects of yatein treatment for 24 h with different concentrations on cell-cycle progression in A549 and CL1-5 cells. The results represent the mean ± SD ($n = 3$). Different letters indicate significant differences among each group in A549 and CL1-5 cells ($p < 0.05$).

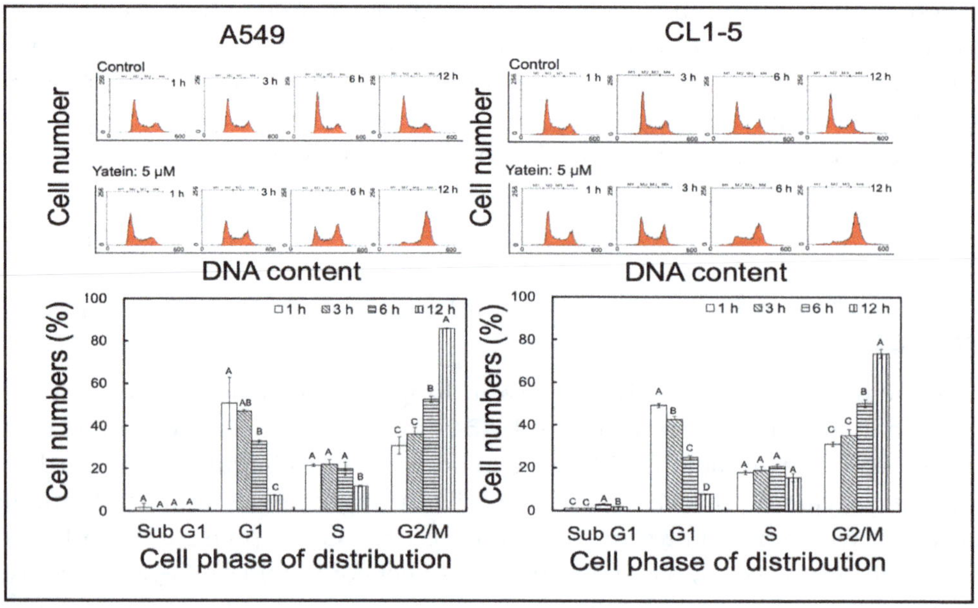

Figure 2. Effect kinetics of 5 μM yatein treatment on cell-cycle progression in A549 and CL1-5 cells. The results represent the mean ± SD (n = 3). Different letters indicate significant differences among each group in A549 and CL1-5 cells ($p < 0.05$).

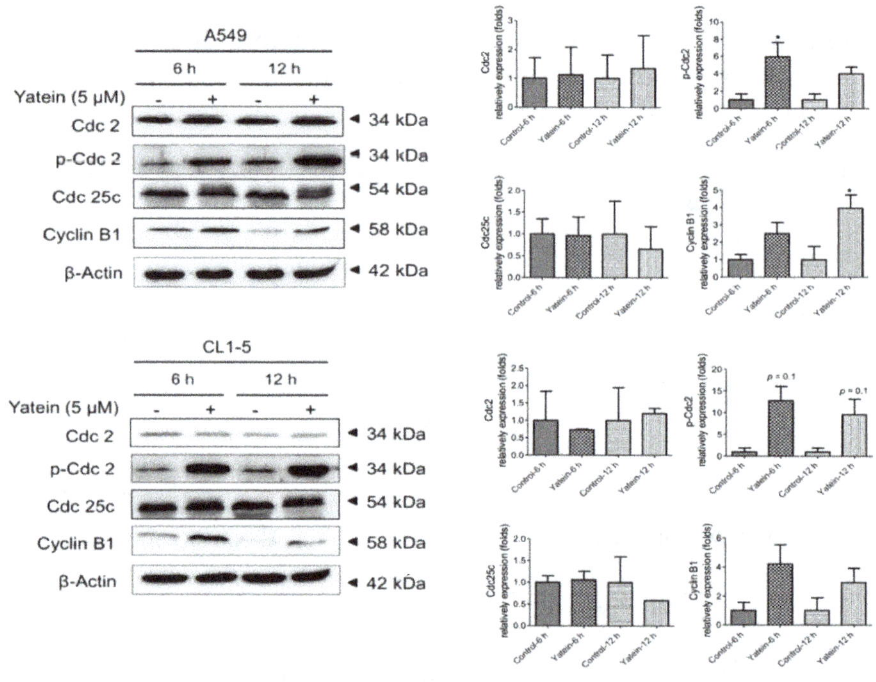

Figure 3. Expression of cell-cycle regulatory proteins in A549 and CL1-5 cells after yatein treatment (5 μM) for 6 h and 12 h. The bands were analyzed using the ImageJ software and normalized to β-actin expression. All data presented are representative of three independent experiments. The quantifications represent the mean ± SEM (n = 2-3). * indicates a significant difference compared with the control group ($p < 0.05$).

2.2. Yatein Induces DNA Damage through Activation of the ATM/ATR Pathway in Human A549 and CL1-5 Cells

DNA damage induces cell-cycle arrest and apoptosis in cancer cells [16]. The ATM/ATR pathway is related to DNA damage process. To address whether yatein induced DNA damage in cells, we examined the effects of yatein treatment on the ATM/ATR pathway. We found that yatein treatment showed an increasing trend of ATM and ATR phosphorylation level in A549 and CL1-5 cells for 6 h and 12 h treatments. However, ATM and ATR expression were not affected (Figure 4A). We next evaluated the expression and phosphorylation of Chk1 and Chk2 in A549 and CL1-5 cells after yatein treatment for 6 and 12 h. Our results revealed that yatein treatment showed an increasing trend of Chk1 and Chk2 phosphorylation level in A549 and CL1-5 cells. These results suggested that yatein induced DNA damage and altered cell-cycle distribution by activating the ATM/Chk2 and ATR/Chk1 DNA repair pathways in A549 and CL1-5 cells. In addition to the activation of the ATM/ATR pathway, we found that yatein treatment affected p53, Wee1, and 14-3-3 σ expression in the A549 cells (Figure 4B). Conversely, yatein did not upregulate the p53 and 14-3-3 σ expression in CL1-5 cells. However, Wee1 expression was increased after yatein treatment for 6 h in CL1-5 cells. These results indicated that the p53 pathway might play an additional role in yatein-induced growth inhibition in A549 cells but not in CL1-5 cells.

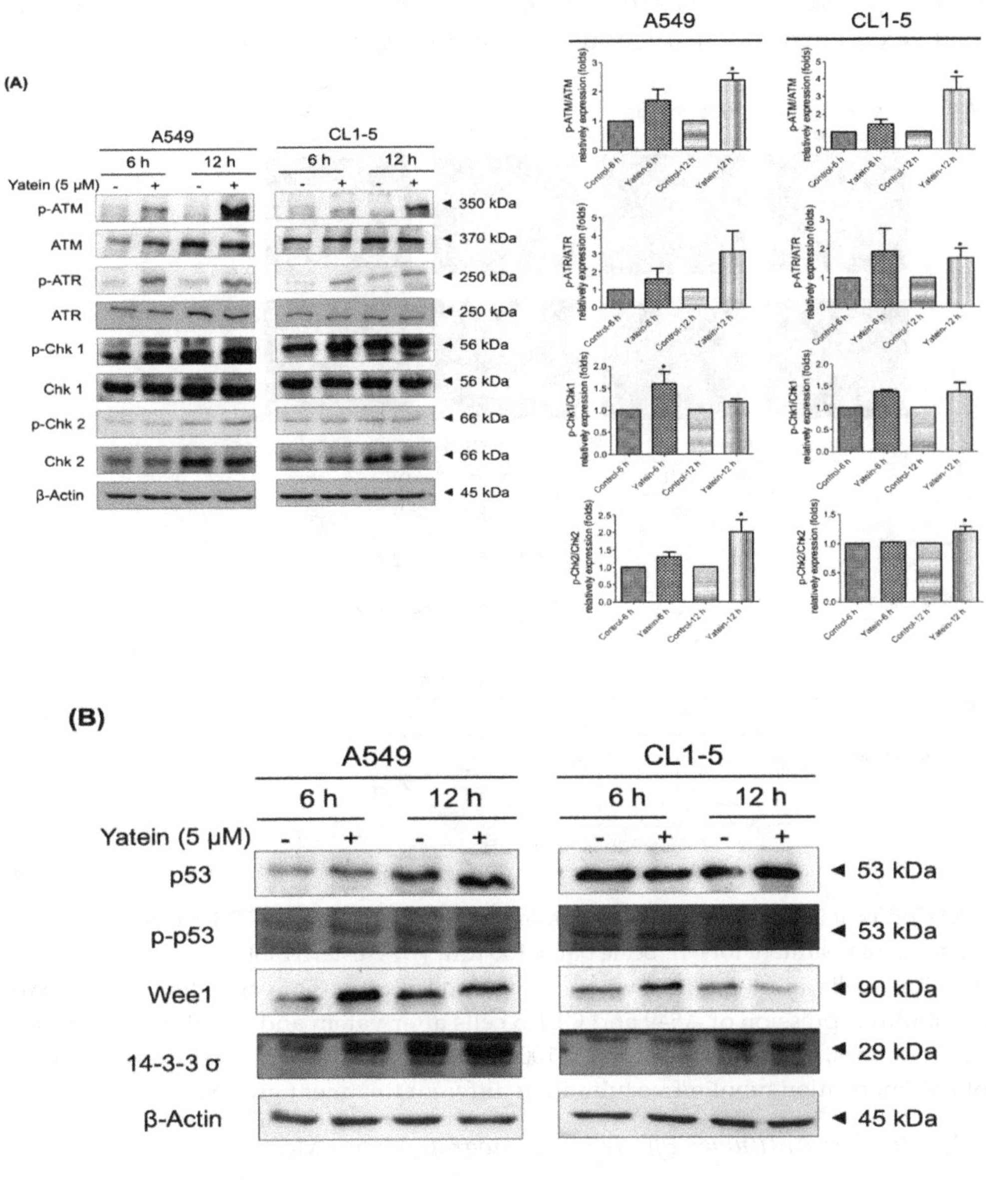

Figure 4. Expression of ATM, ATR, Chk1, and Chk2 (**A**), and p53 related proteins (**B**) in A549 and CL1-5 cells after yatein treatment (5 μM) for 6 and 12 h. All data presented are representative of two to three independent experiments. The quantifications represent the mean ± SEM (n = 2–3). * indicates significant differences compared with the control group in A549 and CL1-5 cells ($p < 0.05$).

2.3. *Yatein Influences Microtubule Dynamics in Human A549 and CL1-5 Cells*

Apart from DNA damage, inhibition of microtubule dynamics is another mechanism that induces G_2/M cell-cycle arrest. For instance, taxol, a well-known anticancer drug, arrests cells in the G_2/M phase by disrupting microtubule polymerization [17]. We assessed microtubule dynamics in yatein-treated A549 and CL1-5 cells using confocal microscopy and western blot analysis. Our confocal microscopy results showed that 5 μM yatein treatment caused a diffusion of green fluorescence (tubulin) in the yatein-treated A549 and CL1-5 cells compared with control cells within 6 h (Figure 5A). In addition, as shown in Figure 5B, yatein decreased tubulin polymerization in a dose-dependent manner in both A549 and CL1-5 cells after 24 h treatment. These results revealed that the effects of yatein on microtubule dynamics were similar to those of colchicine, a microtubule-depolymerizing agent (Figure 5C). Consistently, yatein-treated cells exhibited a similar pattern of tubulin distribution to that of colchicine-treated cells. By contrast, taxol-treated cells demonstrated a higher level of tubulin polymerization compared with the untreated cells. Taken together, our results indicated that yatein and colchicine affected microtubule dynamics by inhibiting tubulin polymerization.

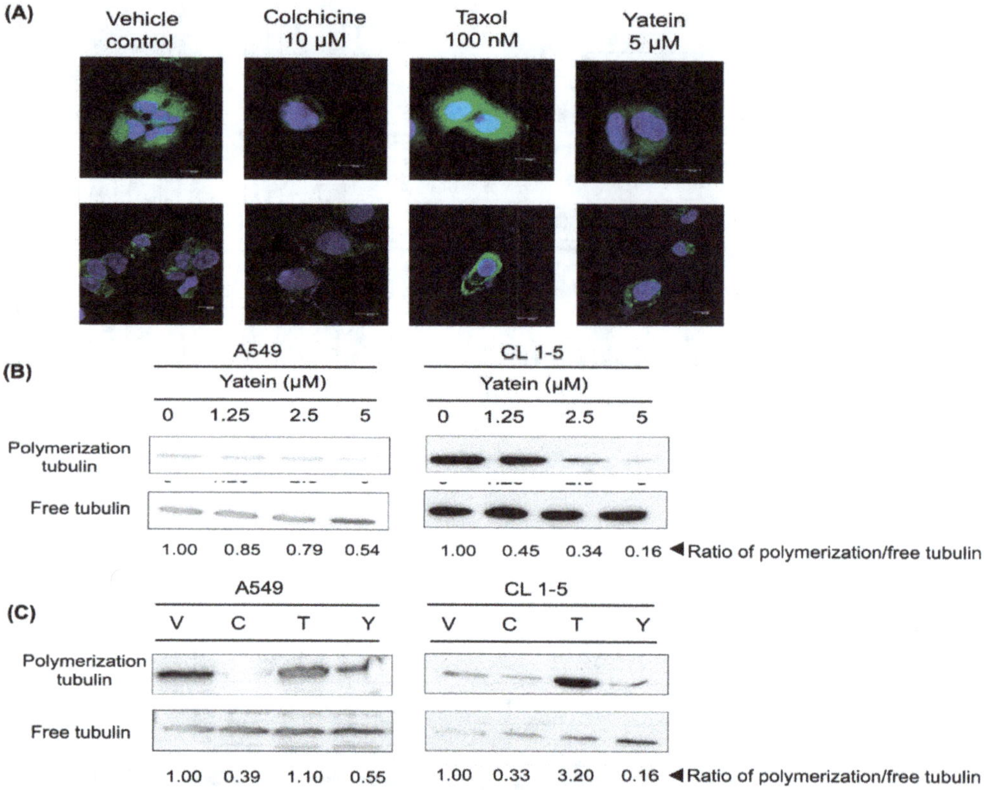

Figure 5. (**A**) Confocal images of tubulin expression of A549 (upper) and CL1-5 (lower) cells after yatein, colchicine, and taxol treatment for 6 h. Scale bar = 100 μm. (**B**) Western blot analysis of tubulin expression of A549 and CL1-5 cells after treatment with various concentrations of yatein for 24 h. (**C**) Western blot analysis of tubulin expression of A549 and CL1-5 cells after yatein and positive control treatment for 24 h. V: Vehicle control, C: 10 μM colchicine, T: 100 nM taxol, Y: 5 μM yatein. The quantitative values are the ratio of polymerization tubulin/free tubulin in different treatment groups.

2.4. *Yatein Exhibits In Vivo Antitumor Effects in a Xenograft Mouse Model*

To validate the growth inhibitory effects of yatein in an in vivo context, we applied a xenograft mouse model using A549 cells. To this end, NOD/SCID mice were inoculated with A549-luc cells for 10 days and were then given 20 mg/kg yatein (i.p.) five times per week for 42 days. Animal body weight, food intake, and tumor growth were monitored and quantified during the experiment. Our results showed that the body weight and food intake of the control and yatein-treated mice did not differ

(Figure 6A,B), suggesting that yatein was well tolerated in the mice. We found that the tumor volumes of the control mice (41.3 mm^3) and yatein-treated mice (38.5 mm^3) were similar in the first 14 days (Figure 6C). However, within the 21-42 days (end of experiment) time window, tumor growth in the yatein-treated mice was significantly slower compared with the control mice ($p < 0.05$). Consistently, In Vivo Imaging System (IVIS) analysis showed that the tumor tissue luminescence in the yatein-treated group (16.5×10^5 photons/s) was lower than that in the vehicle control group (24.0×10^5 photons/s). To confirm that yatein exhibited the same antitumor mechanisms in vivo as observed in vitro, we evaluated cyclin B1 expression and Cdc2 phosphorylation in the tumor tissue in the vehicle control and yatein-treated groups (Figure 6D). We found that both cyclin B1 expression and Cdc2 phosphorylation moderately increased in the yatein-treated group compared with the control group (Figure 6D). Taken together, these results suggested that the induction of cyclin B/Cdc2 complex expression and activation were associated with the antitumor effects of yatein in vivo.

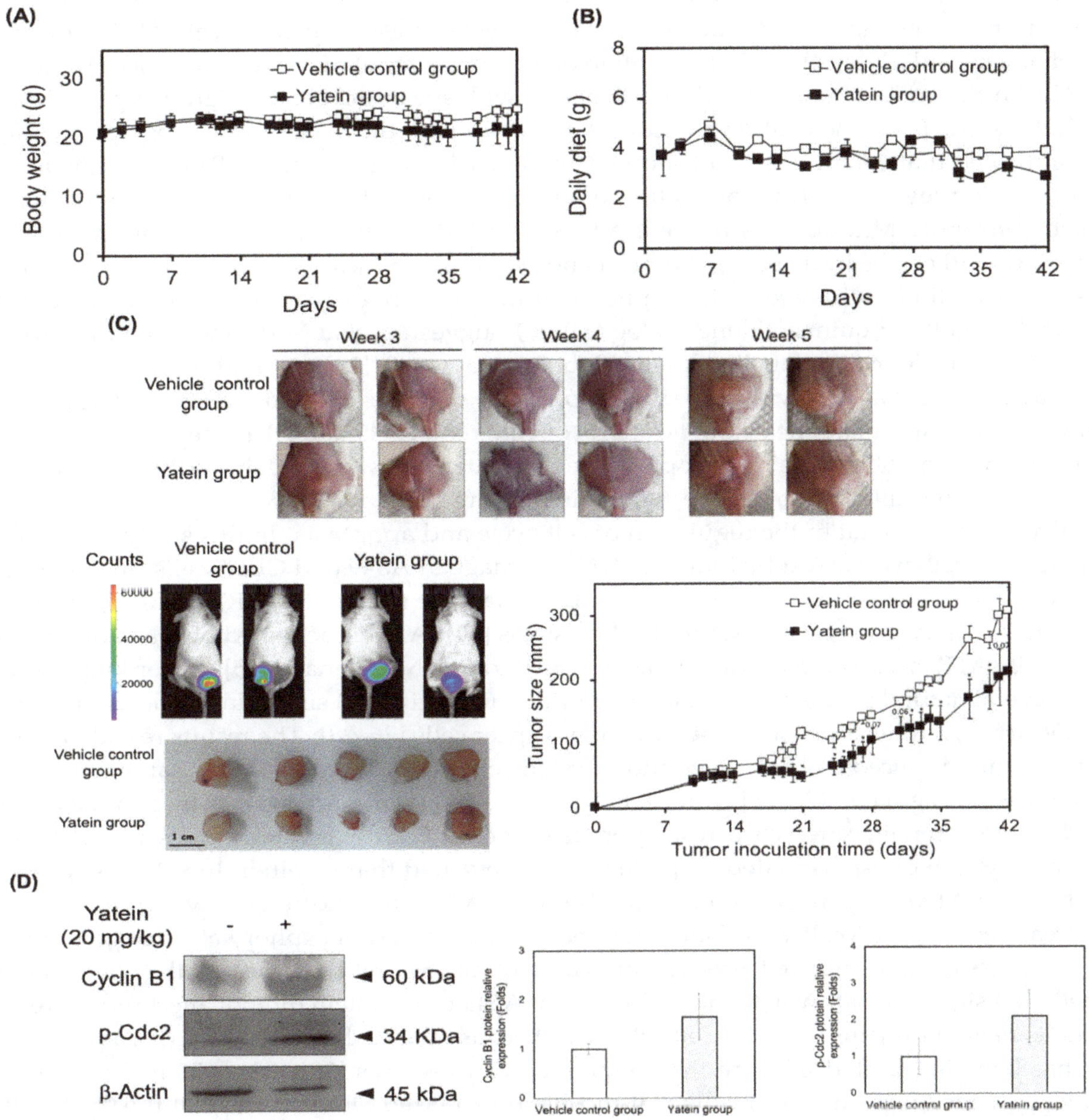

Figure 6. In vivo antitumor effects of yatein. (**A**) Body weight, (**B**) daily diet intake, and (**C**) tumor size and IVIS images of A549-luc cell xenograft mice treated with vehicle or 20 mg/kg of yatein during the experimental period. The results represent the mean ± SEM ($n = 5$). (**D**) Western blot analysis of tumor tissue from the A549-luc xenograft mice (values were mean ± SEM, $n = 3$).

3. Discussion

According to our previous study [15], the IC_{50} values for the 24 h yatein treatment in the A549 and CL1-5 cells were 10.0 and 2.1 μM, respectively. In addition, yatein exhibited excellent growth inhibitory effect in the A549 (IC_{50} values = 3.5 μM) and CL1-5 cells (IC_{50} values = 1.9 μM) after 72 h treatment. Interestingly, yatein was unable to inhibit human nasopharyngeal carcinoma (HONE-1) and human gastric cancer (NUGC) cells growth at a concentration of 50 μg/mL (≅ 125 μM) [10]. In the present study, we found that yatein induced G_2/M cell-cycle arrest in A549 and CL1-5 cells at the first 24 h treatment. Additionally, treatment with yatein for 48 h induced a dose-dependent increase in both early and late stage apoptosis in the A549 and CL1-5 cells [15]. As previously reported, some lignan compounds can inhibit cancer cell growth by inducing cell-cycle arrest. For example, vitexin compound-1 (VB1), a lignan isolated from a plant used in traditional Chinese medicine, namely *Vitex negundo*, inhibits the growth of MDA-MB-435 and SMMC-7721 cells by inducing G_2/M phase cell-cycle arrest after 24 h treatment at a concentration of 10 μM [18]. Similarly, benozofuran lignan shows a dose- and time-dependent induction of G_2/M cell-cycle arrest in Jurkat T-cells [19]. Additionally, the mechanism underlying the effects of yatein on cell-cycle regulation was examined in the present study. Cyclin-dependent kinases (CDKs) collaborate with specific cyclins to tightly regulate cell cycle and cell division. Thus, the CDK/cyclin complex plays a key role in cell-cycle progression [20]. Our results indicated that yatein treatment showed an increasing trend of cyclin B1 expression and Cdc2 phosphorylation level. Aberrant activation of cyclin B1/p-Cdc2 activity is closely associated with mitotic catastrophe. Mitotic catastrophe is a type of cell death that results from mitotic regulation dysfunctions and can be induced by chemical and physical stresses [21]. Liu et al. [22] reported that expression of cyclin B1 and level of Cdc2 phosphorylation were increased in malignant glioma cells treated with a synthetic quinazolinone analog (MJ-66), suggesting that MJ-66 induced G_2/M arrest and mitotic catastrophe in malignant glioma cells. Subramaniam et al. [23] reported that curcumin-induced mitotic catastrophe coupled with increased expression of cyclin B1 and Cdc-2 in MiaPaCa-2 cells. Therefore, we can speculate the cytotoxic effects of yatein on A549 and CL1-5 cells might be partially due to the induction of mitotic catastrophe. The correlation between yatein-induced cell death and mitotic catastrophe still need to be investigated in a future study.

DNA damage is vital in the regulation of cell cycle and apoptosis. In this study, we found that yatein induced cell-cycle arrest by inducing DNA damage in A549 and CL1-5 cells. In general, ATM and ATR kinases are the initiating kinases of the DNA damage response (DDR) signaling pathway that is activated by DNA damage or DNA replication stress [24]. ATM is activated by DNA double-strand breaks, while ATR is activated by various factors related to DNA damage [25]. According to previous studies, several natural products, including berberine, curcumin, and sinularin, induced DNA damage and G_2/M arrest, but not S phase arrest, in various cancer cells [26–28]. The results revealed that these natural products induced DNA damage and arrested cells at G_2/M phase. At the same time, the ATM pathway was up-regulated [26–28]. After ATM activation, several proteins involved in the regulation of ATM on DNA repair, cell-cycle arrest, apoptosis, and other downstream processes, such as Brca1, Chk2, and p53, are phosphorylated [29]. Our results revealed that yatein induced the expression of ATR/Chk1 and ATM/Chk2 in A549 cells. Notably, only ATR/Chk1 expression was upregulated after yatein treatment in CL1-5 cells. We found that the expression and phosphorylation of p53, Wee1, and 14-3-3 σ expression were induced after yatein treatment in A549 cells, suggesting that yatein activated p53-mediated signaling pathway to inhibit growth in A549 cells. Yatein did not affect the expression of p53 and its related proteins in CL1-5 cells; this was because the CL1-5 cell line carries a p53 mutation, which has been implicated in more than 50% of all cancer cases [30]. The p53 mutation causes a defective G_1 checkpoint in cancer cells that results in increased DNA damage at the G_2 checkpoint compared with noncancer cells. Wee1 is a key protein that is closely associated with G_2 checkpoint abrogation and mitotic catastrophe [30,31]. Accordingly, we found that yatein treatment increased Wee1 expression in CL1-5 cells, indicating that Wee1 played a crucial role in the regulation of G_2/M cell-cycle distribution in CL1-5 cells in the context of yatein treatment. On the other hand, we also found yatein is able to induce ROS production in A549 and CL1-5 cells in our previous study [15], suggesting that yatein may induce the oxidative DNA damage. Moreover, our previous results also revealed that the CL1-5 cells were more sensitive for the ROS production than the A549 cells after yatein treatment [15].

Additionally, we showed that yatein affected the microtubule assembly in both A549 and CL1-5 cells after 6 h treatment (Figure 5A) and 24 h treatment (Figure 5B and 5C). The induction of mitotic arrest is associated with dysfunctional microtubule dynamics [32]. Microtubules play vital roles in cell proliferation, trafficking, signaling, and migration [33]. Considering the importance of microtubule dynamics, several small microtubule-targeting molecules have been designed and used as anticancer drugs [30]. Tubulin has three major binding sites: taxane, vinca, and colchicine domains. In this study, we found that yatein exhibited similar effects to that of colchicine, implying that yatein inhibited tubulin polymerization. These results suggested that tubulin polymerization inhibition partially contributed to the ability of yatein to arrest A549 and CL1-5 cells at the G_2/M phase.

The in vivo growth inhibitory effects of yatein on A549 cells were elucidated in this study. Our results revealed that yatein treatment significantly suppressed tumor growth in mice without affecting their body weight and food intake. Additionally, yatein treatment increased cyclin B1 expression and Cdc2 phosphorylation in vivo, indicating that the induction of mitotic catastrophe was involved in the anticancer mechanism of yatein in vivo. Taken together, we found that yatein affected cell-cycle progression and microtubule dynamics, induced DDR, and exhibited anticancer properties in vivo (Figure 7).

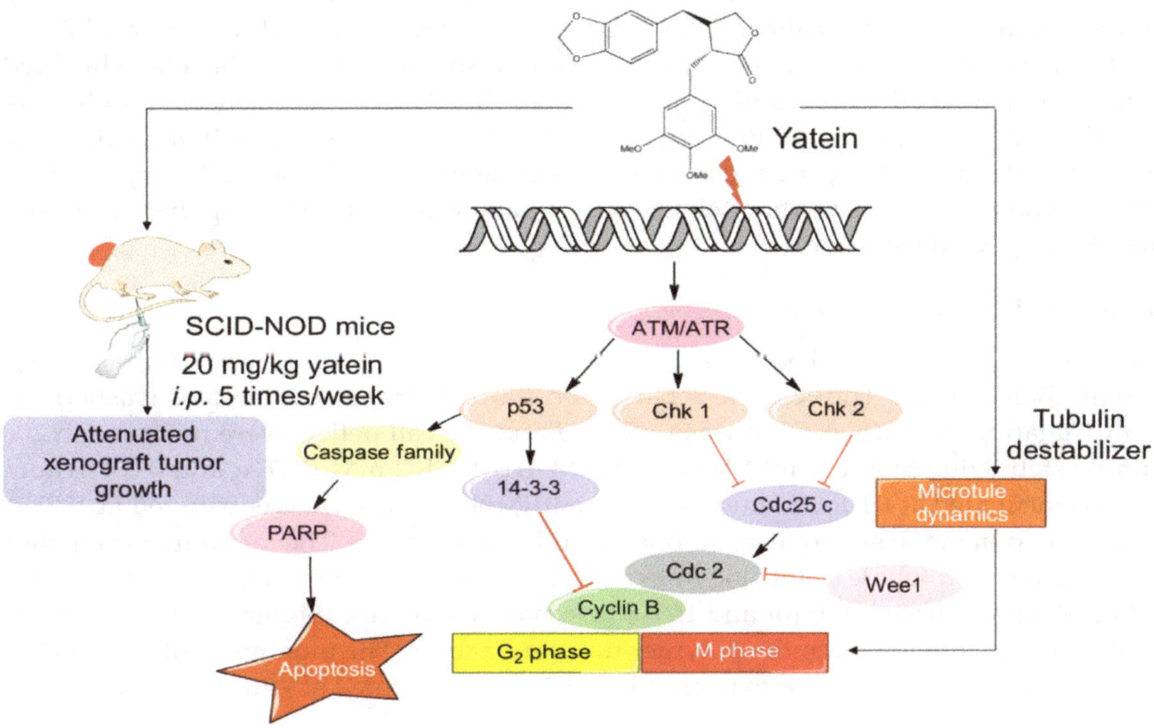

Figure 7. Proposed mechanism of the inhibitory effects of yatein on lung adenocarcinoma cells.

4. Materials and Methods

4.1. Preparation of Yatein

The phytocompound, yatein, was isolated from *C. formosana* leaves extracts. In brief, *C. formosana* leaves were extracted using methanol at room temperature (RT) for one week (twice) to obtain a methanolic extract. The dried samples were further divided to *n*-hexane, ethyl acetate (EtOAc), *n*-butanol, and H_2O fractions using liquid–liquid partition. The *n*-hexane fraction was further fractionated into ten subfractions using normal phase column chromatography (Geduran Si-60, Merck, Darmstadt, Germany). Yatein was isolated and purified from the subfraction 4 by semipreparative high-performance liquid chromatography using a PU-2080 pump (Jasco, Tokyo, Japan) equipped with an RI-2031 detector (Jasco) and a 5 μm Luna silica column (250 mm × 10.0 mm internal diameter; Phenomenex, Torrance, CA, USA). The mobile phase consisted of 30% of EtOAc and 70% of *n*-hexane (*v*/*v*), and the flow rate was 4 mL/min. The retention time of yatein in HPLC analysis was 18.0 min. The purity and the structure elucidation of yatein was conducted by ^{1}H and ^{13}C NMR, and all spectrum data were consistent with literature [34].

4.2. Cell Culture

Human A549 cell line was purchased from Bioresource Collection and Research Center (BCRC 60124) and cultured in RPMI-1640 (Gibco, Gran Island, NY, USA) supplemented with 10% (*v*/*v*) fetal bovine serum (Gibco) and 1% (*v*/*v*) antibiotic–antimycotic agent (Gibco). CL1-5 cell line was provided by Dr. Jeremy J.-W. Chen (National Chung Hsing University, Taichung, Taiwan) and cultured in Dulbecco's modified Eagle's medium (Gibco) supplemented with 10% (*v*/*v*) fetal bovine serum (Gibco) and 1% (*v*/*v*) antibiotic–antimycotic agent (Gibco). The cells were incubated in a 37 °C humidified incubator containing 5% CO_2.

4.3. Cell-Cycle Distribution Analysis

The A549 and CL1-5 cells were seeded onto a 6-well plate at a density of 1×10^5 cells/well and incubated overnight. The cells were then treated with various concentrations of the test samples for the indicated durations. After treatment, the cells were collected and mixed with ice-cold 75% ethanol and then fixed overnight at −20 °C. Then, the cells were washed twice using phosphate-buffered saline (PBS), and then incubated with 200 μL of propidium iodide (PI, BD Bioscience, Franklin Lakes, NJ, USA) solution (containing 1 mg/mL PI, 2 mg/mL RNase A, and 0.5% Triton X-100) for 30 min at RT in the dark. After 30 min, the PI-stained cells were immediately analyzed using a flow cytometer (Accuri 5, Accuri Cytometers, Inc., Ann Arbor, MI, USA). The data were analyzed using the C6 Accuri system software (Accuri Cytometers, Inc.).

4.4. Isolation of Microtubule Proteins

The A549 and CL1-5 cells (1×10^6 cells) were seeded onto culture dishes (10 cm) overnight and treated with 5 μM yatein. The cells were harvested through trypsinization and washed with PBS. After centrifugation, the supernatant was removed and the cell pellets were mixed with 200 μL of microtubule stabilizing buffer (1 mM $MgCl_2$, 2 mM Tris-HCl, 2 mM EGTA, and 0.5% Triton-100 in ddH_2O) and incubated at RT for 20 min. Subsequently, the mixture was centrifuged at 12,000× *g* for 10 min (4 °C) to obtain the supernatant (monomer tubulin fraction). The remaining cell pellets were washed using the microtubule stabilizing buffer and lysed in a radioimmunoprecipitation assay buffer containing 10% proteinase inhibitor and 10% phosphatase inhibitor (Sigma-Aldrich, St. Louis, MO, USA) at 4 °C for 30 min to obtain the polymer tubulin fraction. The monomer tubulin and polymer tubulin fractions were transferred into microtubes (1.5 mL) and stored at −20 °C until further analysis.

4.5. Western Blot Analysis

The expression of proteins in cells were determined using western blot analysis as previously reported [15]. In this study, the primary antibodies were anti-14-3-3 σ (Santa Cruz, Dallas, TX, USA), anti-β-actin (Santa Cruz), anti-ATM (Santa Cruz), anti-ATR (Santa Cruz), anti-Cdc2 (Abcam, Cambridge, MA, USA), anti-Cdc25c (Santa Cruz), anti-Chk1 (Santa Cruz), anti-Chk2 (Santa Cruz), anti-cyclin B1 (Abcam), anti-p53 (Cell Signaling Technology Inc, Danvers, MA, USA), anti-phospho-p53 Ser 15 (Cell Signaling Technology Inc), anti-phospho-ATM (Santa Cruz), anti-phospho-ATR (Santa Cruz), anti-phospho-Cdc2 (Santa Cruz), anti-phospho-Chk1 (Santa Cruz), anti-phospho-Chk2 (Santa Cruz), anti-β-tubulin (Abcam), and anti-Wee1 (Santa Cruz) antibodies. An enhanced chemiluminescence

(ECL, Sigma-Aldrich) system was used for developing signals of the blots, which were analyzed using a LAS3000 system (Fujifilm, Tokyo, Japan).

4.6. *Immunofluorescence*

The A549 and CL1-5 cells (1×10^5 cells) were seeded on a chamber slide for 24 h and treated with colchicine (10 μM), taxol (100 nM), and yatein (5 μM) for 6 h. The cells were washed with PBS and fixed with 1% paraformaldehyde (Sigma-Aldrich) at RT for 30 min. The paraformaldehyde was removed, and the cells were washed thrice with PBS. Next, the cells were blocked using 1% BSA in PBS at 4 °C overnight. After they were washed with PBS, the cells were incubated with the anti-β-tubulin antibody (1:200 in 1% BSA solution) at 4 °C overnight. After washing with PBS, an anti-rabbit-FITC antibody was added to the cells and then incubated overnight. Then, the antibody was rinsed off and the cells were washed thrice using PBS. 4,6-Diamidino-2-phenylindole was added and the cells were incubated for 15 min at RT in the dark. A Leica TCS SP2 confocal spectral microscope (Buffalo, NY, USA) was used to observe immunofluorescence staining of microtubule dynamics.

4.7. *In Vivo Antitumor Activity*

The procedures involving animals were performed according to the guidelines of the Institutional Animal Care and Use Committee of National Chung Hsing University (IACUC no. 107-127). The A549-luc cells were mixed with Matrigel (Sigma-Aldrich) at a 1:1 ratio. The cells were injected subcutaneously into the back of nonobese diabetic and severe combined immunodeficiency (NOD/SCID) mice (male, 6–8 weeks old) at a density of 3.5×10^6 cells/mouse. Tumors were allowed to grow for 10 days and were then treated with an intraperitoneal (i.p.) injection of either 0.5% DMSO in ddH_2O to the mice in the vehicle control group ($n = 5$) or 20 mg/kg of yatein (dissolved in 0.5% DMSO in ddH_2O) to the mice in the yatein group ($n = 5$). The tumor-bearing mice were sacrificed after 42 days. Tumor volume was measured five times/week and calculated using the following formula: Length × width × thickness × 0.5 (mm^3). An IVIS (Caliper lifescience IVIS Spectrum CT) was used to analyze the luminescence of tumor tissue.

4.8. *Statistical Analysis*

Data are expressed as mean ± standard deviation (SD) or mean ± standard error of the mean (SEM). Statistical analysis was performed using the shuffle test or non-parametric Kruskal-Wallis test with Dunn's post hoc tests. A p of < 0.05 was considered statistically significant.

5. Conclusions

The present study demonstrated that yatein suppressed lung adenocarcinoma cancer cells growth by inducing cell-cycle arrest, mitotic catastrophe, and microtubule depolymerization. Yatein induced G_2/M arrest by upregulating the expression of cyclin B1 and Cdc2 phosphorylation in lung adenocarcinoma cancer cells. In addition, mitotic catastrophe and microtubule depolymerization were involved in yatein-mediated lung adenocarcinoma cancer cells growth inhibition. Furthermore, we confirmed the in vivo antitumor effects of yatein using a xenograft mouse model. These findings provide novel insights into the in vitro and in vivo antitumor efficacy of yatein and demonstrate the potential of this phytocompound as an anticancer lead compound for lung adenocarcinoma cancer treatment.

Author Contributions: Conceptualization, S.-T.H., Y.-T.T., and J.-H.W.; methodology, S.-T.H., Y.-T.T. and J.-H.W.; formal analysis, S.-T.H. and C.-C.L.; resources, Y.-T.T. and J.-H.W.; writing—original draft, S.-T.H.; writing—review and editing, C.-C.L., Y.-T.T. and J.-H.W.; supervision, Y.-T.T. and J.-H.W.

References

1. Newman, D.J.; Cragg, G.M. Natural products as sources of new drugs from 1981 to 2014. *J. Nat. Prod.* **2016**, *79*, 629–661. [CrossRef] [PubMed]
2. Visconti, R.; Della Monica, R.; Grieco, D. Cell cycle checkpoint in cancer: a therapeutically targetable double-edged sword. *J. Exp. Clin. Cancer Res.* **2016**, *35*, 153. [CrossRef] [PubMed]
3. Otto, T.; Sicinski, P. Cell cycle proteins as promising targets in cancer therapy. *Nat. Rev. Cancer* **2017**, *17*, 93–115. [CrossRef] [PubMed]
4. Bailon-Moscoso, N.; Cevallos-Solorzano, G.; Romero-Benavides, J.C.; Orellana, M.I. Natural compounds as modulators of cell cycle arrest: application for anticancer chemotherapies. *Curr. Genom.* **2017**, *18*, 106–131. [CrossRef] [PubMed]
5. Chang, H.T.; Cheng, Y.H.; Wu, C.L.; Chang, S.T.; Chang, T.T.; Su, Y.C. Antifungal activity of essential oil and its constituents from *Calocedrus macrolepis* var. formosana Florin leaf against plant pathogenic fungi. *Bioresour. Technol.* **2008**, *99*, 6266–6270.
6. Yen, T.B.; Chang, H.T.; Hsieh, C.C.; Chang, S.T. Antifungal properties of ethanolic extract and its active compounds from *Calocedrus macrolepis* var. formosana (Florin) heartwood. *Bioresour. Technol.* **2008**, *99*, 4871–4877. [CrossRef] [PubMed]
7. Ho, C.L.; Tseng, Y.H.; Wang, E.I.; Liao, P.C.; Chou, J.C.; Lin, C.N.; Su, Y.C. Composition, antioxidant and antimicrobial activities of the seed essential oil of *Calocedrus formosana* from Taiwan. *Nat. Prod. Commun.* **2011**, *6*, 133–136. [CrossRef]
8. Wang, S.Y.; Wu, J.H.; Cheng, S.S.; Lo, C.P.; Chang, H.N.; Shyur, L.F.; Chang, S.T. Antioxidant activity of extracts from *Calocedrus formosana* leaf, bark, and heartwood. *J. Wood Sci.* **2004**, *50*, 422–426. [CrossRef]
9. Yen, P.L.; Wu, C.L.; Chang, S.T.; Huang, S.L.; Chang, H.T. Antioxidative lignans from phytochemical extract of *Calocedrus formosana* Florin. *BioResources* **2012**, *7*, 4122–4131.
10. Chiang, Y.M.; Liu, H.K.; Lo, J.M.; Chien, S.C.; Chan, Y.F.; Lee, T.H.; Su, J.K.; Kuo, Y.H. Cytotoxic constituents of the leaves of *Calocedrus formosana*. *J. Chin. Chem. Soc.* **2013**, *50*, 161–166. [CrossRef]
11. Yuan, S.Y.; Lin, C.C.; Hsu, S.L.; Cheng, Y.W.; Wu, J.H.; Cheng, C.L.; Yang, C.R. Leaf extracts of *Calocedrus formosana* (Florin) induce G2/M cell cycle arrest and apoptosis in human bladder cancer cells. *Evid.-Based Complement. Altern. Med.* **2011**, *2011*, 380923. [CrossRef]
12. Tsai, C.C.; Chen, C.J.; Tseng, H.W.; Hua, K.F.; Tsai, R.Y.; Lai, M.H.; Chao, L.K.; Chen, S.T. Cytomic screening of immuno-modulating activity compounds from *Calocedrus formosana*. *Comb. Chem. High Throughput Screen.* **2008**, *11*, 834–842. [CrossRef]
13. Chao, K.P.; Hua, K.F.; Hsu, H.Y.; Su, Y.C.; Chang, S.T. Anti-Inflammatory activity of sugiol, a diterpene isolated from *Calocedrus formosana* bark. *Planta Med.* **2005**, *71*, 300–305. [CrossRef]
14. Jayakumar, T.; Liu, C.H.; Wu, G.Y.; Lee, T.Y.; Manubolu, M.; Hsieh, C.Y.; Yang, C.H.; Sheu, J.R. Hinokitiol inhibits migration of A549 lung cancer cells via suppression of MMPs and induction of antioxidant enzymes and apoptosis. *Int. J. Mol. Sci.* **2018**, *19*, 939. [CrossRef]
15. Ho, S.T.; Lin, C.C.; Wu, T.L.; Tung, Y.T.; Wu, J.H. Antitumor agent yatein from *Calocedrus formosana* Florin leaf induces apoptosis in non-small-cell lung cancer cells. *J. Wood Sci.*. under review.
16. Sancar, A.; Lindsey-Boltz, L.A.; Ünsal-Kaçmaz, K.; Linn, S. Molecular mechanisms of mammalian DNA repair and the DNA damage checkpoints. *Annu. Rev. Biochem.* **2004**, *73*, 39–85. [CrossRef]
17. Bacus, S.S.; Gudkov, A.V.; Lowe, M.; Lyass, L.; Yung, Y.; Komarov, A.P.; Keyomarsi, K.; Yarden, Y.; Seger, R. Taxol-Induced apoptosis depends on MAP kinase pathways (ERK and p38) and is independent of p53. *Oncogene* **2001**, *20*, 147. [CrossRef]
18. Xin, H.; Kong, Y.; Wang, Y.; Zhou, Y.; Zhu, Y.; Li, D.; Tan, W. Lignans extracted from *Vitex negundo* possess cytotoxic activity by G2/M phase cell cycle arrest and apoptosis induction. *Phytomedicine* **2013**, *20*, 640–647. [CrossRef]
19. Manna, S.K.; Bose, J.S.; Gangan, V.; Raviprakash, N.; Navaneetha, T.; Raghavendra, P.B.; Babajan, B.; Kumar, C.S.; Jain, S.K. Novel derivative of benzofuran induces cell death mostly by G2/M cell cycle arrest through p53-dependent pathway but partially by inhibition of NF-Kappab. *J. Biol. Chem.* **2010**, *285*, 22318–22327. [CrossRef]
20. Satyanarayana, A.; Kaldis, P. Mammalian cell-cycle regulation: several Cdks, numerous cyclins and diverse compensatory mechanisms. *Oncogene* **2009**, *28*, 2925. [CrossRef]

21. Vakifahmetoglu, H.; Olsson, M.; Zhivotovsky, B. Death through a tragedy: mitotic catastrophe. *Cell Death Differ.* **2008**, *15*, 1153. [CrossRef] [PubMed]
22. Liu, W.T.; Chen, C.; Lu, I.C.; Kuo, S.C.; Lee, K.H.; Chen, T.L.; Song, T.S.; Lu, Y.L.; Gean, P.W.; Hour, M.J. MJ-66 induces malignant glioma cells G2/M phase arrest and mitotic catastrophe through regulation of cyclin B1/Cdk1 complex. *Neuropharmacology* **2014**, *86*, 219–227. [CrossRef] [PubMed]
23. Subramaniam, D.; Ramalingam, S.; Linehan, D.C.; Dieckgraefe, B.K.; Postier, R.G.; Houchen, C.W.; Jensen, R.A.; Anant, S. RNA binding protein CUGBP2/CELF2 mediates curcumin-induced mitotic catastrophe of pancreatic cancer cells. *PLoS ONE* **2011**, *6*. [CrossRef] [PubMed]
24. Maréchal, A.; Zou, L. DNA damage sensing by the ATM and ATR kinases. *Cold Spring Harb. Perspect. Biol.* **2013**, *5*, 012716. [CrossRef] [PubMed]
25. Smith, J.; Tho, L.M.; Xu, N.; Gillespie, D.A. The ATM-Chk2 and ATR-Chk1 pathways in DNA damage signaling and cancer. *Adv. Cancer Res.* **2010**, *108*, 73–112.
26. Sahu, R.P.; Batra, S.; Srivastava, S.K. Activation of ATM/Chk1 by curcumin causes cell cycle arrest and apoptosis in human pancreatic cancer cells. *Br. J. Cancer* **2009**, *100*, 1425–1433. [CrossRef]
27. Wang, Y.; Liu, Q.; Liu, Z.; Li, B.; Sun, Z.; Zhou, H.; Zhang, X.; Gong, Y.; Shao, C. Berberine, a genotoxic alkaloid, induces ATM-Chk1 mediated G2 arrest in prostate cancer cells. *Mutat. Res.* **2012**, *734*, 20–29. [CrossRef]
28. Chung, T.W.; Lin, S.C.; Su, J.H.; Chen, Y.K.; Lin, C.C.; Chan, H.L. Sinularin induces DNA damage, G2/M phase arrest, and apoptosis in human hepatocellular carcinoma cells. *BMC Complement Altern. Med.* **2017**, *17*, 62. [CrossRef]
29. Shiloh, Y. ATM and related protein kinases: Safeguarding genome integrity. *Nat. Rev. Cancer* **2003**, *3*, 155–168. [CrossRef]
30. Schmidt, M.; Rohe, A.; Platzer, C.; Najjar, A.; Erdmann, F.; Sippl, W. Regulation of G2/M transition by inhibition of WEE1 and PKMYT1 kinases. *Molecules* **2017**, *22*, 2045. [CrossRef]
31. Ashwell, S. Chapter 10—Checkpoint Kinase and Wee1 inhibitors as anticancer therapeutics. In *DNA Repair in Cancer Therapy*; Kelley, M.R., Ed.; Academic Press: San Diego, CA, USA, 2012; pp. 211–234.
32. Cotugno, R.; Fortunato, R.; Santoro, A.; Gallotta, D.; Braca, A.; De Tommasi, N.; Belisario, M.A. Effect of sesquiterpene lactone coronopilin on leukaemia cell population growth, cell type-specific induction of apoptosis and mitotic catastrophe. *Cell Prolif.* **2011**, *45*, 53–65. [CrossRef] [PubMed]
33. Dumontet, C.; Jordan, M.A. Microtubule-Binding agents: a dynamic field of cancer therapeutics. *Nat. Rev. Drug Discov.* **2010**, *9*, 790–803. [CrossRef] [PubMed]
34. Ikeda, R.; Nagao, T.; Okabe, H.; Nakano, Y.; Matsunaga, H.; Katano, M.; Mori, M. Antiproliferative constituents in umbelliferae plants. III. Constituents in the root and the ground part of *Anthriscus sylvestris* Hoffm. *Chem. Pharm. Bull.* **1998**, *46*, 871–887. [PubMed]

6

Anti-tumor Activity and Epigenetic Impact of the Polyphenol Oleacein in Multiple Myeloma

Giada Juli [1], Manuela Oliverio [2], Dina Bellizzi [3], Maria Eugenia Gallo Cantafio [1], Katia Grillone [1], Giuseppe Passarino [3], Carmela Colica [4], Monica Nardi [2], Marco Rossi [1], Antonio Procopio [2], Pierosandro Tagliaferri [1], Pierfrancesco Tassone [1,*] and Nicola Amodio [1,*]

1 Department of Experimental and Clinical Medicine, *Magna Graecia* University of Catanzaro, 88100 Catanzaro, Italy
2 Department of Health Science, *Magna Graecia* University of Catanzaro, 88100 Catanzaro, Italy
3 Department of Biology, Ecology and Earth Sciences (DiBEST), University of Calabria, 87036 Arcavacata di Rende, Italy
4 CNR, IBFM UOS of Germaneto, *Magna Graecia* University of Catanzaro, 88100, Catanzaro Italy
* Correspondence: tassone@unicz.it (P.T.); amodio@unicz.it (N.A.)

Abstract: Olive oil contains different biologically active polyphenols, among which oleacein, the most abundant secoiridoid, has recently emerged for its beneficial properties in various disease contexts. By using in vitro models of human multiple myeloma (MM), we here investigated the anti-tumor potential of oleacein and the underlying bio-molecular sequelae. Within a low micromolar range, oleacein reduced the viability of MM primary samples and cell lines even in the presence of bone marrow stromal cells (BMSCs), while sparing healthy peripheral blood mononuclear cells. We also demonstrated that oleacein inhibited MM cell clonogenicity, prompted cell cycle blockade and triggered apoptosis. We evaluated the epigenetic impact of oleacein on MM cells, and observed dose-dependent accumulation of both acetylated histones and α-tubulin, along with down-regulation of several class I/II histone deacetylases (HDACs) both at the mRNA and protein level, providing evidence of the HDAC inhibitory activity of this compound; conversely, no effect on global DNA methylation was found. Mechanistically, HDACs inhibition by oleacein was associated with down-regulation of Sp1, the major transactivator of HDACs promoter, *via* Caspase 8 activation. Of potential translational significance, oleacein synergistically enhanced the in vitro anti-MM activity of the proteasome inhibitor carfilzomib. Altogether, these results indicate that oleacein is endowed with HDAC inhibitory properties, which associate with significant anti-MM activity both as single agent or in combination with carfilzomib. These findings may pave the way to novel potential anti-MM epi-therapeutic approaches based on natural agents.

Keywords: experimental therapeutics; HDAC; multiple myeloma; oleacein

---

1. Introduction

Multiple myeloma (MM) is a clonal B cell malignancy characterized by the accumulation of tumor plasma cells (PCs) in the bone marrow (BM), where different cell types establish a complex microenvironment that supports survival, proliferation and drug-resistance of the malignant clone. The last few years have witnessed a rapid development of drugs for the treatment of this malignancy, leading to increased extent and frequency of response and to the improvement in median overall survival of patients. However, despite such therapeutic advancements, MM eventually evolves into a drug-resistant phase leading to patients' death [1]. This finding has stimulated continuous investigation on new therapeutic options, as single agents or in combination with established anti-MM drugs. In this regard, natural compounds have recently emerged as novel chemopreventive and/or therapeutic tools able to target oncogenic pathways involved in the pathogenesis of human malignancies. Significant anti-inflammatory, anti-oxidant and cytotoxic effects of natural agents have been demonstrated also in MM, either by epidemiologic or animal studies, and even by clinical trials [2]. Several natural compounds from various plants, fungi and marine organisms have been shown to target epigenetic events underpinning tumorigenesis, such as DNA methylation, histone modifications (methylation, acetylation and phosphorylation), and non-coding RNAs [3], known to be deeply dysregulated and representing valuable therapeutic targets in MM [2].

Polyphenols are important constituents of several plants and vegetables, recognized as powerful anti-oxidants endowed with anti-inflammatory, antimicrobial and antitumor activities [4]. Indeed, a major source of polyphenols is represented by extra virgin olive oil (EVOO), whose polyphenolic fraction includes simple phenols (tyrosol and hydroxytyrosol), secoiridoids (oleuropein, oleocanthal and oleacein), and lignans. EVOO-derived secoiridoids, characterized by the presence of elenoic acid or its derivatives in their molecular structure, have been shown to prevent obesity, osteoporosis, and neurodegeneration. Oleocanthal has shown anti-tumor activity in different types of tumors, including MM, hepatocellular carcinoma, breast, prostate, pancreatic cancers and melanoma [5–9]. The most abundant secoiridoid of EVOO is the dialdehydic form of elenolic acid conjugated with 3,4-(dihydroxyphenyl)ethanol (3,4-DHPEA-EDA), also known as oleacein, whose anti-oxidant, anti-inflammatory, and anti-microbial properties have recently emerged [10], while its effects on tumor biology are still poorly defined.

We here aimed to investigate the anti-tumor potential of oleacein against MM. Our results highlight a previously unknown epigenetic impact of oleacein on MM cells, with potential implications for the management of MM and possibly other malignancies.

2. Results

2.1. *Inhibitory Effects of Oleacein on MM Cell Viability and Survival*

Oleacein, whose chemical structure is reported in Figure 1A, was obtained by a green semi-synthetic modification of oleuropein as previously reported [11]. By using a panel of eight different MM cell lines carrying the major cytogenetic aberrations of MM, we sought to analyze the impact of oleacein on cell viability. MM cells were exposed to increasing doses of oleacein, and cell viability was assessed by Cell Titer Glo (CTG) assay. Noteworthy, a dose-dependent inhibition of cell viability was observed 48 h after oleacein treatment, with IC50s ranging from 5.0 to 20.0 μM (Figure 1B); conversely, oleacein did not affect the viability of PBMCs from healthy donors (Figure 1C), suggesting a favorable therapeutic index. We next evaluated the effects of oleacein on MM cells in the presence of the BM *milieu*, which is known to trigger drug-resistance [1]. Importantly, the inhibitory effect of oleacein was maintained even when MM cell lines, or primary $CD138^+$ cells purified from MM patients, were cultured in the presence of HS-5 stromal cells, thus suggesting that oleacein can overcome BM microenvironment-mediated pro-survival effects (Figure 1D). In addition, oleacein drastically suppressed the clonogenicity of MM cells in methylcellulose cultures (Figure 1E). Collectively, these data unveil an inhibitory activity of oleacein on MM cell viability and survival.

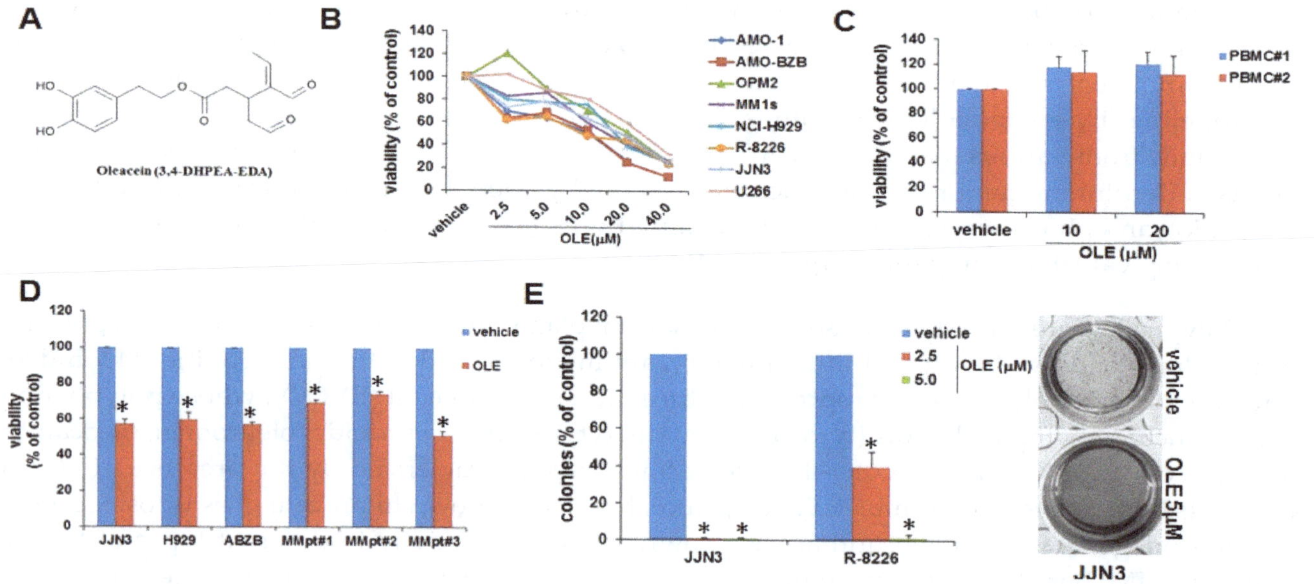

Figure 1. Effects of oleacein on multiple myeloma (MM) cell survival. (**A**) Chemical structure of oleacein. (**B**) Cell viability of MM cell lines as determined by Cell Titer Glo (CTG) assay 48 h after treatment with increasing doses of oleacein or vehicle (DMSO). (**C**) CTG assay performed on peripheral blood mononuclear cells (PBMCs) from three different healthy donors treated with oleacein for 48 h. (**D**) CTG assay in MM cell lines and primary CD138^{+} cells from three MM patients (MM pt#1, #2 and#3) co-cultured on HS-5 stromal cells and treated for 48 h with 5.0μM oleacein. (**E**) Colony formation assay performed on MM cell lines treated for 14 days with oleacein; representative pictures of JJN3 colonies at day 14 are shown in the right panel (5× magnification). * $p < 0.05$ as compared to vehicle-treated cells.

2.2. Oleacein Triggers Cell Cycle Arrest and Apoptosis

To unravel the biological sequelae of oleacein in MM, we first analyzed by flow cytometry the cell cycle profile of oleacein-treated cells after propidium iodide staining. As shown in Figure 2A, oleacein increased the percentage of hypodiploid cells (sub-G0 phase), and also induced the accumulation of cells in the G0/G1 phase; WB analysis showed a dose-dependent increase of cell cycle inhibitors $p27^{KIP1}$ and $p21^{CIP1}$ protein expression (Figure 2B), strengthening the capability of oleacein to trigger cell cycle blockade.

In order to confirm apoptosis induction, we performed Annexin V/7-AAD staining on MM cell lines after oleacein treatment. We found an increase in late apoptotic events, which ranged from 20 to 30% after treatment with oleacein 5.0 and 10.0 μM, respectively (Figure 2C); the increase in cleaved PARP1, caspase-3 and caspase-8 on oleacein-treated MM cell lines, as shown by Western Blot (WB), further confirmed apoptosis induction (Figure 2D); no activation of caspase-7 and -9 was observed (Supplementary Figure S1), thus indicating that oleacein predominantly activates the extrinsic apoptotic pathway. These results therefore indicate that oleacein may elicit anti-MM activity through modulation of cell cycle and apoptosis.

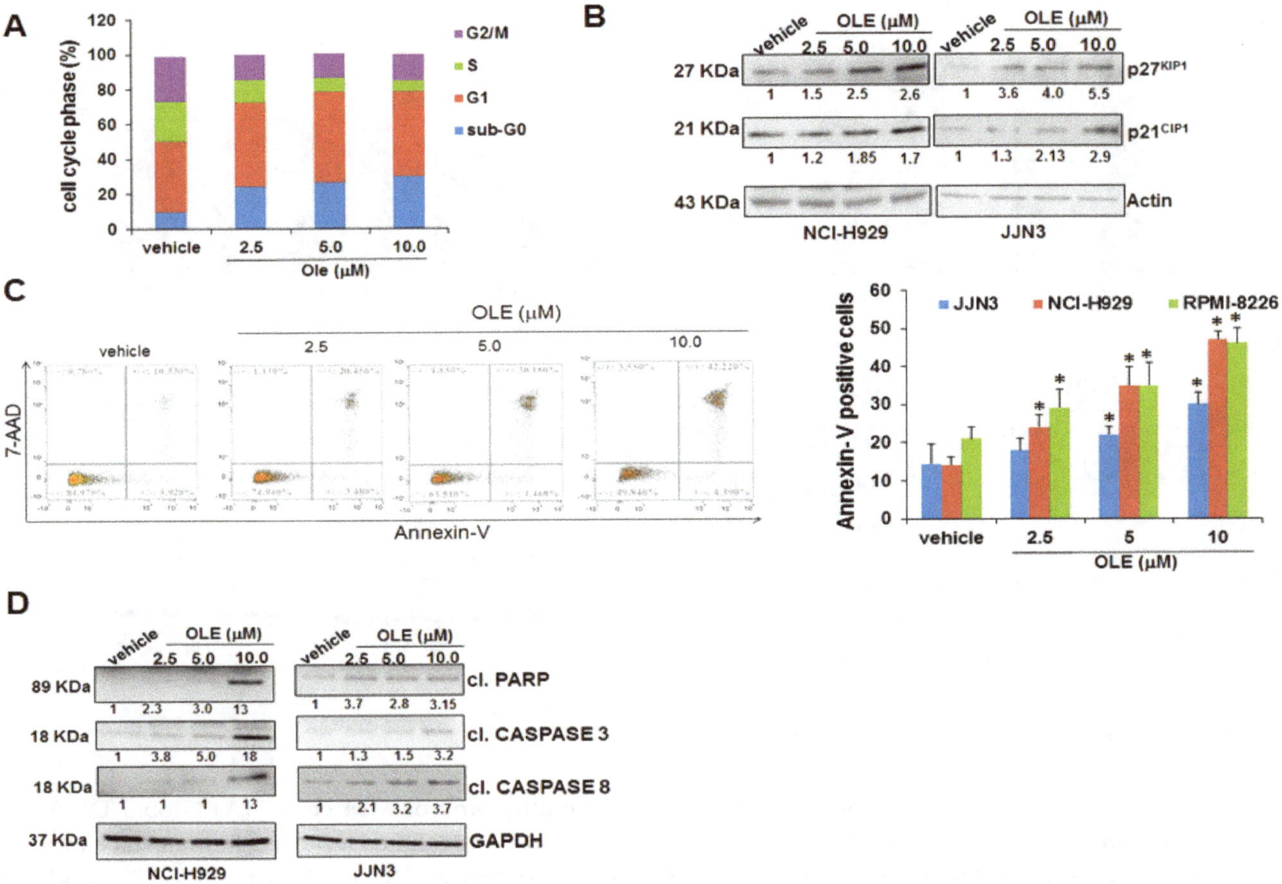

Figure 2. Oleacein triggers cell cycle blockade and apoptosis. (**A**) Cell cycle analysis was performed on NCI-H929 cells by PI staining, 24 h after treatment with oleacein or vehicle (DMSO). (**B**)Western Blot (WB) analysis of $p27^{KIP1}$ and $p21^{CIP1}$ in whole cell lysates from MM cells after treatment with oleacein for 24 h; actin was used as loading control. (**C**) Annexin V/7-AAD staining of MM cells after treatment with oleacein for 48 h; a representative experiment on NCI H929 cells is shown on the left side. (**D**) WB of PARP1, cleaved caspase-3 and cleaved caspase-8 in NCI-H929 and JJN3 cell lines after 24 h of oleacein treatment; GAPDH was used as loading control. * $p < 0.05$ as compared to vehicle-treated cells.

2.3. HDAC Inhibitory Activity of Oleacein in MM

Aberrant epigenetic patterns are common in MM, where they are frequently associated with disease onset and/or progression to advanced stages [12–14]. A large body of literature has highlighted the capability of several natural compounds to revert the altered epigenome of MM cells by counteracting key oncogenic epigenetic regulators [2]. On this basis, we investigated the epigenetic impact of oleacein on MM cells, by analyzing its effects both on global DNA methylation (GDM) and histone acetylation, the two major epigenetic mechanisms dysregulated in MM. Oleacein did not significantly modify the whole content of methylated cytosines in DNA from NCI-H929 and JJN3 cell lines (Figure 3A); in line with the latter finding, no significant changes in mRNA or protein levels of DNA methyltransferases (DNMT1, DNMT3A and DNMT3B) were observed upon oleacein treatment, as shown by QRT-PCR (Figure 3B) and WB analyses (Figure 3C). Conversely, oleacein induced a significant increase in acetylated histone H3, histone H4 (Figure 3D) and α-tubulin (Figure 3E). Collectively, these findings suggest that oleacein is able to modulate the acetylome of MM cells.

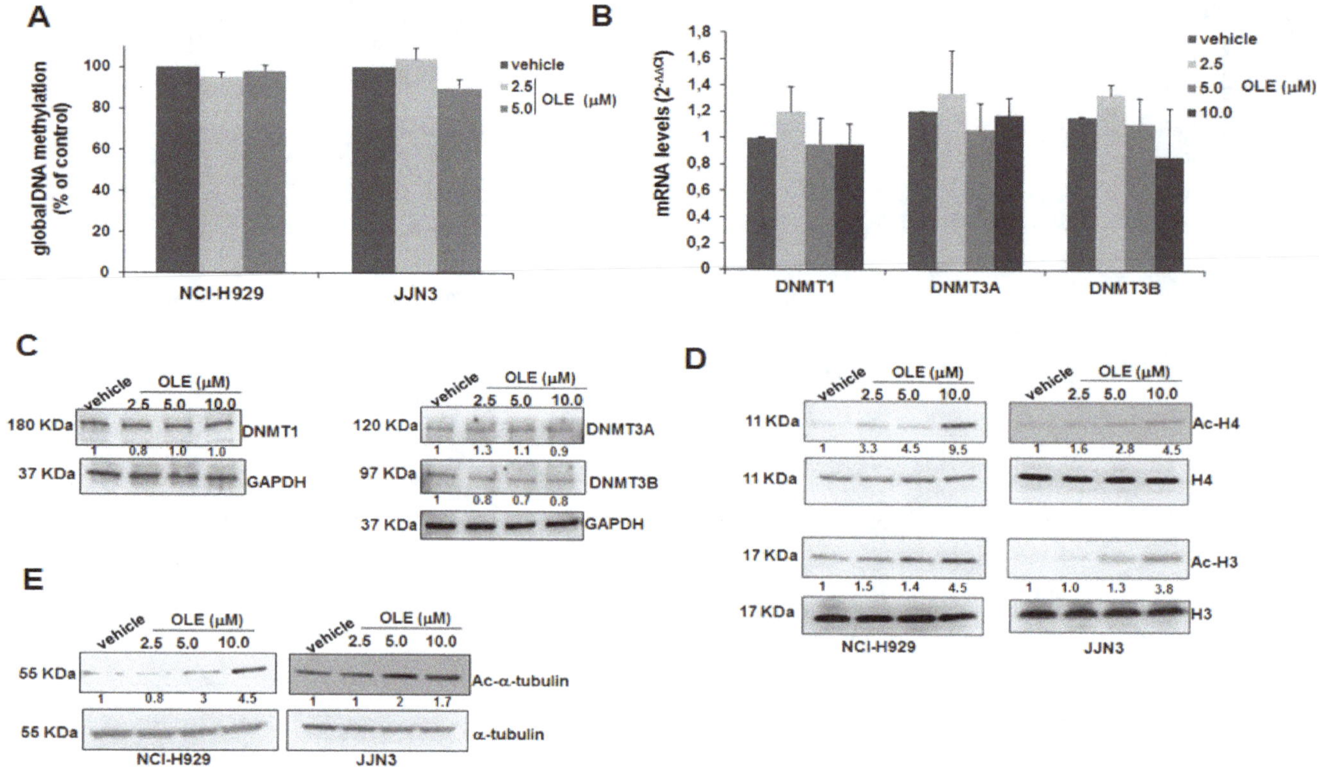

Figure 3. Oleacein affects the acetylome but not the methylome of MM cells. (**A**) Global DNA methylation was measured in MM cells treated for 24 h with oleacein, as reported in materials and methods. Quantitative Real Time PCR (QRT-PCR) (**B**) and WB analysis (**C**) of DNMT1, DNMT3A and DNMT3B in JJN3 cells treated for 24 h with oleacein; GAPDH was used as loading control. WB analysis of acetylated histone H3, histone H3, acetylated histone H4, histone H4 (**D**) and acetylated α-tubulin (**E**) in NCI-H929 and JJN3 cells treated with oleacein for 24 h; GAPDH was used as loading control.

Aberrant expression and/or activity of HDACs drive malignant transformation of tumor cells, thus making HDACs valuable therapeutic targets in MM [13,15]. We analyzed, in oleacein-treated JJN3 cells, the mRNA and protein expression of HDACs with established oncogenic role in MM. Intriguingly, oleacein induced down-regulation of several class I/II HDACs, namely HDAC1/2/3/4/6, both at mRNA (Figure 4A) and protein level (Figure 4B); moreover, biochemical fractionation experiments indicated that oleacein reduced both the nuclear and the cytoplasmic fraction of class II HDAC4 and HDAC6, which are known to shuttle between the nucleus and the cytoplasm (Figure 4C). To understand whether oleacein could act as a canonic HDAC inhibitor, we carried out an in vitro HDAC activity assay using JJN3 nuclear extracts. Incubation with oleacein did not induce any change in the HDAC activity recovered from nuclear extracts, differently from trichostatin A (TSA) or SAHA (Supplementary Figure S2), that were used as positive controls. This finding suggests that the impact of oleacein on the acetylome of MM cells does not occur via enzymatic HDAC inhibition. We therefore explored additional mechanisms accounting for oleacein effects on HDACs, and hypothesized that oleacein could transcriptionally regulate HDACs *via* Sp1. In fact, Sp1, a ubiquitous transcription factor endowed with oncogenic activity in hematologic and solid malignancies [12,13,16,17], was proven to act as a transcriptional activator of HDACs [18]. Interestingly, oleacein treatment induced down-regulation of Sp1 (Figure 4D), and this effect occurred in a caspase 8-dependent fashion, since it was abrogated by Z-IETD-FMK, a selective caspase 8 inhibitor (Figure 4E). These results indicate that oleacein effects on HDACs expression might be mediated by Sp1.

Sp1 is involved in negative feedback loops with miRNAs, like miR-29b [19–21] and miR-22 [22], both acting as tumor suppressors in MM [23,24]. As expected, oleacein-induced Sp1 inhibition was paralleled by the upregulation of miR-29b and miR-22 (Supplementary Figure S3), thus strengthening the role of Sp1 pathway's inhibition in the anti-MM activity of oleacein.

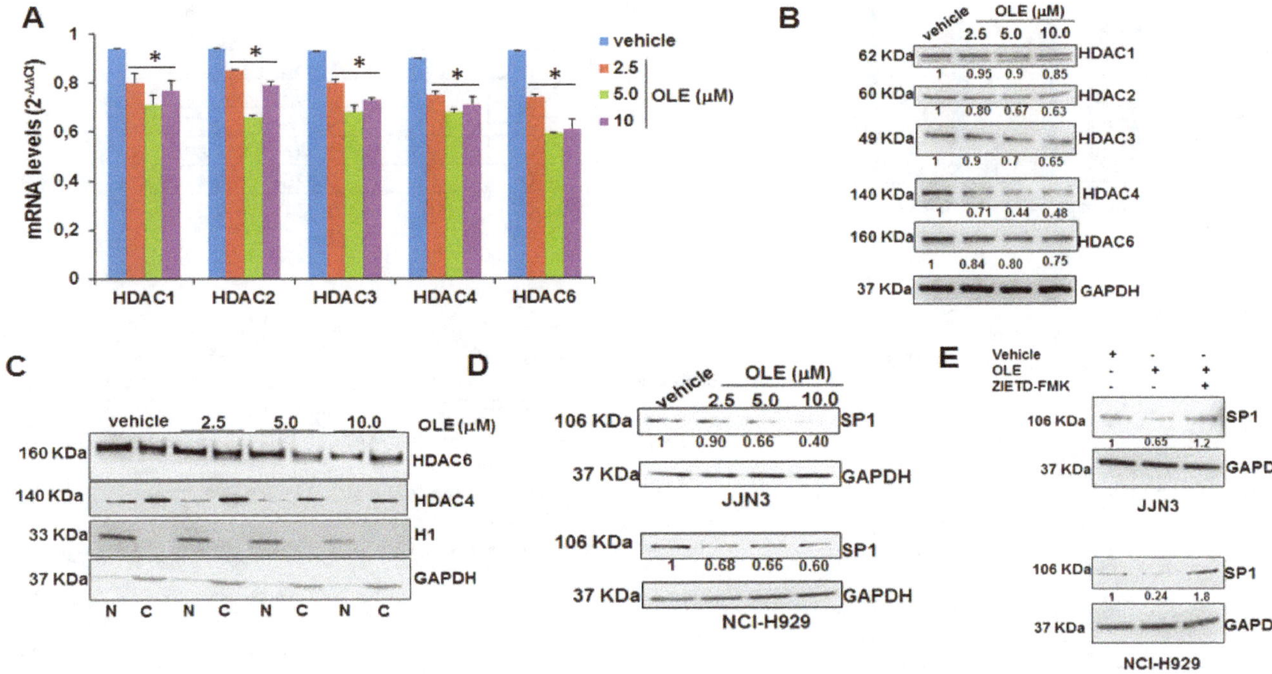

Figure 4. Oleacein targets HDACs. QRT-PCR (**A**) and WB analysis (**B**) of HDAC1, HDAC2, HDAC3, HDAC4, HDAC6 in JJN3 cells treated with oleacein for 24 h; GAPDH was used as loading control. (**C**) WB analysis of HDAC4 and HDAC6 in nuclear (N) and cytoplasmic (C) protein fractions from JJN3 cells treated for 24 h with oleacein; histone H1 and GAPDH were used as nuclear and cytoplasmic marker, respectively. (**D**) WB analysis of Sp1 in JJN3 cells treated with oleacein for 24 h. (**E**) WB analysis of Sp1 in JJN3 cells treated with 5.0 μM oleacein with or without 20.0 μM Z-ITED-FMK; GAPDH was used as loading control. * $p < 0.05$ as compared to vehicle-treated cells.

2.4. Oleacein Enhances the Anti-MM Activity of Carfilzomib

HDAC inhibitors (HDACi) are part of the therapeutic armamentarium against MM, and clinical studies have shown promising therapeutic activity of pan- or selective-HDACi when used within combination regimens [13]. On this basis, we investigated whether, similarly to pan-HDACi, oleacein treatment could trigger synergistic anti-MM activity in combination with clinically-relevant proteasome inhibitors. With this aim, NCI-H929 cells were treated with different concentrations of oleacein with or without bortezomib or carfilzomib, and subsequently cell viability was analyzed by CTG; the occurrence of synergism was assessed by Calcusyn. Interestingly, oleacein synergistically enhanced the effects of carfilzomib (CI < 1.0) on the inhibition of cell viability (Figure 5A), while combination with bortezomib was generally antagonistic (CI > 1.0; Supplementary Figure S4). Annexin V-7AAD staining of NCI-H929-treated cells indicated a higher apoptotic rate when oleacein was combined with carfilzomib, as compared to single agent treatment (Figure 5B). Accordingly, WB analysis showed increased cleavage of caspase 3 and superior Sp1 downregulation upon oleacein *plus* carfilzomib combination, thus confirming enhancement of apoptosis; moreover, oleacein *plus* carfilzomib enhanced downregulation of HDAC2, HDAC3, HDAC4 and HDAC6, with respect to single-agent treatment, which associated with increased histone H4 acetylation (Figure 5C). Collectively, these results indicate that the combination of olecein with carfilzomib results in significant acetylome derangement and apoptosis triggering of MM cells.

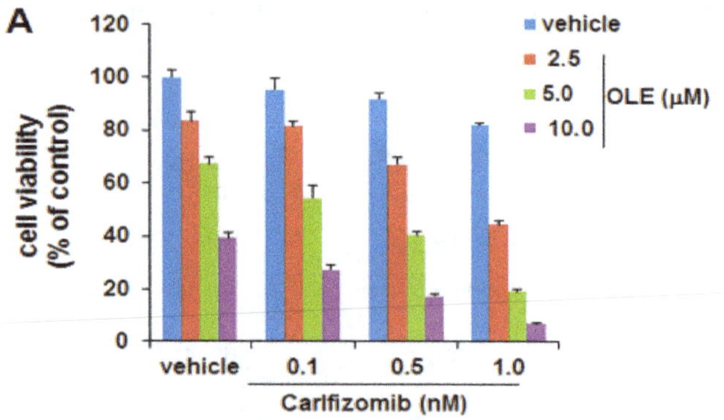

Oleacein	Carfilzomib	Fa	CI
2.5	0.1	0.184	**0.94**
2.5	0.5	0.328	**0.66**
2.5	1	0.555	**0.38**
5.0	0.1	0.456	**0.74**
5.0	0.5	0.596	**0.54**
5.0	1	0.81	**0.27**
10.0	0.1	0.724	**0.68**
10.0	0.5	0.825	**0.47**
10.0	1	0.931	**0.23**

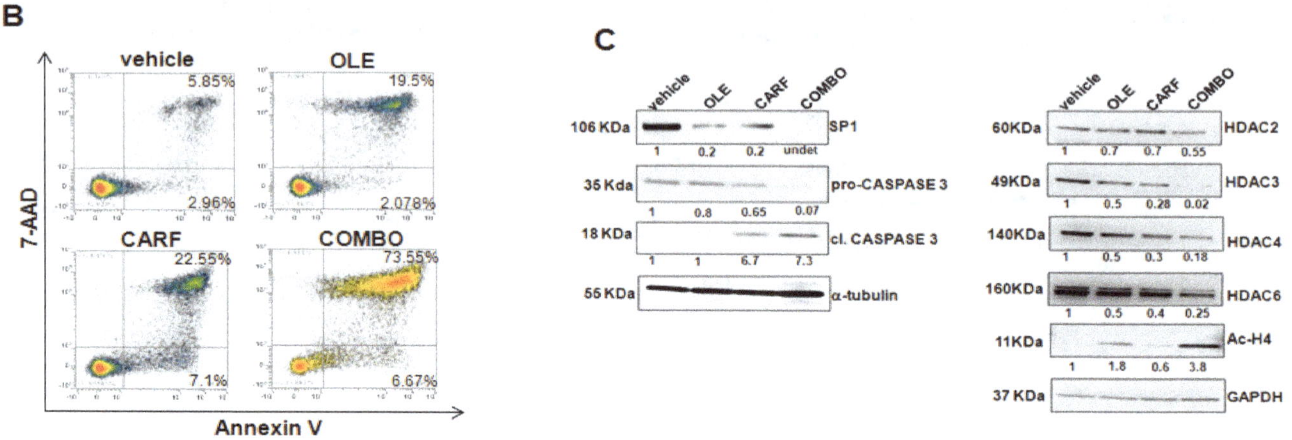

Figure 5. Oleacein enhances the anti-MM activity of carfilzomib. (**A**) CTG assay was performed on NCI-H929 cells treated with oleacein (2.5, 5.0 or 10.0 μM) and carfilzomib (0.1, 0.5 and 1.0 nM). Results are expressed as percentage of the viability of vehicle-treated cells. The right panel reports values of fraction affected (Fa) and combination indexes (CI) in a triplicate experiment, as calculated by the Calcusyn software. (**B**) Annexin V/7-AAD staining of NCI-H929 cells after treatment with vehicle (DMSO), 5.0 μM oleacein and 1.0 nM carfilzomib for 24 h; a representative FACS experiment is reported. (**C**). WB analysis of pro-Caspase 3, cleaved caspase 3, SP1, HDAC2, HDAC3, HDAC4, HDAC6, and acetylated histone H4 in NCI-H929 cells treated with carfilzomib (1.0 nM), oleacein (5.0 μM) or a combination of the two; α-tubulin or GAPDH were used as loading controls.

3. Discussion

Naturally occurring compounds endowed with anti-tumor activity have been found in different sources, such as vegetables, fruits, herbs and fermented products. These agents may act either by preventing the onset of primary cancer, or by antagonizing the evolution of pre-malignant and malignant lesions towards more aggressive stages. Noteworthy, experimental findings on a variety of natural compounds, including curcumin, resveratrol, celastrol and many others, have demonstrated significant advantages for the management of MM [2]. The molecular mechanisms underlying the anti-tumor activity of such compounds are diverse and only partially understood, with inhibition of oncogenic signal transduction pathways and modulation of the cellular epigenome being the most well documented. Regarding the epigenetic-modulating effects, it has been demonstrated that several natural agents, by targeting DNMTs [25], HDACs [26] or non-coding-RNAs [27], may revert aberrant epigenetic patterns implicated in the pathogenesis of human neoplasias, including MM [2].

Polyphenols found in the EVOO, a major component of mediterranean diet, have demonstrated to be protective against several diseases, including those of cardiovascular and metabolic origin [28]. The pro-active ingredient oleuropein and its derivative hydroxytyrosol have been widely studied, demonstrating many beneficial effects, both in vitro and in vivo, in experimental preclinical models [29]. Moreover, many studies have disclosed remarkable anti-tumor activity of oleuropein and hydroxytyrosol against several types of cancers [30]. However, the amount of oleuropein in the EVOO is too low to fully explain the beneficial effects deriving from EVOO assumption with diet. In fact, the endogenous β-glucosidase released during the olive oil extraction process hydrolyzes oleuropein, generating a series of degradation products, all of which are less hydrophilic than the original natural secoiridoids, and therefore more soluble in the oily matrix extracted from the drupes. Thus, EVOO is scarce in oleuropein and much more abundant in its degradation product oleacein [31], thus making it one of the most plausible effectors of the biological activity of EVOO [11,32].

Oleacein can be obtained by a simple and environmentally friendly method, starting from the easily available natural oleuropein [11]. Recent preclinical studies have highlighted anti-microbial [33], anti-inflammatory [34], and protective effects of oleacein against diet-dependent metabolic alterations [35]; conversely, its anti-antitumor activity remains poorly characterized. We here provided the first evidence of the anti-tumor activity of oleacein against MM cells: importantly, oleacein triggered cell cycle arrest and apoptosis and reduced clonogenicity, without exerting any toxic effect on healthy PBMCs, thus suggesting a favorable therapeutic index of this agent. Moreover, oleacein cytotoxic effects were also observed against primary MM cells co-cultured with BM-derived stromal cells, demonstrating the capability of oleacein to overcome BM microenvironment-dependent drug resistance.

We sought to shed light on the molecular mechanisms underlying oleacein anti-tumor activity in MM. To this aim, we focused on epigenetic mechanisms, known to be a major target of several natural agents, and whose dysregulation has been largely implicated in the pathogenesis of MM [14]. Indeed, aberrant expression of effectors of the epigenetic machinery, including DNMTs [36], HDACs [13], polycomb genes [37,38] and non-coding RNAs [39,40], has been reported in MM and has been harnessed in the context of novel anti-tumor strategies [41].

Collectively, our data indicate a strong increase in acetylation of histones and of α-acetyl-tubulin upon oleacein treatment, while no effect on GDM could be observed. This finding highlights a novel HDAC inhibitory activity of oleacein in MM. We attempted to characterize the mechanisms underlying such HDAC inhibitory effects, and found out that oleacein could transcriptionally inhibit HDACs expression likely *via* targeting of Sp1, a known transactivator of HDACs' promoter. Since previous findings indicated that bortezomib-evoked transcriptional repression of HDACs by Sp1 occurs in a caspase 8-dependent fashion [18], we investigated whether oleacein effect on Sp1 could be similarly mediated by caspase 8. In agreement with this hypothesis, oleacein-induced Sp1 down-regulation was abrogated by the caspase 8 inhibitor Z-IETD-FMK.

Dysregulated transcription factors may drive down-regulation of tumor suppressor miRNAs in MM [12,40,42]. By establishing molecular feedback loops, Sp1, a pleiotropic transcription factor endowed with oncogenic activity in human malignancies [17], was shown to negatively affect the expression of miRNAs [40]. We have previously reported that miRNA dysregulation features prominently in the pathobiology of MM, with certain miRNAs, such as miR-125a-5p [43], miR-21 [44], miR-221 [45] and miR-17-92 cluster [46], highly expressed in MM and acting as oncogenes, while others such as miR-29b [20], miR-22 [24] and miR-125b [47], behave as tumor suppressors.

Consistent with inhibition of Sp1, oleacein triggered upregulation of tumor suppressive miRNAs, namely miR-29b [20] and miR-22 [24], which are known to be negatively regulated by this transcription factor [19,22]. These findings underscore the ability of oleacein to trigger a tumor suppressive miRNA network likely contributing to its cytotoxicity against MM cells.

Non-selective HDAC inhibitors, such as romidepsin, vorinostat and panobinostat, have shown a remarkable anti-MM effect in preclinical and clinical studies, with significant efficacy, along with reduced side effects, when given within combination regimens [13]; amongst pan-HDACi, panobinostat has been approved by FDA for MM treatment [48]. Having demonstrated its pan-HDAC inhibitory activity, and taking into account the promising clinical data which emerged from MM patients treated with proteasome inhibitors and pan-HDACi combination therapies, we also explored whether oleacein could enhance the anti-tumor activity of bortezomib or carfilzomib. Notably, when combined with carfilzomib, oleacein synergistically enhanced its in vitro cytotoxicity, with superior Sp1 and HDACs down-regulation and a resultant increase in apoptosis of MM cells. A follow-up investigation is planned to evaluate the anti-tumor effect of oleacein-based treatments in the context of validated in vivo preclinical models of human MM.

4. Materials and Methods

4.1. Chemicals

A green semi-synthetic procedure was carried out to purify oleacein from Coratina cultivar olive leaves of Olea Europaea L. as reported; in detail, oleacein was directly extracted from a water solution of oleuropein in the presence of NaCl under microwave assistance at 180 °C; the crude extract was purified by flash chromatography on silica gel (eluent mixture: $CHCl_3$/MeOH 95:5 v/v) [49]. The purity was determined by RP-HPLC, HRMS-ESI, ^{1}H-and ^{13}C-NMR, as previously reported [11]. Bortezomib and carfilzomib were purchased from Selleckchem (Houston, TX, USA) as DMSO stock-solutions.

4.2. Cell Cultures

MM cell lines NCI-H929, RPMI-8226, U266, MM1s and JJN3 were purchased from DSMZ, which certified authentication performed by short tandem repeat DNA typing; the bone marrow stromal cell line HS-5 was purchased from the American Type Culture Collection (Rockville, MD, USA); AMO-1 and AMO-BZB cells were kindly provided by Dr. C. Driessen (University of Tubingen, Tubingen, Germany). The most relevant characteristics of the MM cell lines used are reported in Supplementary Table S1. All these cell lines were immediately frozen and used from the original stock within 6 months. Human MM cell lines were cultured in RPMI-1640 media containing 10% FBS, 2 μmol/L glutamine, 100 U/mL penicillin, and 100 μg/mL streptomycin (GIBCO; Life Technologies, Carlsbad, CA, USA) and tested for mycoplasma contamination. Peripheral blood mononuclear cells (PBMCs) and CD138^{+} cells from BM of MM patients were isolated by Ficoll-hypaque (Lonza Group, Basel, Switzerland), followed by anti-CD138 microbeads (Miltenyi Biotec, Bergish Gladbach, Germany) selection, in accordance with the Declaration of Helsinki following informed consent and Institutional Review Board (University of Catanzaro, Catanzaro, Italy) approval, as previously reported (institutional approval: n.120/2015) [50]; the purity of immunoselected cells was assessed by flow cytometry using a phycoerythrin-conjugated CD138 monoclonal antibody (BD Pharmingen, San Jose, CA, USA; clone DL-101) and was higher than 95%. In co-culture experiments, primary CD138^{+} MM cells (2.5×10^5 cells) were plated in 24-well plates, and left separated from HS-5 stromal cells (2.5×10^5 cells) growing adherent to the plate by a transwell insert of 0.4 μm pore size (Corning, New York, NY, USA).

4.3. Cell Viability, Apoptosis and Cell Cycle Assay

Cell viability was evaluated by Cell Titer-Glo (CTG; Promega, Madison, Wisconsin, USA), as previously reported [12]. For colony formation assay, 200 cells were plated in triplicate in 1 mL of mixture composed of 1.1% methylcellulose (MethoCult™ STEMCELL Technologies, Cambridge, UK) in RPMI-1640 + 10% FBS. Crystal violet-stained colonies were scored after 2 weeks under an inverted microscope (Leica DM IL LED, Wetzlar, Germany) at 5× magnification using a grid. Apoptosis was evaluated by flow cytometric (FACS) analysis following Annexin V-7AAD staining (BD Pharmingen, San Jose, CA, USA). Drug interactions were assessed by CalcuSyn 2.0 software (Biosoft, Novosibirsk, Russia), which is based on the Chou-Talalay method. When combination index (CI) = 1, this equation represents the conservation isobologram and indicates additive effects; CI < 1 indicates synergism; CI > 1 indicates antagonism. Cell cycle distribution was evaluated by FACS analysis on MM cells previously treated with oleacein for 24 h, after staining with Propidium Iodide (PI). Cells were collected, washed twice with phosphate-buffered saline (PBS) and fixed in cold 70% ethanol at −20 °C. Before FACS analysis, cells were washed with PBS and stained in 50 μg/mL PI, 100 μg/mL RNase, 0.05% Nonidet P-40 for 1 h at room temperature in the dark. Cell cycle profiles were obtained using Attune NxT Flow Cytometer (Thermo Fisher Scientific, Waltham, MA, USA).

4.4. Western Blot and Antibodies

Whole cell protein extracts were prepared using NP40 lysis buffer containing Halt Protease Inhibitor cocktail (Invitrogen, Thermo Scientific, Carlsbad, CA, USA), separated using 4–12% Novex Bis-Tris SDS-acrylamide gels (Invitrogen), and electrotransferred on nitrocellulose membranes (Bio-Rad, Hercules, CA, USA), as described [39]. Then, nitrocellulose membranes were blocked with milk and probed over-night with primary antibodies at 4 °C; then membranes were washed three times in PBS-Tween and incubated with a secondary antibody conjugated with horseradish peroxidase for 2 h at room temperature. Chemiluminescence was detected using SuperSignal West Pico PLUS Chemiluminescent Substrate (Thermo Scientific). Western blot (WB) was performed using Cell Signaling antibodies: PARP (#9532), -Caspase-8 (#9746), -Caspase-3 (#9665), AcH3-Lysin 8 (K9) (#9649P), SP1 (#9389S), HDAC1 (#5356T), HDAC2 (#5113P), HDAC3 (3949P), HDAC4 (#7628S), HDAC6 (#7558P), histone H4 (#2935), histone H3 (#4499), α-tubulin (#2125). Ac-α tubulin (sc-23950), Ac-H4 Ser1/Lys 5/Lys8/Lys Lys 12 (sc-34263), Actin (sc-1616) and -GAPDH (sc-25778) were from Santa Cruz Biotechnology (Dallas, TX, USA); Dnmt1 (ab 13537), Dnmt3a (ab 13888) and Dnmt3b (ab 2851) were from abcam (Cambridge, UK). Densitometric analysis of blots was performed by LI-COR Image Studio Digits Ver 5.0 (Bad Homburg, Germany), expressed as a relative protein unit after normalization with appropriate housekeeping, and reported under each blot. Whole blots of all experiments presented in this study are reported as Supplementary Figures S5–S9.

4.5. Reverse Transcription and Quantitative Real Time PCR (qRT-PCR)

Total RNA was extracted from cells using TRIzol® reagent (Gibco, Life Technologies, Carlsbad, CA, USA), following the manufacturer's instructions. The RNA quantity and quality were assessed through NanoDrop® ND-1000 Spectrophotometer (Waltham, MA, USA). To evaluate transcript changes, 1000 ng of total RNA was reverse-transcribed to cDNA using the "High Capacity cDNA Reverse Transcription Kit" (Applied Biosystems, Carlsbad, CA, USA). The following single-tube TaqMan assays (Applied Biosystems, Carlsbad, CA, USA) were used to detect and quantify genes using the Viia7 DX real time PCR instrument (Life Technologies, Waltham, MA, USA): DNMT1 (Hs00154749_m1), DNMT3a (Hs01027166_m1), DNMT3b (Hs00171876_m1), HDAC1 (Hs02621185_s1), HDAC2 (Hs00231032_m1), HDAC3 (Hs00187320_m1), HDAC4 (Hs01041638_m1), HDAC6 (Hs00195869_m1), and GAPDH (Hs02786624 g1). miRNA expression levels were determined by TaqMan RT-PCR, using the single-tube TaqMan miRNA assays (hsa-miR-29b, assay ID 000413; hsa-miR-22, assay ID 000398, Applied Biosystems) to quantify mature miRNAs, by the use of the StepOne Thermocycler (Thermo Fisher Scientific, Waltham, MA, USA) and the sequence detection system, as previously reported [51]; miRNAs expression levels were normalized on RNU44 (assay ID 001094). Comparative real-time polymerase chain reaction (RT-PCR) was performed in triplicate.

4.6. HDAC Activity Assay

Nuclear extracts prepared using NE-PER Nuclear and Cytoplasmic Extraction Reagents kit (Thermo Scientific, catalog #78833) were mixed with Oleacein or DMSO, and then HDAC activity was determined according to the manufacturer's instructions (BioVision, Zurich, Switzerland; catalog #K331-100). Trichostatin A (TSA) and SAHA were used as positive controls.

4.7. Quantification of Global 5-Methylcytosine Levels

Global DNA methylation levels were determined by using 5-mC DNA ELISA kit (Zymo Research, Irvine, CA, USA) as described [52]. Briefly, 100ng of genomic DNA, brought to final volume to 100 μL with 5-mC coating buffer, was denatured at 98 °C for 5min, put in ice for 10′ and then coated on the surface of the ELISA plate wells. After incubation at 37 °C for 1 h, the wells were washed thrice with 200 μL of 5-mC ELISA buffer and then incubated at 37 °C for 1 h with an antibody mix consisting of anti-5-mC (1:2000) and secondary (1:1000) antibodies. Then, the antibody mix was removed from the wells through three consecutive washes with 200μL of 5-mC ELISA buffer. One-hundred microliters of HRP developer was added to each well and incubated at room temperature for 1 h. Absorbance at 405nm was measured using an ELISA plate reader. The percentage of 5-mC was calculated using the second-order regression equation of the standard curve that was constructed by using mixtures of the fully unmethylated and methylated control DNAs, provided by the manufacturer, to generate standards of known 5-mC percentage (0, 5, 10, 25, 50, 75 and 100%).

4.8. Statistical Analysis

Each experiment was performed at least three times, and values were reported as mean ± standard deviation. Data were analyzed using Student's t tests for two group comparisons or a one-way analysis of variance (ANOVA) for multiple comparisons using the Graphpad software (GraphPad Software, La Jolla, CA, USA). p-value < 0.05 was considered significant.

5. Conclusions

Our results indicate that oleacein, the most abundant EVOO secoiridoid, elicits significant anti-tumor activity by promoting cell cycle arrest and apoptosis, either as a single agent or in combination with the proteasome inhibitor carfilzomib. Moreover, our data highlight an epigenetic impact of oleacein in MM, as demonstrated by the impairment of the MM acetylome, likely *via* Sp1-dependent transcriptional inhibition of HDACs. Altogether, these findings provide the molecular rationale for potential epi-therapeutic anti-MM strategies based on natural agents.

Supplementary Materials:
Figure S1: WB of pro-caspase 7, cleaved caspase 7, pro-caspase 9 and cleaved caspase 9 in NCI-H929 cells after 24 h of oleacein treatment, Figure S2: HDAC activity was determined in JJN3 cells treated with oleacein, as reported in materials and methods; TSA was used as positive control. Results are expressed as percentage of HDAC activity as compared to DMSO-treated cells, Figure S3: miR-29b and miR-22 expression levels were determined by qRT-PCR in JJN3 cells treated for 24 h with oleacein; miRNA expression was normalized on RNU44, Figure S4: CTG assay was performed on NCI-H929 cells treated with oleacein (2.5, 5.0 or 10.0 μM) and bortezomib (1.0, 2.0 and 5.0 nM). Results are expressed as percentage of the viability of vehicle-treated cells. The right panel reports values of fraction affected (Fa) and combination indexes (CI) in a triplicate experiment, as calculated by the Calcusyn software, Figure S5: whole blots for Figure 2, Figure S6: whole blots for Figure 3, Figure S7: whole blots for Figure 4, Figure S8: whole blots for Figure 5, Figure S9: whole blots for Figure S1. Table S1: Characteristics of the MM cell lines used in this study.

Author Contributions: Data curation, K.G. and M.N.; Formal analysis, M.R.; Investigation, G.J., M.O., D.B. and N.A.; Methodology, M.E.G.C., G.P. and A.P.; Resources, P.T.; Software, C.C.; Writing—original draft, P.T. (Pierosandro Tagliaferri), P.T. (Pierfrancesco Tassone) and N.A.; Writing—review & editing, N.A.

Acknowledgments: We thank Ivana Criniti for editorial and laboratory assistances.

References

1. Anderson, K.C. Progress and Paradigms in Multiple Myeloma. *Clin. Cancer Res.* **2016**, *22*, 5419–5427. [CrossRef] [PubMed]
2. Raimondi, L.; De Luca, A.; Giavaresi, G.; Barone, A.; Tagliaferri, P.; Tassone, P.; Amodio, N. Impact of natural dietary agents on multiple myeloma prevention and treatment: Molecular insights and potential for clinical translation. *Curr. Med. Chem.* **2018**. [CrossRef] [PubMed]
3. Aggarwal, R.; Jha, M.; Shrivastava, A.; Jha, A.K. Natural Compounds: Role in Reversal of Epigenetic Changes. *Biochemistry* **2015**, *80*, 972–989. [CrossRef] [PubMed]
4. Pandey, K.B.; Rizvi, S.I. Plant polyphenols as dietary antioxidants in human health and disease. *Oxid. Med. Cell Longev.* **2009**, *2*, 270–278. [CrossRef] [PubMed]

5. Akl, M.R.; Elsayed, H.E.; Ebrahim, H.Y.; Haggag, E.G.; Kamal, A.M.; El Sayed, K.A. 3-O-[N-(p-fluorobenzenesulfonyl)-carbamoyl]-oleanolic acid, a semisynthetic analog of oleanolic acid, induces apoptosis in breast cancer cells. *Eur. J. Pharmacol.* **2014**, *740*, 209–217. [CrossRef] [PubMed]
6. Khanfar, M.A.; Bardaweel, S.K.; Akl, M.R.; El Sayed, K.A. Olive Oil-derived Oleocanthal as Potent Inhibitor of Mammalian Target of Rapamycin: Biological Evaluation and Molecular Modeling Studies. *Phytother. Res.* **2015**, *29*, 1776–1782. [CrossRef] [PubMed]
7. LeGendre, O.; Breslin, P.A.; Foster, D.A. (-)-Oleocanthal rapidly and selectively induces cancer cell death via lysosomal membrane permeabilization. *Mol. Cell. Oncol.* **2015**, *2*, e1006077. [CrossRef] [PubMed]
8. Scotece, M.; Gomez, R.; Conde, J.; Lopez, V.; Gomez-Reino, J.J.; Lago, F.; Smith, A.B., 3rd; Gualillo, O. Oleocanthal inhibits proliferation and MIP-1alpha expression in human multiple myeloma cells. *Curr. Med. Chem.* **2013**, *20*, 2467–2475. [CrossRef] [PubMed]
9. Fogli, S.; Arena, C.; Carpi, S.; Polini, B.; Bertini, S.; Digiacomo, M.; Gado, F.; Saba, A.; Saccomanni, G.; Breschi, M.C.; et al. Cytotoxic Activity of Oleocanthal Isolated from Virgin Olive Oil on Human Melanoma Cells. *Nutr. Cancer* **2016**, *68*, 873–877. [CrossRef]
10. Naruszewicz, M.; Czerwinska, M.E.; Kiss, A.K. Oleacein. translation from Mediterranean diet to potential antiatherosclerotic drug. *Curr. Pharm. Des.* **2015**, *21*, 1205–1212. [CrossRef]
11. Costanzo, P.; Bonacci, S.; Cariati, L.; Nardi, M.; Oliverio, M.; Procopio, A. Simple and efficient sustainable semi-synthesis of oleacein [2-(3,4-hydroxyphenyl) ethyl (3S,4E)-4-formyl-3-(2-oxoethyl)hex-4-enoate] as potential additive for edible oils. *Food Chem.* **2018**, *245*, 410–414. [CrossRef] [PubMed]
12. Fulciniti, M.; Amodio, N.; Bandi, R.L.; Cagnetta, A.; Samur, M.K.; Acharya, C.; Prabhala, R.; D'Aquila, P.; Bellizzi, D.; Passarino, G.; et al. miR-23b/SP1/c-myc forms a feed-forward loop supporting multiple myeloma cell growth. *Blood Cancer J.* **2016**, *6*, e380. [CrossRef]
13. Cea, M.; Cagnetta, A.; Gobbi, M.; Patrone, F.; Richardson, P.G.; Hideshima, T.; Anderson, K.C. New insights into the treatment of multiple myeloma with histone deacetylase inhibitors. *Curr. Pharm. Des.* **2013**, *19*, 734–744. [CrossRef] [PubMed]
14. Amodio, N.; D'Aquila, P.; Passarino, G.; Tassone, P.; Bellizzi, D. Epigenetic modifications in multiple myeloma: Recent advances on the role of DNA and histone methylation. *Expert Opin. Ther. Targets* **2017**, *21*, 91–101. [CrossRef] [PubMed]
15. Imai, Y.; Hirano, M.; Kobayashi, M.; Futami, M.; Tojo, A. HDAC Inhibitors Exert Anti-Myeloma Effects through Multiple Modes of Action. *Cancers* **2019**, *11*. [CrossRef]
16. Fulciniti, M.; Amodio, N.; Bandi, R.L.; Munshi, M.; Yang, G.; Xu, L.; Hunter, Z.; Tassone, P.; Anderson, K.C.; Treon, S.P.; et al. MYD88-independent growth and survival effects of Sp1 transactivation in Waldenstrom macroglobulinemia. *Blood* **2014**, *123*, 2673–2681. [CrossRef]
17. Safe, S.; Abbruzzese, J.; Abdelrahim, M.; Hedrick, E. Specificity Protein Transcription Factors and Cancer: Opportunities for Drug Development. *Cancer Prev. Res.* **2018**, *11*, 371–382. [CrossRef]
18. Kikuchi, J.; Wada, T.; Shimizu, R.; Izumi, T.; Akutsu, M.; Mitsunaga, K.; Noborio-Hatano, K.; Nobuyoshi, M.; Ozawa, K.; Kano, Y.; et al. Histone deacetylases are critical targets of bortezomib-induced cytotoxicity in multiple myeloma. *Blood* **2010**, *116*, 406–417. [CrossRef]
19. Amodio, N.; Di Martino, M.T.; Foresta, U.; Leone, E.; Lionetti, M.; Leotta, M.; Gulla, A.M.; Pitari, M.R.; Conforti, F.; Rossi, M.; et al. miR-29b sensitizes multiple myeloma cells to bortezomib-induced apoptosis through the activation of a feedback loop with the transcription factor Sp1. *Cell Death Dis.* **2012**, *3*, e436. [CrossRef]
20. Amodio, N.; Stamato, M.A.; Gulla, A.M.; Morelli, E.; Romeo, E.; Raimondi, L.; Pitari, M.R.; Ferrandino, I.; Misso, G.; Caraglia, M.; et al. Therapeutic Targeting of miR-29b/HDAC4 Epigenetic Loop in Multiple Myeloma. *Mol. Cancer Ther.* **2016**, *15*, 1364–1375. [CrossRef]
21. Amodio, N.; Rossi, M.; Raimondi, L.; Pitari, M.R.; Botta, C.; Tagliaferri, P.; Tassone, P. miR-29s: A family of epi-miRNAs with therapeutic implications in hematologic malignancies. *Oncotarget* **2015**, *6*, 12837–12861. [CrossRef] [PubMed]
22. Xia, S.S.; Zhang, G.J.; Liu, Z.L.; Tian, H.P.; He, Y.; Meng, C.Y.; Li, L.F.; Wang, Z.W.; Zhou, T. MicroRNA-22 suppresses the growth, migration and invasion of colorectal cancer cells through a Sp1 negative feedback loop. *Oncotarget* **2017**, *8*, 36266–36278. [CrossRef] [PubMed]

23. Raimondi, L.; De Luca, A.; Morelli, E.; Giavaresi, G.; Tagliaferri, P.; Tassone, P.; Amodio, N. MicroRNAs: Novel Crossroads between Myeloma Cells and the Bone Marrow Microenvironment. *Biomed. Res. Int.* **2016**, *2016*, 6504593. [CrossRef] [PubMed]
24. Caracciolo, D.; Di Martino, M.T.; Amodio, N.; Morelli, E.; Montesano, M.; Botta, C.; Scionti, F.; Talarico, D.; Altomare, E.; Gallo Cantafio, M.E.; et al. miR-22 suppresses DNA ligase III addiction in multiple myeloma. *Leukemia* **2019**, *33*, 487–498. [CrossRef] [PubMed]
25. Saldivar-Gonzalez, F.I.; Gomez-Garcia, A.; Chavez-Ponce de Leon, D.E.; Sanchez-Cruz, N.; Ruiz-Rios, J.; Pilon-Jimenez, B.A.; Medina-Franco, J.L. Inhibitors of DNA Methyltransferases From Natural Sources: A Computational Perspective. *Front. Pharmacol.* **2018**, *9*, 1144. [CrossRef]
26. Singh, A.K.; Bishayee, A.; Pandey, A.K. Targeting Histone Deacetylases with Natural and Synthetic Agents: An Emerging Anticancer Strategy. *Nutrients* **2018**, *10*. [CrossRef] [PubMed]
27. Huang, D.; Cui, L.; Ahmed, S.; Zainab, F.; Wu, Q.; Wang, X.; Yuan, Z. An overview of epigenetic agents and natural nutrition products targeting DNA methyltransferase, histone deacetylases and microRNAs. *Food Chem. Toxicol.* **2019**, *123*, 574–594. [CrossRef]
28. Bulotta, S.; Celano, M.; Lepore, S.M.; Montalcini, T.; Pujia, A.; Russo, D. Beneficial effects of the olive oil phenolic components oleuropein and hydroxytyrosol: Focus on protection against cardiovascular and metabolic diseases. *J. Transl. Med.* **2014**, *12*, 219. [CrossRef]
29. Barbaro, B.; Toietta, G.; Maggio, R.; Arciello, M.; Tarocchi, M.; Galli, A.; Balsano, C. Effects of the olive-derived polyphenol oleuropein on human health. *Int. J. Mol. Sci.* **2014**, *15*, 18508–18524. [CrossRef]
30. Fabiani, R. Anti-cancer properties of olive oil secoiridoid phenols: A systematic review of in vivo studies. *Food Funct.* **2016**, *7*, 4145–4159. [CrossRef]
31. Flemmig, J.; Rusch, D.; Czerwinska, M.E.; Rauwald, H.W.; Arnhold, J. Components of a standardised olive leaf dry extract (Ph. Eur.) promote hypothiocyanite production by lactoperoxidase. *Arch. Biochem. Biophys.* **2014**, *549*, 17–25. [CrossRef] [PubMed]
32. Nardi, M.; Bonacci, S.; De Luca, G.; Maiuolo, J.; Oliverio, M.; Sindona, G.; Procopio, A. Biomimetic synthesis and antioxidant evaluation of 3,4-DHPEA-EDA [2-(3,4-hydroxyphenyl) ethyl (3S,4E)-4 formyl-3-(2-oxoethyl)hex-4-enoate]. *Food Chem.* **2014**, *162*, 89–93. [CrossRef] [PubMed]
33. Koutsoni, O.S.; Karampetsou, K.; Kyriazis, I.D.; Stathopoulos, P.; Aligiannis, N.; Halabalaki, M.; Skaltsounis, L.A.; Dotsika, E. Evaluation of total phenolic fraction derived from extra virgin olive oil for its antileishmanial activity. *Phytomedicine* **2018**, *47*, 143–150. [CrossRef] [PubMed]
34. Filipek, A.; Czerwinska, M.E.; Kiss, A.K.; Wrzosek, M.; Naruszewicz, M. Oleacein enhances anti-inflammatory activity of human macrophages by increasing CD163 receptor expression. *Phytomedicine* **2015**, *22*, 1255–1261. [CrossRef] [PubMed]
35. Lombardo, G.E.; Lepore, S.M.; Morittu, V.M.; Arcidiacono, B.; Colica, C.; Procopio, A.; Maggisano, V.; Bulotta, S.; Costa, N.; Mignogna, C.; et al. Effects of Oleacein on High-Fat Diet-Dependent Steatosis, Weight Gain, and Insulin Resistance in Mice. *Front. Endocrinol.* **2018**, *9*, 116. [CrossRef] [PubMed]
36. Amodio, N.; Leotta, M.; Bellizzi, D.; Di Martino, M.T.; D'Aquila, P.; Lionetti, M.; Fabiani, F.; Leone, E.; Gulla, A.M.; Passarino, G.; et al. DNA-demethylating and anti-tumor activity of synthetic miR-29b mimics in multiple myeloma. *Oncotarget* **2012**, *3*, 1246–1258. [CrossRef]
37. Rizq, O.; Mimura, N.; Oshima, M.; Saraya, A.; Koide, S.; Kato, Y.; Aoyama, K.; Nakajima-Takagi, Y.; Wang, C.; Chiba, T.; et al. Dual Inhibition of EZH2 and EZH1 Sensitizes PRC2-Dependent Tumors to Proteasome Inhibition. *Clin. Cancer Res.* **2017**, *23*, 4817–4830. [CrossRef]
38. Stamato, M.A.; Juli, G.; Romeo, E.; Ronchetti, D.; Arbitrio, M.; Caracciolo, D.; Neri, A.; Tagliaferri, P.; Tassone, P.; Amodio, N. Inhibition of EZH2 triggers the tumor suppressive miR-29b network in multiple myeloma. *Oncotarget* **2017**, *8*, 106527–106537. [CrossRef]
39. Amodio, N.; Stamato, M.A.; Juli, G.; Morelli, E.; Fulciniti, M.; Manzoni, M.; Taiana, E.; Agnelli, L.; Cantafio, M.E.G.; Romeo, E.; et al. Drugging the lncRNA MALAT1 via LNA gapmeR ASO inhibits gene expression of proteasome subunits and triggers anti-multiple myeloma activity. *Leukemia* **2018**, *32*, 1948–1957. [CrossRef]
40. Amodio, N.; Di Martino, M.T.; Neri, A.; Tagliaferri, P.; Tassone, P. Non-coding RNA: A novel opportunity for the personalized treatment of multiple myeloma. *Expert Opin. Biol. Ther.* **2013**, *13*, S125–137. [CrossRef]

41. Rossi, M.; Amodio, N.; Di Martino, M.T.; Tagliaferri, P.; Tassone, P.; Cho, W.C. MicroRNA and multiple myeloma: From laboratory findings to translational therapeutic approaches. *Curr. Pharm. Biotechnol.* **2014**, *15*, 459–467. [CrossRef] [PubMed]
42. Calura, E.; Bisognin, A.; Manzoni, M.; Todoerti, K.; Taiana, E.; Sales, G.; Morgan, G.J.; Tonon, G.; Amodio, N.; Tassone, P.; et al. Disentangling the microRNA regulatory milieu in multiple myeloma: Integrative genomics analysis outlines mixed miRNA-TF circuits and pathway-derived networks modulated in t(4;14) patients. *Oncotarget* **2016**, *7*, 2367–2378. [CrossRef] [PubMed]
43. Leotta, M.; Biamonte, L.; Raimondi, L.; Ronchetti, D.; Di Martino, M.T.; Botta, C.; Leone, E.; Pitari, M.R.; Neri, A.; Giordano, A.; et al. A p53-dependent tumor suppressor network is induced by selective miR-125a-5p inhibition in multiple myeloma cells. *J. Cell. Physiol.* **2014**, *229*, 2106–2116. [CrossRef]
44. Pitari, M.R.; Rossi, M.; Amodio, N.; Botta, C.; Morelli, E.; Federico, C.; Gulla, A.; Caracciolo, D.; Di Martino, M.T.; Arbitrio, M.; et al. Inhibition of miR-21 restores RANKL/OPG ratio in multiple myeloma-derived bone marrow stromal cells and impairs the resorbing activity of mature osteoclasts. *Oncotarget* **2015**, *6*, 27343–27358. [CrossRef] [PubMed]
45. Gulla, A.; Di Martino, M.T.; Gallo Cantafio, M.E.; Morelli, E.; Amodio, N.; Botta, C.; Pitari, M.R.; Lio, S.G.; Britti, D.; Stamato, M.A.; et al. A 13 mer LNA-i-miR-221 Inhibitor Restores Drug Sensitivity in Melphalan-Refractory Multiple Myeloma Cells. *Clin. Cancer Res.* **2016**, *22*, 1222–1233. [CrossRef] [PubMed]
46. Morelli, E.; Biamonte, L.; Federico, C.; Amodio, N.; Di Martino, M.T.; Gallo Cantafio, M.E.; Manzoni, M.; Scionti, F.; Samur, M.K.; Gulla, A.; et al. Therapeutic vulnerability of multiple myeloma to MIR17PTi, a first-in-class inhibitor of pri-miR-17-92. *Blood* **2018**, *132*, 1050–1063. [CrossRef] [PubMed]
47. Morelli, E.; Leone, E.; Cantafio, M.E.; Di Martino, M.T.; Amodio, N.; Biamonte, L.; Gulla, A.; Foresta, U.; Pitari, M.R.; Botta, C.; et al. Selective targeting of IRF4 by synthetic microRNA-125b-5p mimics induces anti-multiple myeloma activity in vitro and in vivo. *Leukemia* **2015**, *29*, 2173–2183. [CrossRef]
48. Fenichel, M.P. FDA approves new agent for multiple myeloma. *J. Natl. Cancer Inst.* **2015**, *107*, djv165. [CrossRef]
49. Procopio, A.; Alcaro, S.; Nardi, M.; Oliverio, M.; Ortuso, F.; Sacchetta, P.; Pieragostino, D.; Sindona, G. Synthesis, biological evaluation, and molecular modeling of oleuropein and its semisynthetic derivatives as cyclooxygenase inhibitors. *J. Agric. Food Chem.* **2009**, *57*, 11161–11167. [CrossRef]
50. Amodio, N.; Gallo Cantafio, M.E.; Botta, C.; Agosti, V.; Federico, C.; Caracciolo, D.; Ronchetti, D.; Rossi, M.; Driessen, C.; Neri, A.; et al. Replacement of miR-155 Elicits Tumor Suppressive Activity and Antagonizes Bortezomib Resistance in Multiple Myeloma. *Cancers* **2019**, *11*. [CrossRef]
51. Di Sanzo, M.; Chirillo, R.; Aversa, I.; Biamonte, F.; Santamaria, G.; Giovannone, E.D.; Faniello, M.C.; Cuda, G.; Costanzo, F. shRNA targeting of ferritin heavy chain activates H19/miR-675 axis in K562 cells. *Gene* **2018**, *657*, 92–99. [CrossRef] [PubMed]
52. Guarasci, F.; D'Aquila, P.; Mandala, M.; Garasto, S.; Lattanzio, F.; Corsonello, A.; Passarino, G.; Bellizzi, D. Aging and nutrition induce tissue-specific changes on global DNA methylation status in rats. *Mech. Ageing Dev.* **2018**, *174*, 47–54. [CrossRef] [PubMed]

7

Molecular Insights into Potential Contributions of Natural Polyphenols to Lung Cancer Treatment

Qingyu Zhou [1,*], Hua Pan [2] and Jing Li [3]

[1] Department of Pharmaceutical Sciences, Taneja College of Pharmacy, University of South Florida, Tampa, FL 33612, USA
[2] Department of Cardiovascular Sciences, Mossani College of Medicine, University of South Florida, Tampa, FL 33612, USA; huapan@health.usf.edu
[3] Karmanos Cancer Institute, Wayne State University School of Medicine, Detroit, MI 48201, USA; bb8374@wayne.edu
* Correspondence: qzhou1@usf.edu

Abstract: Naturally occurring polyphenols are believed to have beneficial effects in the prevention and treatment of a myriad of disorders due to their anti-inflammatory, antioxidant, antineoplastic, cytotoxic, and immunomodulatory activities documented in a large body of literature. In the era of molecular medicine and targeted therapy, there is a growing interest in characterizing the molecular mechanisms by which polyphenol compounds interact with multiple protein targets and signaling pathways that regulate key cellular processes under both normal and pathological conditions. Numerous studies suggest that natural polyphenols have chemopreventive and/or chemotherapeutic properties against different types of cancer by acting through different molecular mechanisms. The present review summarizes recent preclinical studies on the applications of bioactive polyphenols in lung cancer therapy, with an emphasis on the molecular mechanisms that underlie the therapeutic effects of major polyphenols on lung cancer. We also discuss the potential of the polyphenol-based combination therapy as an attractive therapeutic strategy against lung cancer.

Keywords: lung cancer; natural polyphenols; anticancer activities; molecular mechanisms

---

1. Introduction

Lung cancer is the second most common cancer in both men and women and is the leading cause of cancer mortality in the United States [1], with an overall five-year survival rate of 19.4% (https://seer.cancer.gov/statfacts/html/lungb.html). The two main types of lung cancer are small cell lung cancer (SCLC) and non-small cell lung cancer (NSCLC), which account for about 15% and 85% of all lung cancer cases, respectively [2]. Tobacco smoking is the principal cause of lung cancer [3]. Secondhand smoking, chronic exposure to various occupational and environmental lung carcinogens, and previous lung diseases can also increase the risk of lung cancer [4–9]. Historically, intakes of fruits, non-starchy vegetables, whole grains, and herbs abundant in certain phytochemicals are thought to be protective against lung cancer. Epidemiological and experimental evidence suggests that natural bioactive compounds can act as chemopreventive agents to delay, suppress or reverse carcinogenic progression to advanced lung cancer through various mechanisms, including antioxidant/anti-inflammatory activities, modulation of biotransformation enzymes, anti-proliferative effect, and modulation of the immune system [10–18]. In addition, natural products that are derived from a variety of sources, including phytochemicals [19–21], hormones [22,23], and nutrients [24–26], have been shown to reduce the side effects and toxicities that are associated with chemotherapy and radiation therapy for lung cancer.

Although the consumption of fruits, vegetables, and natural products with a high content in anticancer natural compounds are generally considered to be beneficial in preventing and combating lung cancer, bioactive compounds from foods, or natural product extracts are not ready for uniform adoption into complementary and integrative therapy use due to inconclusive or negative results from clinical trials [27–33]. Over the past two decades, the rapid evolution of medical research and technologies has led to significant breakthroughs in our understanding of the molecular and genetic alterations that drive cancer development and progression. Consequently, the undergoing transition from the empirical trial-and-error medicine to precision medicine according to the unique genetic mapping of individual patients has stimulated considerable research activities in the area of natural bioactive compounds. With the advent of improved cellular and molecular experimental systems, significant progression has been made in unraveling the molecular mechanisms that underlie the antitumor properties of individual natural compounds. In this review, we focus on the compelling evidence from in vitro and in vivo studies demonstrating the ability of natural polyphenols, one of the most important groups of phytochemicals, to suppress lung cancer progression through the induction of tumor cell death and inhibition of aberrantly activated pro-proliferative and pro-survival signaling pathways. Our purpose is to highlight the potential of natural polyphenols to be developed and integrated into standard therapeutic strategies to improve clinical outcomes for patients with advanced lung cancer.

2. Mutations and Dysregulated Signaling Pathways in Lung Cancer

Lung cancer arises through a multistep process that is driven by the sequential accumulation of genetic mutations and epigenetic modifications, which leads to uncontrolled cell proliferation and inactivation of programmed cell death (apoptosis) [34–36]. As a lung tumor grows in size, the angiogenic switch is triggered so that the existing vascular network expands to form new blood vessels (angiogenesis) that are intended to sustain the nutrient and oxygen supply in the growing tumor [37–39]. Subsequently, lung tumor cells can acquire the ability to invade the surrounding tissues, intravasate into the circulatory system, travel to distant tissue sites, extravasate, and develop a secondary tumor at distant sites (metastasis) [40,41]. A typical lung cancer contains approximately 200 nonsynonymous mutations, some of which are considered "driver mutations" that play a dominant-acting role in tumor growth and progression [42]. For example, activating mutations in the Kirsten rat sarcoma viral oncogene homolog (KRAS) and epidermal growth factor receptor (EGFR) genes and rearrangements in the anaplastic lymphoma kinase (ALK) or ROS proto-oncogene 1 receptor tyrosine kinase (ROS1) genes are identified as oncogenic drivers in certain subtypes of NSCLC [43–47], so are the inactivating mutations in tumor protein p53 (TP53) and retinoblastoma 1 (RB1) genes in SCLC [48,49]. Most driver mutations are gain-of-function mutations that result in the overexpression of oncogenes or mutant proteins with dysregulated activities. For example, constitutive activation of EGFR or K-RAS that is due to mutation subsequently upregulates the Mitogen-activated protein kinase kinase (MEK)/extracellular signal-regulated kinase (ERK) and phosphoinositide 3-kinase (PI3K)/v-akt murine thymomaviral oncogene (AKT) signaling pathways, which triggers a cascade of downstream effectors promoting tumor growth, angiogenesis, and metastasis [50,51]. The p53 tumor suppressor gene is a transcription factor that activates a number of target genes to restrict aberrant cell growth through the induction of senescence, cell cycle arrest, or apoptosis [52,53]. The high expression of p53 protein is a favorable prognostic factor in a subset of patients with NSCLC [54], whereas the exon 8 mutation of p53 gene reduces the responsiveness to tyrosine kinase inhibitors (TKIs) and worsens prognosis in EGFR-mutant NSCLC patients [55]. It is well accepted that the inactivation of apoptosis plays an important role in lung carcinogenesis and resistance to treatment [56,57]. There are two main apoptotic pathways [58]. The extrinsic apoptotic pathway is initiated by the activation of multiple death receptors, such as Fas, tumor necrosis factor receptors (TNFRs), and TNF-related apoptosis-inducing ligand receptors (TRAILRs), and it proceeds through caspase-8 [59], while the intrinsic pathway is activated by mitochondrial outer membrane permeabilization (MOMP), followed by the release of cytochrome c to the cytoplasm and recruitment of pro-caspase 9 to cytochrome c [60]. The Bcl-2 family proteins, including pro-apoptotic members (such as Bad, Bak, Bax, Bcl-Xs, BID, Bik, Bim, HRK, Noxa, and PUMA) and anti-apoptotic members (such as Bcl-2, Bcl-W, Bcl-Xl, Bfl-1, and MCL-1) also regulate the intrinsic pathway [61]. The extrinsic and intrinsic pathways converge on the effector caspases (e.g., Caspases 3, 6, and 7), which are capable of cleaving hundreds of substrates, including nuclear proteins, plasma membrane proteins, and mitochondrial proteins, to trigger cell death [62]. Given that the evasion of apoptosis is one of the prominent hallmarks of cancer [63], an ideal therapeutic strategy to effectively induce apoptosis and avoid the "death by a thousand cuts" in lung cancer would be to restore p53 function and facilitate caspase activation [64,65].

3. Classification and Structures of Natural Polyphenols

Polyphenols are a large group of nature compounds present in plant-based foods and beverages, including fruits, vegetables, whole grains, tea, and wine. So far, more than 10,000 polyphenolic compounds have been identified [66]. Polyphenols can be classified into four main groups, including phenolic acids, flavonoids, stilbenes, and lignans, based on the number of aromatic rings, the structural elements connecting these rings to one another, and the substituents that are bound to the rings (Figure 1) [67,68]. Phenolic acids contain a single benzene rings and they can be further divided into two main subclasses, hydroxybenzoic acid and hydroxycinnamic acid derivatives that are based on the C6–C1 and C6–C3 backbones, respectively [69]. Flavonoids share a common structure with two aromatic rings (A and B) that are connected by three carbon atoms that form an oxygenated heterocycle (ring C), which is also known as the flavan nucleus or 1,3-diphenylpropane structure (C6-C3-C6 carbon skeleton) [69]. Flavonoids can be divided into six major subclasses, including flavonols, flavones, flavonones or dihydroflavones, isoflavones, anthocyanidins, flavanols, or catechins based on the variations in hydroxyl/methoxy group placements on the ring structures [68,70]. Natural stilbenes are structurally characterized by the presence of 1,2-diphenylethylene nucleus (C6–C2–C6 carbon skeleton) [71]. Lignans are a diverse group of optically active phenylpropanoid dimers, in which the two phenylpropane units are connected by the center carbon (C-8/C-8′) of their side chains [72].

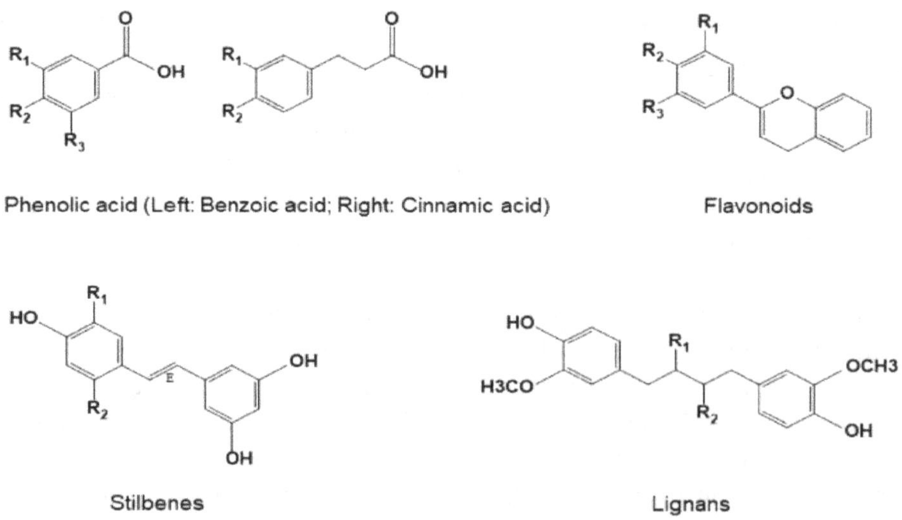

Figure 1. Chemical structures of different classes of natural polyphenols.

The structure-activity relationships of many natural polyphenols in terms of their anticancer potential have been documented. The basic chemical structure of polyphenols contains one or more aromatic rings with one or more hydroxyl groups attached. The presence of functional phenolic hydroxyl groups makes polyphenols excellent hydrogen bond donors that confer high affinities for proteins and nuclear acids [73]. Therefore, the number and position of hydroxyl groups can have a decisive impact on the cellular bioactivities of polyphenols, which are central to their antitumoral, antimutagenic, pro-apoptotic, and antioxidant effects [74–76]. Considerable efforts have been devoted to the characterization of structure-activity relationships that provide the basis of rational design of polyphenol analogs with improved anticancer effect, given that the polyphenol core represents an attractive chemical structure towards new anticancer agents. For example, the cytotoxic activity is enhanced in phenols with low bond dissociation energy (BDE) values or large negative $\sigma+$ values since the inhibitory effect of simple phenols on fast-growing murine leukemia cells is related to the O–H BDE that is required to form a phenoxy radical and the brown variation of the Hammett electronic parameter ($\sigma+$) [77,78].

Structure-activity relationship (SAR), quantitative structure-activity relationship (QSAR), and docking approaches have been used to delineate the structural mechanisms that underlie the correlation between the binding affinity of polyphenol compounds for a specific oncogenic molecule and the expected anticancer activities [76]. For example, gossypol, a polyphenol that is derived from cotton seeds, is an effective inhibitor of Bcl-2, Bcl-xL, and MCL-1 with the inhibitor constant (Ki) values at sub-micromolar levels [79,80]. The elimination of the two reactive aldehydes from gossypol based on a model of the docked structure of the compound into Bcl-xL resulted in a semisynthetic analog of gossypol, namely apogossypol, which showed superior efficacy and markedly reduced toxicity in Bcl-2-transgenic mice as compared with gossypol [81,82]. A couple of studies by Wang's group have demonstrated that gossypol forms a hydrogen bonding network with residues Arg146 and Asn143 in Bcl-2 through its aldehyde group and the adjacent hydroxyl groups on one of its naphthalene rings, while the isopropyl group on the same naphthalene ring is inserted into a hydrophobic pocket in Bcl-2 [83,84]. Based on the predicted binding model, a simplified pyrogallol-based analogue of gossypol was designed to mimic the hydrogen bonding and part of the hydrophobic interactions between gossypol and Bcl-2. Moreover, modification to the isopropyl group of pyrogallol resulted in not only improved binding affinities for Bcl-2 and Mcl-1, but also an increased cytotoxic effect on the MDA-MB-231 and PC-3 cancer cell lines with the inhibitory concentration IC50 values at sub-nanomolar levels [85].

A molecular docking study on the interaction between tea catechins and hepatocyte growth factor receptor (Met) has revealed that the gallate-containing catechins, including (−)-epicatechin gallate (ECG), (−)-epigallocatechin gallate (EGCG), and gallocatechin gallate (GCG), favorably fit into the Met binding site with hydrogen bonding being established between the aromatic hydroxyl groups of the gallate moiety and the backbone –NH of two Met kinase active sites, i.e., Met1160 and Pro1158, whereas tea catechins without the gallate group, including (−)-catechin (CAT), (−)-epicatechin (EC), and (−)-epigallocatechin (EGC), did not interact with Met1160, but exhibit affinity for the backbone –NH of Asp1222, which suggests that the gallate group is a key structure feature for binding of tea catechins to the active sites of Met kinase domain [86] The findings of the molecular docking study were confirmed by the Met kinase activity assay, which showed that ECG, EGCG, and GCG had inhibitory effects on Met kinase activity, while the other tea catechins had little or no effect [86]. Another potential molecular target of tea catechins is the proteasome, which is known to mediate the degradation of many intracellular proteins that are involved in carcinogenesis and tumor progression [87]. The SAR studies by Dou's group showed that the ester bond-containing tea polyphenols, such as ECG, GCG, EGCG, and catechin-3-gallate (CG), were strong inhibitors for the chymotrypsin-like activity of the purified 20S proteasome with IC50 values at nanomolar levels, whereas the tea polyphenols without the gallate ester function, such as EGC, EC, gallocatechin (GC), and CAT, were unable to inhibit the proteasomal chymotrypsin-like activity [88,89].

4. Molecular Underpinnings of Polyphenols in Lung Cancer Treatment

The use of bioactive natural polyphenols for therapeutic prevention and intervention is an evolving strategy in the management of cancer. A thorough understanding of the mechanisms of action is imperative for integrating those polyphenols into standard oncology care. In this section, we primarily focus on the recent advances in understanding the antitumor actions of natural polyphenols in lung cancer (Figure 2). The preclinical studies were identified through a literature review that was conducted on PubMed using the key terms polyphenol and lung cancer (Table 1). Only original studies credibly investigating molecular mechanisms underlying the antitumor potential of natural polyphenols and their analogues were included.

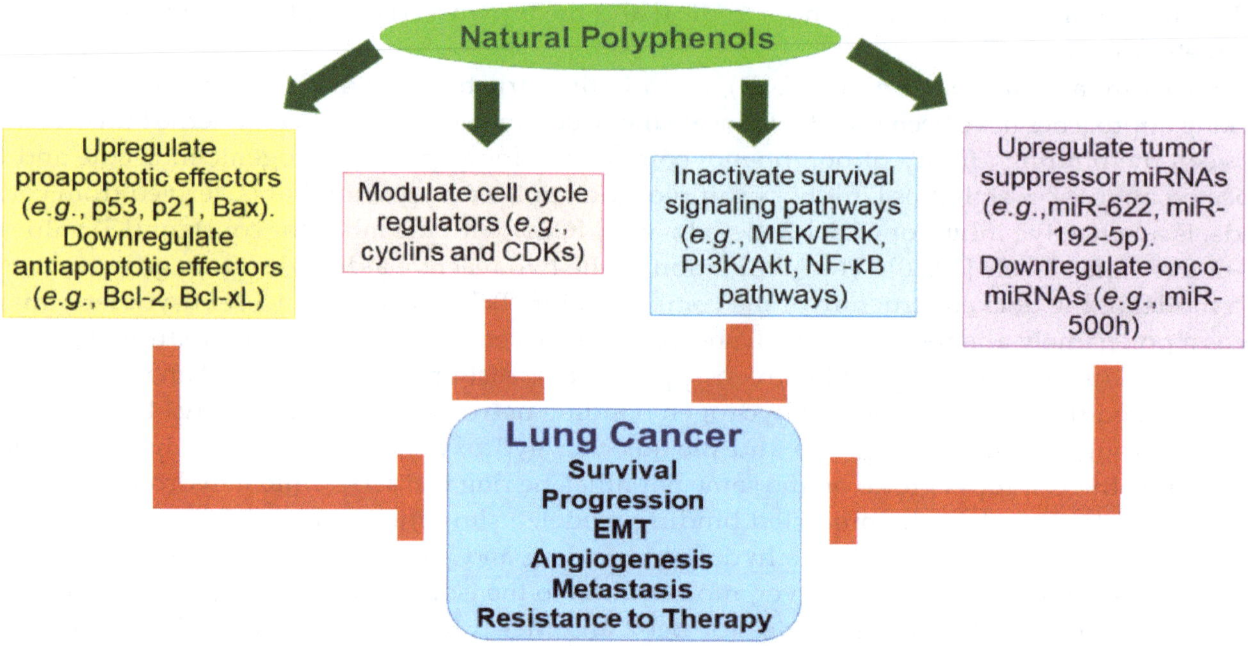

Figure 2. The role of bioactive natural polyphenols in lung cancer therapy.

Table 1. Preclinical Studies on the Mechanisms Underlying the Antitumor Activities of Natural Polyphenols.

Polyphenol Compounds or Extracts	Mechanisms	In Vitro and/or In Vivo Models	References
Resveratrol	Induction of apoptosis by up-regulation of p53 and p21, activation of the caspases and disruption of the mitochondrial membrane complex. Cell cycle arrest at the G_1 phase. Alterations in expressions of cyclin A, chk1, CDC27, and Eg5. Anti-tumor effect mediated by transforming growth factor-β pathway, particularly through the Smad proteins. i.e., down-regulation of the Smad activators 2 and 4 and up-regulation of the repressor Smad 7	A549 human NSCLC cell line	[90]
Resveratrol	Induction of apoptosis as a result of mitochondrial depolarization, release of cytochrome c from the mitochondrial compartment to the cytoplasm, apoptosis-inducing factor translocation from the mitochondrial compartment to the nucleus, and altered protein levels of Bcl-2, Bcl-xL and Bax	H446 human SCLC cells	[91]
Resveratrol	Induction of TRAIL-mediated apoptosis through suppression of NF-κB and downregulation of anti-apoptotic factors Bcl-2 and Bcl-xl	A549 and HCC15 human NSCLC cells	[92]
Resveratrol	Suppressed M2-like polarization of tumor associated macrophages and inhibited STAT3 activity	A549 and H1299 human NSCLC cells. Lewis lung cancer (LLC) s.c. xenograft model (Intraperitoneal (i.p.) administration) [a]	[93]
Resveratrol	Resveratrol enhancing the effects of cisplatin on inhibition of cancer cell proliferation, induction of cell apoptosis, depolarization of mitochondrial membrane potential, release of cytochrome c, upregulation of Bax, downregulation of Bcl-2	H520 and H838 human NSCLC cell lines	[94]
Resveratrol	Upregulation of p21 and TRAIL receptor 1 and 2 expression, and downregulation of Bcl2, cyclin D, NF-κB and IKK1 expression	A549 human NSCLC cell line	[95]
Resveratrol	Increase in production of hydrogen peroxide (H_2O_2), activation of Bid, PARP and caspase 8, and downregulation of pEGFR, pAkt, c-FLIP and NF-κB protein expression	H460 human NSCLC cells	[96]
Resveratrol	Suppress of tumor cell growth via an apoptosis-independent mechanism involving induction of premature senescence by increasing P53 and p21 expression and ROS production and decreasing EF1A expression	A549 and H460 human NSCLC cell lines	[97]
Resveratrol	Enhancing ionizing radiation through increased production of ROS, and induction of DNA double-strand breaks and senescence induction	A549 and H460 human NSCLC cell lines	[98]
Resveratrol	Resveratrol overcoming gefitinib resistance by increasing the intracellular gefitinib concentration through inhibition of CYP1A1 and ABCG2 and by inducing cell apoptosis, autophagy, cell cycle arrest and senescence through increase in expression of cleaved caspase-3, LC3B-II, p53 and p21	PC9/G human NSCLC cells	[99]
Resveratrol	Resveratrol-enhanced erlotinib-mediated apoptosis through decreasing survivin expression and induction of PUMA expression	H460, A549, PC-9 and H1975 human NSCLC cell lines	[100]

Table 1. *Cont.*

Polyphenol Compounds or Extracts	Mechanisms	In Vitro and/or In Vivo Models	References
Resveratrol	Resveratrol-enhanced etoposide-Induced cytotoxicity through down-regulating ERK1/2 and AKT-mediated X-ray repair cross-complement group 1 (XRCC1) protein expression	H1703 and H1975 human NSCLC cell lines	[101]
Resveratrol	Modulation of the expression of specific miRNAs with potential target genes involved in apoptosis, cell cycle regulation, cell proliferation, and differentiation	A549 human NSCLC cell line	[102]
Resveratrol	Upregulation of miR-622 leading to suppression of K-Ras mRNA translation without affecting its accumulation levels	16HBE-T human bronchial epithelial cell line and H460 human NSCLC cell line.	[103]
Resveratrol	Inhibition of lung cancer progression by downregulating miR-500h, which subsequently leads to downregulation of PP2A expression, inactivation of AKT/NF-kB and downregulation of FOXC2	CL1-5, A549, H322, H520 and H1435 human NSCLC cell lines	[104]
Resveratrol	Induction of G2/M cell cycle arrest through downregulation of checkpoint protein cyclin B1. Induction of apoptosis by increasing p53 and p21 expression and the release of cytochrome c in the cytosol	A549 human NSCLC cell line	[105]
Resveratrol	Inhibition of A549 cell proliferation through the reduction of the ratio of Bcl-2/Bax through activation of p53, thus activating the caspase-3- dependent apoptotic cascade and induces apoptosis	A549 human NSCLC cells.	[106]
Resveratrol	Attenuated A549 cell-induced platelet secretion and angiogenic responses in vitro and suppressed A549 lung cancer metastasis and angiogenesis in vivo through inhibition of platelets-mediated angiogenic responses induced by [106] adenosine diphosphate (ADP) through increased cGMP generation and cGMP-mediated vasodilator-stimulated phosphoprotein phosphorylation along with reduced intracellular Ca^{2+} mobilization	A549 human NSCLC cells, and A549 subcutaneous (s.c.) xenograft tumors in nude mice (i.p. administration) [a]	[107]
Resveratrol	Anticancer effects attributable to inhibition of STAT-3 Signaling	A549 human NSCLC cells	[108]
Resveratrol	Inhibition of anchorage-dependent and -independent growth of NSCLC cells by decreasing EGFR and downstream kinases Akt and ERK1/2 activation, and subsequent impairment of hexokinase II (HK2)-mediated glycolysis by inhibiting HK2 expression mediated by the Akt signaling pathway	H460, H1650 and HCC827 human NSCLC cells. H460 s.c. xenograft model (i.p. administration) [a]	[109]
Resveratrol	Synergism between Resveratrol and Metformin attributable to the suppression of DNA damage based on the downregulation of γH2AX/p53/p-chk2, inhibition of cell cycle progression via modulation of cyclin E/cdk2, Rb, p21 cyclin B1/cdk1 and plk1/cdc25c and enhancement of DNA repair indicated by the upregulation of p53R2	A549 human NSCLC cells	[110]
Resveratrol	Inhibition of the release of IL-6 and VEGF for co-cultured A549 lung cancer cells and adipose-derived mesenchymal stem cells	Co-cultured A549 human lung cancer cells and adipose-derived mesenchymal stem cells	[111]
Resveratrol	Induction of cell cycle arrest in the G0/G1 phase by downregulating the expression levels of cyclin D1, cyclin-dependent kinase (CDK)4 and CDK6, and upregulating the expression levels of the CDK inhibitors, p21 and p27	A549 human NSCLC cell line	[112]

Table 1. *Cont.*

Polyphenol Compounds or Extracts	Mechanisms	In Vitro and/or In Vivo Models	References
Resveratrol	miR-200c sensitized tumor cell response to resveratrol by targeting reversion-inducing cysteine-rich protein with Kazal motifs (RECK), followed by activation of the JNK signaling pathway and ER stress	H460 human NSCLC cell line	[113]
Resveratrol	Suppression of invasion and metastasis through reversal of TGF-β1-induced EMT through increasing E-cadherin expression and repressing Fibronectin, Vimentin, Snail1 and Slug expression	A549 human NSCLC cell line	[114]
Resveratrol	Enhancing the radiosensitivity through NF-κB inhibition and S-phase arrest	NCI-H838 human NSCLC cell line	[115]
Resveratrol	Anti-metastasis effect attributable to the inhibition of expression of MMP-9/MMP-2 by suppression of HO-1, which in part results from the suppression of NF-κB-dependent signaling pathway	A549 human NSCLC cell line	[116]
Resveratrol	Inhibition of the proliferation of SPC-A-1/CDDP cells, induction of apoptosis and cell cycle arrest at phase between G0-G1 and S phase or at the G2/M phase by downregulating survivin	Human multidrug-resistant SPC-A-1/CDDP cells	[117]
Resveratrol	Anti-proliferative effect associated with inhibition of the phosphorylation of the retinoblastoma protein (pRB) and induction of cyclin-dependent kinase (Cdk) inhibitor p21WAF1/CIP. Induction of apoptosis associated with activation of caspase-3, shift in Bax/Bcl-xL ratio and inhibition of transcriptional activity of NF-κB	A549 human NSCLC cell line	[118]
Resveratrol loaded gelatin nanoparticles	Induction of cell death through inhibition of cell cycle progression and constitutive NF-κB activation by altering the expression of p53, p21, caspase-3, Bax, Bcl-2 and NF-κB	H460 human NSCLC cell line	[119]
SS28 (a synthetic Resveratrol analog)	Inhibition of Tubulin polymerization during cell division to cause cell cycle arrest at G2/M phase of the cell cycle	A549 human NSCLC cell line	[120]
4,4′-Dihydroxy-*trans*-stilbene (DHS) (a resveratrol analog)	Inhibition on anchorage-dependent or -independent cell growth, leading to impairment of the cell cycle progression with reduction of cell numbers arresting at the G1 phase	Murine Lewis lung carcinoma (LLC) cell line	[121]
Curcumin and resveratrol alone or in combination	Improvement of lung histoarchitecture and ultrahistoarchitecture during benzopyrene-induced lung carcinogenesis in mice	3,4-Benzopyrene-induced mouse lung carcinoma model (Oral (p.o.) administration) [a]	[122]
Resveratrol and dibenzoylmethane	Induction of apoptosis through activation of caspase-9 and caspase-3 and subsequent cleavage of PARP	A549 and CH27 human NSCLC cell lines	[123]
Heyneanol A (HA) (A tetramer of resveratrol)	Induction of caspase-mediated cancer cell apoptosis by inducing cleavage of caspase-9 and caspase-3 and suppression of basic fibroblast growth factor (bFGF)-induced tumor angiogenesis.	In vivo Lewis lung tumor model (i.p. administration) [a]	[124]
EGCG, ECG, EGC and EC	Induction of apoptosis through a p53-dependent pathway.	A549 human NSCLC cell line	[125]
EGCG	Induction of G2-M arrest. Incorporation into cytosol and nuclei	PC-9 human NSCLC cell line	[126]

Table 1. *Cont.*

Polyphenol Compounds or Extracts	Mechanisms	In Vitro and/or In Vivo Models	References
EGCG	EGCG inhibited cell growth through decreasing the phosphorylation of Akt and ERK irrespective of EGFR-, ALK- or ROS1-dependency. The antiangiogenic effect of EGCG might be attributable to the inhibition of HIF-1α	PC-9, RPC-9, H1975, H2228 and HCC78 human NSCLC cell lines (EGFR- or fusion gene-driven tumor cells) and xenograft models (p.o. administration) [a]	[127]
EGCG	Downregulation of gene expression of NF-κB inducing kinase (NIK), death-associated protein kinase 1 (DAPK 1), RhoB and tyrosine-protein kinase (SKY), and upregulation of the retinoic acid receptor alpha1 gene expression	PC-9 human NSCLC cell line	[128]
EGCG	Induction of miRNA profile changes, which modulate several regulatory networks associated to AKT, NF-κB, MAP kinases, and cell cycle	4-(Methylnitrosamino)-1-(3-pyridyl)-1-butanone (NNK) induced mouse lung cancer (p.o. administration) [a]	[129]
EGCG	Co-treatment with celecoxib synergistically inducing apoptosis by upregulation of growth arrest and DNA damage-inducible 153 (GADD153) through the ERK signaling pathway	A549, ChaGo K-1 and PC-9 human NSCLC cell lines	[130]
EGCG	Co-treatment of EGCG with cisplatin resulting in proliferation inhibition, cell cycle arrest in G1 phase, increase in apoptosis along with inhibition of DNA methyltransferase (DNMT) activity and histone deacetylase (HDAC) activity, reversal of hypermethylated status and downregulated expression of *GAS1*, *TIMP4*, *ICAM1* and *WISP2* genes	Cisplatin-resistant A549 (A549/DDP) human NSCLC cell line and A549/DDP xenograft tumor model (i.p. administration)	[131]
EGCG and Luteolin	Enhanced antitumor effect attributable to ATM (ataxia telangiectasia mutated) kinase-dependent Ser15 phosphorylation of p53 as a consequence of DNA double strand break	H292, A549 and H460 human NSCLC cell lines expressing wild-type p53; A549 xenograft tumor model (p.o. administration) [a]	[132]
Tea polyphenols	Upregulation of p53 expression and downregulation of Bcl-2 expression with no influence on H-Ras and c-Myc expressions	NCI-H460 human NSCLC cell line	[133]
Black tea polyphenols	Inhibition of Cox-1 and induction of caspase-3 and caspase-7 expression	3,4-Benzopyrene induced mouse lung tumor model	[134]
Black tea polyphenols	Suppressing cell proliferation and inducing apoptosis	3,4-Benzopyrene induced mouse lung tumor model	[135]
Green tea polyphenols	Preventive effect against lung cancer by upregulating p53 and downregulating Bcl-2	3,4-Benzopyrene induced rat lung tumor model	[136]
Tea polyphenols	Increase in p53 expression and decrease in Bcl-2 expression	3,4-Benzopyrene-induced rat lung carcinoma model	[137]

Table 1. *Cont.*

Polyphenol Compounds or Extracts	Mechanisms	In Vitro and/or In Vivo Models	References
Tea polyphenols	Inhibition of Akt and cyclooxygenase-2 expression, and inactivation of nuclear factor-kappa B via blocking phosphorylation and subsequent degradation of IkappaB alpha	Diethylnitrosoamine- induced mouse lung tumor model (p.o. administration) [a]	[138]
Green tea polyphenols	TAM67-mediated changes in gene expression involving the downregulation of activator protein-1 (AP-1)	H1299 human NSCLC cell line and SPON 10 mouse lung tumor cell line	[139]
Green tea extracts	Modulation of the expression of 14 proteins involved in calcium-binding, cytoskeleton and motility, metabolism, detoxification, or gene regulation	A549 human NSCLC cell line	[140]
Green tea polyphenols	Synergistic antitumor effect with atorvastatin attributable to increased apoptosis, reduced Mcl-1 level and increased cleaved caspase-3 and cleaved poly(ADP)-ribose polymerase (PARP)	H1299 and H460 human NSCLC cell lines. 4-(Methylnitrosaminao)-1-(3-pyridyl)-1-butanone induced mouse lung tumor model (p.o. administration) [a]	[141]
Green tea extract	Induction of protective autophagy	A549 human NSCLC cell line	[142]
Thymoquinone (TQ)	Upregulation of Bax and downregulation of Bcl-2 expression and increase in the Bax/Bcl-2 ratio. Decrease in the expression of cyclin D, NF-κB and IKK1 and increase in the expression of p21 and TRAIL receptor 1 and 2 expression	A549 human NSCLC cell line	[95]
Curcumin	Induction of apoptosis through p53-independent pathway by downregulation of Bcl-2 and Bcl-xL expression	A549 and H1299 human NSCLC cell lines	[143]
Curcumin	Induction of cell cycle arrest at the G1/S phase and apoptosis through up-regulation of *GADD45* and *GADD153*	PC-9 human NSCLC cell line	[144]
Curcumin	Induction of cell cycle arrest at the G2/M phase and apoptosis through upregulation of Bax and Bad expression, downregulation of Bcl-2, Bcl-xL and XIAP expression, increase in ROS, intracellular Ca^{2+} and endoplasmic reticulum stress, activation of GRP78 and GADD153 proteins and FAS/caspase-8 pathway	H460 human NSCLC cell line	[145]
Curcumin	Induction of apoptosis through a mitochondria-dependent mechanism as manifested by the decrease in the mitochondrial membrane potential, releasing cytochrome c from mitochondria to cytoplasm	A549 human NSCLC cell line	[146]
Curcumin	Induction of apoptosis via the ROS-mediated mitochondrial pathway accompanied by increased Bax expression and decreased expression of Bcl-2 and Bcl-xL	H446 human SCLC cell line	[147]
Curcumin	Inhibition of tumor cell proliferation and induction of apoptosis through upregulation of miR-192-5p and suppression of the PI3K/Akt signaling pathway	A549 human NSCLC cell line	[148]
Curcumin	Enhancing autophagy and apoptosis through inaction of PI3K/mTOR signaling pathway	A549 and H1299 human NSCLC cell lines	[149]

Table 1. *Cont.*

Polyphenol Compounds or Extracts	Mechanisms	In Vitro and/or In Vivo Models	References
Curcumin	Induction of autophagy leading to suppression of tumor cell proliferation.	A549 human NSCLC cell line	[150]
Curcumin	Inhibition of tumor cell invasion and metastasis through attenuating GLUT1/MT1-MMP/MMP2 pathway	A549 human NSCLC cell line and xenograft tumor model (i.p. administration) [a]	[151]
Curcumin	Inhibition of tumor cell metastasis through inhibition of the adiponectin/NF-κB/MMPs signaling pathway	A549 human NSCLC cell line and xenograft tumor model (i.p. administration) [a]	[152]
A501 (Curcumin analogue)	Induction of cell cycle arrest at the G2/M phase and apoptosis through decreasing the expression of cyclinB1, cdc-2, Bcl-2, while increasing the expression of p53, cleaved caspase-3 and Bax	A549 and H460 human NSCLC cell lines	[153]
Curcumin and gefitinib	Potentiating the antitumor effect of gefitinib in gefitinib-resistant tumor cells through induction of endogenous EGFR protein degradation and downregulation of EGFR and AKT protein expression. Reduction of the gefitinib-induced villi damage and apoptosis in mouse intestine through attenuating gefitinib-induced p38 activation	CL1-5, A549 and H1975 human NSCLC cell lines and xenograft models (p.o. administration) [a]	[154]
Curcumin and carboplatin	Synergistic antitumor activity mediated by multiple mechanisms involving suppression of NF-kB via inhibition of the Akt/IKKα pathway, enhancement of ERK1/2 activity and downregulation of MMP-2 and MMP-9 expression	A549 human NSCLC cell line	[155]
Quercetin	Induction of cell cycle arrest at the G2/M phase and apoptosis through increased expression of cyclin B1 and phosph-cdc2 (T161), survivin, total p53, phosphor-p53 (S15) and p21 proteins	A549 and H1299 human NSCLC cell lines	[156]
Quercetin	Induction of apoptosis through activation of MEK-ERK pathway, inactivation of Akt and alteration in the expression of Bcl-2 family	A549 human NSCLC cell line	[157]
Quercetin	Proapoptosis activity through multiple mechanisms including upregulated the expression of genes associated with the death pathway, the JNK pathway, the IL1 receptor pathway, the caspase cascade, the NF-κB pathway and cell cycle arrest, and downregulated the expression of genes related to cell proliferation	H460 human NSCLC cell line	[158]
Quercetin	Anti-invasion activity through inhibition of monocarboxylate transporter 1	A110L human lung cancer cell line	[159]
Quercetin	Targeting aurora B kinase	A549 human NSCLC cell line and xenograft model (i.p. administration) [a]	[160]
Quercetin	Trigger Bcl-2/Bax-mediated apoptosis, necrosis and mitotic catastrophe. Inhibition of cell migration through disassembly of microfilaments, microtubules and vimentin filaments and inhibition of vimentin and N-cadherin expression	A549 human NSCLC cell line	[161]

Table 1. *Cont.*

Polyphenol Compounds or Extracts	Mechanisms	In Vitro and/or In Vivo Models	References
Quercetin	Suppression of in vitro cell migration/invasion and in vivo bone metastasis through inhibition of Snail-dependent Akt activation and Snail-independent ADAM9 expression pathways	A549 and HCC827 human NSCLC cell lines and A549 xenograft model (i.p. administration) [a]	[162]
Quercetin and chrysin	Suppressed the secretion of cytokines, IL-1β, IL-6, TNF-α and IL-10, and decreased the phosphorylation of IKKβ and IκB, the nuclear level of p65 (NF-κB) as well as the expression of MMP-9 in A549cells exposed to nickel	A549 human NSCLC cell line	[163]
Quercetin and trichostatin A	Enhancing the antitumor activity of trichostatin A through upregulation of p53 expression	A549 and H1299 human NSCLC cell lines and A549 xenograft model (i.p. administration) [a]	[164]
Quercetin and gemcitabine	Promoting apoptosis and sensitizing tumor response to gemcitabine via inhibition of HSP70 expression	A549 and H4650 human NSCLC cell lines	[165]
Caffeic acid phenethyl ester (CAPE)	Upregulation of Bax, p21 and TRAIL receptor 1 and 2 expression, and downregulation of cyclin D expression	A549 human NSCLC cell line	[95]
Pterostilbene	Exhibition of p53-dependent chemotherapeutic effects through the ATM/CHK/p53 tumor suppressive pathway leading to cell senescence	Precancerous human bronchial epithelial cell lines, HBECR and HBECR/p53i, with normal p53 and suppressed p53 expression, respectively	[166]
Bakuchiol	Increase in reactive oxygen species production, decrease in mitochondrial membrane potential (ΔΨm), cell cycle arrest at S phase, caspase 9/3 activation, p53 and Bax up-regulation, and Bcl-2 downregulation	A549 human NSCLC cell line	[167]
Chlorogenic acid (CGA)	Decrease in hypoxia-induced HIF-1α protein level and suppression of the transcriptional activity of HIF-1α under hypoxic conditions, leading to antiangiogenic activity through inhibition of HIF-1α/AKT pathway and decrease in VEGF expression	A549 human NSCLC cell line	[168]
Fisetin	Inhibition of cell growth through concomitant suppression of PI3K/Akt and mTOR signaling	A549 and H1792 human NSCLC cell lines	[169]
Fisetin	Enhancing cisplatin cytotoxicity in cisplatin-resistant cells by modulation of the MAPK/survivin/caspase pathway	A549 human NSCLC cell line	[170]
Fisetin	Synergistic interaction between paclitaxel and fisetin due to the induction of mitotic catastrophe probably through the promotion of multipolar spindle formation. Mitotic catastrophe induced protective autophagy against apoptosis, which then switched to the autophagic cell death	A549 human NSCLC cell line	[171]
Liquiritin, isoliquiritin and isoliquirigenin	Induction of apoptosis and cell cycle at the G2/M phase by increasing p53, p21 and BAX expression and decreasing PCNA, MDM2, p-GSK-3β, p-Akt, p-c-Raf, p-PTEN, caspase-3, pro-caspase-8, pro-caspase-9, PARP and Bcl-2 expression	A549 human NSCLC cell line	[172]

Table 1. *Cont.*

Polyphenol Compounds or Extracts	Mechanisms	In Vitro and/or In Vivo Models	References
Eucalyptus globulus Labill	Cell cycle arrest in the G0/G1 phase. Increase in the expression of p53, p21 and cyclin D1 proteins	NCI-H460 human NSCLC cell line	[173]
Polyphenols isolated from	Suppressed cell migration by targeting MMP-9. Induced cell apoptosis through intrinsic apoptosis pathways, accompanied by increasing the expression of Bax and caspase-3	A549 human NSCLC cell line	[174]
Rosemary extract	Reduced total and phosphorylated/activated Akt, mTOR and p70S6K levels	A549 human NSCLC cell line	[175]
Salvianolic acid A	Salvianolic acid A enhanced sensitivity to cisplatin through suppression of the c-met/AKT/mTOR signaling pathway	A549 human lung cancer cisplatin resistance cell line (A549/DDP)	[176]
Red wine	Inhibition of basal and EGF-stimulated Akt and Erk signals and enhancement of total and phosphorylated levels of p53, leading to inhibition of A549 cell proliferation and clonogenic survival	A549 human NSCLC cell line	[15]
Magnolol and polyphenol mixture (PM) derived from Magnolia officinalis	Induction of cell apoptosis by arresting the cell cycle in the G0/G1 phase while simultaneously activating various pro-apoptotic signals, including TRAIL-R2 (DR5), Bax, caspase 3, cleaved caspase 3, and cleaved PARP	A549 and H1299 human NSCLC cell lines	[177]
Pomegranate juice	Attenuated the formation of lung nodules and reduced PHH3 (marker of mitotic activity) and HIF-1α expression	Two-month-old adult male AJ mice (p.o. administration) [a]	[178]
Polyphenolic compounds of Achyranthes aspera (PCA) extract	Downregulation of the expression of pro-inflammatory cytokines IL-1β, IL-6 and TNF-α, TFs, NF-κB and Stat3, and upregulation of the expression of pro-apoptotic proteins Bax and p53. Increase in the activities and expression of antioxidant enzymes GST, GR, CAT, and SOD. Decrease in the activity and expression of LDH enzymes	Urethane-induced mouse lung cancer in vivo model (p.o. administration) [a]	[179]
Bilberry extract (BE), genistein (GEN), delphinidin-3-O-glucoside (D3G), delphinidin (DE), gallic acid (GA), and phloroglucinol aldehyde (PGA)	Antagonistic interactions of BE, D3G, DEL and GEN with erlotinib. No effect of GA on erlotinib, while synergistic interaction of PGA with erlotinib. Mechanism unknown	A431 human epithelial cell line	[180]

Note: a. The route of administration for individual natural polyphenols evaluated in in vivo studies.

4.1. Resveratrol

Resveratrol (3,5,4′-trihydroxy-*trans*-stilbene) is a naturally occurring stilbene phytoalexin that was first isolated from the white hellebore *Veratrum grandiflorum* in the 1940's [181]. It has a wide spectrum of biological activities that confer various health-promoting effects, such as antioxidant, anti-inflammatory, antidegenerative, cardioprotective, and anticarcinogenic properties [182,183]. The anticancer activities of resveratrol are often associated with modulating enzymes that are responsible for metabolism of carcinogens, activating or inhibiting molecular targets, and signaling pathways that control cancer development and progression [184–186]. In lung cancer, considerable progress has been made in understanding the mechanisms by which resveratrol inhibits cell proliferation, induces apoptosis and cell cycle arrest, and suppresses invasion and metastasis (Figure 3), which highlights the potential of resveratrol to be used as a complementary treatment to augment the efficacy of existing therapies, and providing the insight into the development of novel synthetic resveratrol analogues with improved therapeutic efficacy and reduced side-effects.

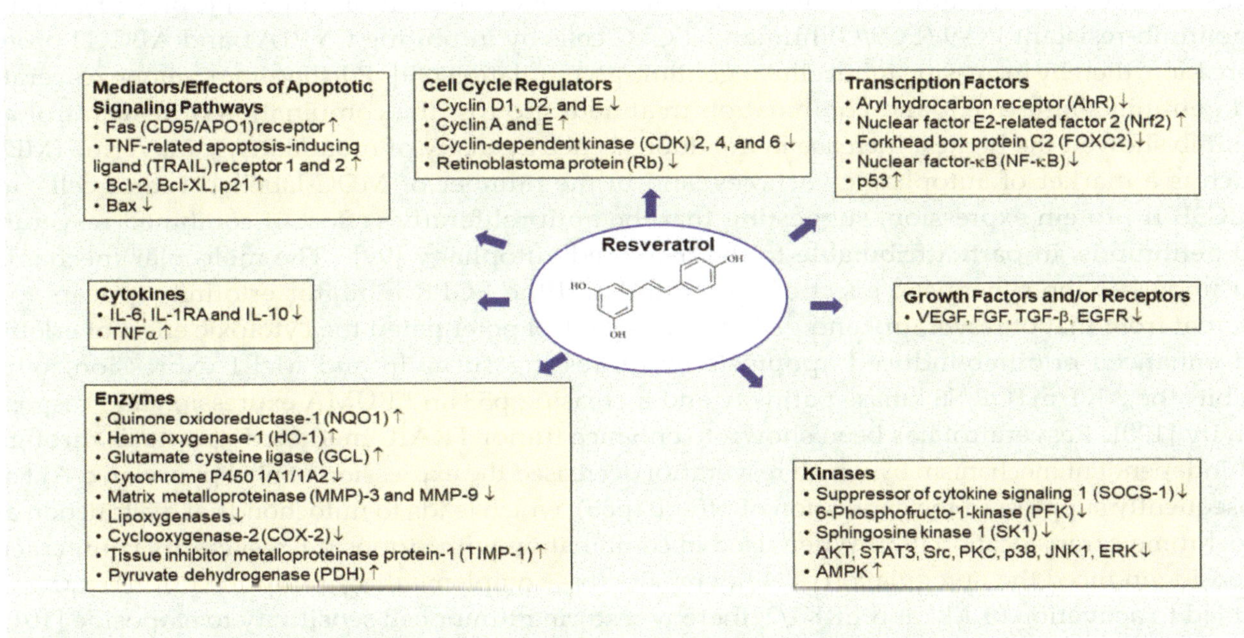

Figure 3. Molecular Mechanisms of Antitumor Activities of Resveratrol in Lung Cancer.

The in vitro anti-proliferative effect of resveratrol is often associated with the induction of cell cycle arrest and apoptosis although the molecular underpinnings may vary among individual lung cancer cell lines. The results of the high-throughput immunoblotting (PowerBlot) and microarray gene expression profiling have revealed that the growth inhibitory effect of resveratrol was mediated by the transforming growth factor-β (TGF-β)/Smad pathway through the downregulation of the TGF-β pathway activators, Smad 2 and Smad 4, and the upregulation of the repressor Smad 7. Moreover, resveratrol-induced apoptosis and G1 phase cell cycle arrest was attributable to the activation of the caspases, the loss of mitochondrial permeability transition, and the increase in the expression of pro-apoptotic tumor suppressor p53 and cyclin-dependent kinase inhibitors p21 and p27 at both the gene and protein levels [90]. Similar results have been documented by others, which indicate that resveratrol-induced apoptosis is associated with increased expression of p53, Bax, and cleaved caspase-3 and decreased expression of Bcl-2 [91–95]. Resveratrol has also been shown to induce apoptosis through the downregulation of cellular FLICE (FADD-like interleukin-1 beta-converting enzyme) inhibitory protein (c-FLIP), which leads to a decrease in phospho-Akt, phospho-EGFR and NF-κB protein expression and an increase in the cleavage and upregulation of Bid, PARP, and caspase-8 and the production of hydrogen peroxide (H_2O_2) [96]. Besides the induction of apoptosis, resveratrol-induced premature senescence is another mechanism that is associated with its anticancer activities [97,98]. Resveratrol-induced premature senescence is correlated with increased DNA double strand breaks (DSBs) and reactive oxygen species (ROS) production in lung cancer cells [97]. When A549 and H460 cells underwent ionizing radiation and resveratrol co-treatment, resveratrol enhanced ionizing radiation-induced premature senescence and increased the ROS production in those cells [98].

The ability of resveratrol to induce apoptosis and cell cycle arrest in lung cancer cells renders it an ideal candidate for combination cancer therapy with the potential to provide additive anticancer efficacy and counteract the onset of acquired drug resistance in the treatment of lung cancer. Resveratrol has been shown to potentiate the growth inhibitory effect of cisplatin through induction of cell apoptosis, which was preceded by the depolarization of mitochondrial membrane potential, opening of the mitochondrial permeability transition pore, release of cytochrome *c*, upregulation of Bax expression, and downregulation of Bcl-2 expression [94]. Preclinical evaluation of the synergistic effect of resveratrol and the EGFR inhibitor gefitinib in a panel of human NSCLC cell lines demonstrated that resveratrol increased the sensitivity to gefitinib in all the cell lines tested, regardless of their EGFR mutation status. Moreover, resveratrol enhanced the inhibitory effect of gefitinib on EGFR phosphorylation in gefitinib-resistant PC-9 (PC9/G) human NSCLC cells by inhibiting CYP1A1 and ABCG2 protein expression, thereby increasing intracellular gefitinib accumulation [99]. Furthermore, among resveratrol and gefitinib single agent and combination treatment groups, the combination of resveratrol and gefitinib showed the highest increase in the fluorescence intensity of monodansylcadaverine (MDC), which is a marker of autophagic vacuoles, and in the number of MDC-labelled tumor cells, and in LC3B II protein expression, suggesting that the antiproliferative effect of combined resveratrol and gefitinib is, in part, attributable to the increased autophagy [99]. The molecular mechanism that underlies the synergistic effect of resveratrol and the EGFR inhibitor erlotinib appears to be different from that of resveratrol and gefitinib. Resveratrol potentiated the cytotoxic effect of erlotinib and enhanced erlotinib-induced apoptosis by repressing survivin and Mcl-1 expression, which inhibits the AKT/mTOR/S6 kinase pathway and increasing p53 and PUMA expression and caspase 3 activity [100]. Resveratrol has been shown to enhance tumor TRAIL-mediated apoptosis through a p53-independent mechanism by which resveratrol decreased the expression of phosphorylated Akt and subsequently suppressed the expression of NF-κB (p65), which leads to mitochondrial dysfunction and cytochrome c translocation [92]. When used in combination with etoposide, resveratrol counteracted etoposide-induced the upregulation of X-ray repair cross-complementing group 1 (XRCC1) expression that led to activation of Akt and ERK1/2, thereby restoring tumor cell sensitivity to etoposide [101].

Several studies have identified modulation of microRNAs (miRNAs) as one of the key mechanisms by which resveratrol exerts its antitumor activities in lung cancer [102–104]. Bae and coworkers identified 71 miRNAs with considerable changes in their expression levels in resveratrol-treated A549 cells while using microarray analysis [102]. Further analysis revealed that 25 of the 71 miRNAs target genes possessing experimentally confirmed function in apoptosis (97 genes), cell cycle regulation (20 genes), cell proliferation and differentiation (28 genes) [102]. Several recent studies have demonstrated the cell line-dependent functional link between the antitumor activities of resveratrol and resveratrol-regulated miRNA expression. In a study by Han et al., resveratrol treatment resulted in the upregulation of miR-622 in 16HBE-T human bronchial epithelial cells and H460 cells [103]. miR-622 was considered to be a tumor suppressor, as an increase in the expression level of miR-622 inhibited the cell proliferation and colony formation, induced cell cycle arrest at G0 phase, and delayed tumor growth in nude mice. Moreover, increase in miR-622 expression reduced K-Ras protein expression levels but had no effect on K-Ras mRNA level, suggesting miR-622 exerts its antitumor activity via targeting K-Ras [103]. In another study, Yu and coworkers examined the role of miR-520h in mediating the antitumor effect of resveratrol in CL1-4 and A549 lung cancer cells. Resveratrol was shown to induce the mesenchymal-epithelial transition (MET) by increasing the expression of protein phosphatase 2A catalytic subunit (PP2A/C) and reducing the expression of FOXC2, phospho-Akt, and p65. As the increased expression of PP2A/C was associated with downregulation of miR-520h [187], and treatment with resveratrol decreased miR-520h expression in A549 cells, it is suggested that resveratrol-induced MET and its inhibitory effect on lung cancer cell migration and invasion are attributable to its ability to inhibit miR-520h expression and activate PP2A/C, which in turn suppresses Akt-mediated activation of the NF-κB pathway, which promotes the malignant behaviors of lung cancer cells [104].

Based on the identified structure-activity relationship, analogues of resveratrol have been synthesized and tested for their antitumor activities in lung cancer cell lines. A synthetic resveratrol named BCS (3,4,5-trimethoxy-4V-bromo-*cis*-stilbene), in which the hydroxyl group of resveratrol is substituted by the methoxy group, was about 1100 times more potent than resveratrol in the growth inhibition of A549 cells (IC_{50}; 0.03 μM vs. 33 μM) [105]. The anti-proliferative effect of BCS was highly associated with cell cycle arrest at G2/M phase and the induction of apoptosis possibly through a mitochondrial-mediated pathway, as manifested by the elevated expression levels of p53 and p21, and the release of cytochrome c in the cytosol [105]. SS28 ((E)-1,2,3-trimethoxy-5-(4-methylstyryl)benzene (6 h)) is a resveratrol-based tubulin inhibitor that exerts its antiproliferative activity by binding to its cellular target tubulin to disrupt the microtubule dynamics [120]. SS28 treatment induces G2/M cell cycle arrest by inhibiting tubulin polymerization during cell division and it leads to apoptosis via the intrinsic (mitochondrial) pathway, as indicated by the loss of mitochondrial membrane potential and activation of Caspase 9 and Caspase 3 [120]. Another resveratrol analogue, 4,4′-dihydroxy-*trans*-stilbene (DHS), significantly suppressed tumor growth and angiogenesis in C57BL/6 mice bearing Lewis lung carcinoma (LLC) and inhibited the anchorage-dependent or -independent LLC cell growth in both mouse and zebrafish lung cancer invasion models [121]. In addition, the results of the in vitro study showed that DHS inhibited LLC cell proliferation, migration, and invasion, and induced the accumulation of hypodiploid cells in the sub-G1 phase, which suggests that the antitumor effect of DHS is via inhibiting DNA synthesis and driving cells towards the apoptotic pathway [121].

4.2. Tea Catechins

Catechins belong to a family of flavonoids and they are the main component of green tea in which catechins comprise 80–90% of the flavonoids, with EGCG being the most abundant catechin (up to 60%) and EGC being the second most abundant (up to 20%), followed by ECG (up to 14%) and EC (about 6%) [188,189]. With a structure of two benzene rings (the A- and B-rings) and a dihydropyran heterocycle (the C-ring) with a hydroxyl or galloyl group over carbon 3, catechins have four possible diasteroisomers. Two isomers with *trans* configuration are called catechin ((+)-catechin and (−)-catechin), and two with *cis* configuration, called epicatechin ((+)-epicatechin and (−)-epicatechin) [190]. The number and configuration of hydroxyl groups on the B ring are the most important determinants of the antioxidant ability of catechins, while the presence of the galloyl group might further increase the antioxidant action [191–193].

The mechanism underlying the inhibitory effects of tea catechins, especially EGCG, on lung cancer progression have been extensively investigated [194–197]. In general, the growth inhibition effect of EGCG is superior to EGC, ECG, and EC [125], and it is associated with the induction of G_2-M arrest [126] and activation of p53-dependent transcription [125]. EGCG treatment has been shown to effectively inhibit the in vitro and in vivo growth of fusion gene- or EGFR-driven lung cancer cells such as H2228 and HCC78 cells that harbor the EML4-ALK fusion gene and SLC34A2-ROS1 fusion gene, respectively, and PC-9, RPC-9, and H1975 cells that harbor $EGFR^{19DEL}$, $EGFR^{19DEL + T790M}$, and $EGFR^{L858R + T790M}$ mutations, respectively [127], which suggests that EGCG has a broad growth inhibitory effect independent of the EGFR mutation status and the ALK or ROS1 fusion status. Although the results of the in vitro study showed that the anti-proliferative activity of EGCG was attributable to the suppressed phosphorylation of EGFR, ALK, and ROS1, and their downstream proteins, Akt and ERK, the in vivo growth inhibitory effect of EGCG in xenograft tumors was associated with the inhibition of HIF-1α expression and reduction tumor angiogenesis, which suggests that tumor response to EGCG is influenced by the tumor microenvironment [127].

The results from a human cancer cDNA expression array study showed that EGCG downregulated the expression of 12 genes and upregulated the expression of four genes out of the 163 genes examined [128]. Among the 12 downregulated genes, two genes (NF-κB inducing kinase (NIK) and death-associated protein kinase 1 (DAPK1)) are associated with apoptosis, two genes (MAP kinase p38γ and CDC 25B/M-phase inducer phosphatase 2) associated with cell cycle, two genes (envoplakin and synapse-associated protein 102 (SAP102)) related to cell-cell interaction, three genes (Rho B, T-lymphoma invasion and metastasis inducing protein 1 (TIAM1) and Cdc42 GTPase-activating protein (Cdc42GAP)) related to the Rho family of small GTPase and regulator, tyrosine–protein kinase (SKY) gene, dishevelled 1 gene, and *EGFR* gene [128]. The four EGCG-upregulated genes included retinoblastoma binding protein (RBQ1), *VEGF*, retinoic acid receptor α1 (RAR-α1), and insulin-like growth factor-binding protein 3 (IGFBP 3) genes [128]. It is noteworthy that high levels of IGFBP 3 in plasma are associated with reduced lung cancer risk [198].

A line of evidence has shown changes in miRNA expression in response to EGCG treatment in lung tumor cell lines and 4-(methylnitrosamino)-1-(3-pyridyl)-1-butanone (NNK)-induced mouse lung tumors [129,199]. EGCG treatment resulted in increased miR-210 expression, leading to reduced proliferation and anchorage-independent growth in CL13 mouse lung adenocarcinoma cells and H460 and H1299 human NSCLC cells [199]. Moreover, EGCG increased the activity of both mouse and human miR-210 gene promoters in H1299 and H460 cells that were transfected with the 2 kb of mouse and 600 bp of human miR-210 gene promoter driven luciferase reporters [199]. Furthermore, the activity of HRE-luciferase in response to EGCG was increased from 2000–4500 U to 8000–40,000 U with the addition of HIF-1a expression vector, and an increased HIF-1α protein expression was observed in EGCG-treated lung cancer cells, which suggests that the upregulation of miR-210 by EGCG is mediated through the HRE in the promoter of miR-210 and stabilization of HIF1α [199]. The involvement of miRNA-mediated gene regulation in antitumor activities of EGCG has also been demonstrated to modulate miRNA expression in 4-(methylnitrosamino)-1-(3-pyridyl)-1-butanone (NNK)-induced mouse lung tumor model [200]. The results of the miRNA microarray showed that 12 miRNAs were upregulated in response to the EGCG treatment, while 9 miRNAs were downregulated. ECGC treatment was found to induce changes in the expression of 21 mRNAs in NNK-induced mouse lung tumors. Moreover, a group of 26 genes were identified as potential targets of the EGCG-regulated miRNAs. Changes in the expression levels of those genes were inversely correlated to changes in the expression levels of the corresponding miRNAs [200]. Further analysis of the role of the 26 miRNA targeted genes revealed an interaction network that is centralized by IGFBP5 and is involved in the regulation of Akt, MAP kinases, NF-κB, and cell cycle [200], which is consistent with the documented mechanisms of inhibitory effects of EGCG on cell cycle and inflammation [194,201]. It was noted that EGCG-induced the upregulation of miR-210 in cultured lung tumor cells was not one of the 26 miRNAs which expression levels were significantly altered in response to EGCG treatment in vivo. This discrepancy could be due to differences in the oxidative stress levels and EGCG-binding proteins between in vitro cultured cells and primary tumors, and in EGCG bioavailability and the elimination half-life between the in vitro and in vivo systems [200].

EGCG has been proved to be beneficial in combination with cancer preventive and chemotherapeutic agents [130,131]. Cotreatment of EGCG with celecoxib, a cyclooxygenase-2 selective inhibitor, synergistically induced apoptosis through the upregulation of *GADD153* gene expression and activation of the mitogen-activated protein kinase (MAPK) signaling pathway [130]. EGCG in combination with cisplatin significantly inhibited cell proliferation and induced cell cycle arrest in G1 phase and apoptosis in cisplatin-resistant A549 cells and suppressed the growth of cisplatin-resistant A549 xenograft tumors [131]. The mechanism of resensitization of tumor cells to cisplatin by EGCG is linked to the inhibition of DNA methyltransferase (DNMT) activity and histone deacetylase (HDAC) activity, reversal of hypermethylated status, and downregulated expression of the GAS1, TIMP4, ICAM1, and WISP2 gene [131]. The combined treatment of EGCG and another dietary polyphenol, luteolin, resulted in synergistic/additive apoptotic and growth inhibitory effects in both in vitro and in vivo lung tumor models. It was noted that p53 wildtype lung cancer cell lines showed greater sensitivity to co-treatment with EGCG and luteolin than p53-mutant or p53-null cell lines, and the combination effectively increased stabilization and ATM-dependent S15 phosphorylation of p53 and mitochondrial translocation of p53. Those results suggest that p53 is required for apoptosis that is induced by the combination of EGCG and luteolin [132].

Similar to EGCG, green tea extract has been demonstrated to exert anticancer activities across a spectrum of lung cancer cell lines and in vivo tumor models through different mechanisms, including the induction of apoptosis through upregulation of p53 expression and downregulation of Bcl-2 expression [133–137], and the inhibition of tumorigenesis through inhibition of cyclooxygenase-2, inactivation of Akt and NF-κB and degradation of IκBα [138], and through the induction of dominant-negative activator protein 1 (*TAM67*) and inhibition of activator protein-1 (AP-1) pathway [139]. The results of the proteomic analysis of A549 cells treated with green tea exact reveals 14 proteins with a ≥2-fold change in the expression level are involved in calcium-binding, cytoskeleton and motility, metabolism, detoxification, or gene regulation [140]. In particular, green tea extract was found to upregulate the expression of lamin A/C, which regulates actin polymerization in nucleus, which leads to decreased cell motility and growth and increased apoptosis [140]. Combination of polyphenon E (a standardized green tea polyphenol preparation) and atorvastatin, an inhibitor of 3-hydroxy-3-methylglutaryl CoA reductase that is commonly used for the treatment of hypercholesterolemia, synergistically inhibited 4-(methylnitrosaminao)-1-(3-pyridyl)-1-butanone induced lung tumorigenesis in mice and the tumor cell proliferation through enhanced apoptosis, which implicates that the combined use of green tea polyphenols and atorvastatin might be beneficial in lung cancer prevention and therapy [141].

4.3. Curcumin

Curcumin is a bioactive phytochemical in the dietary spice turmeric and it has potential anticancer activity against various types of cancer, including lung cancer [202,203]. The results from the in vitro studies have demonstrated that curcumin treatment inhibits tumor cell growth by inducing apoptosis through a variety of p53-independent and mitochondria-dependent pathways [143–147]. In a study by Wu et al., curcumin treatment in cultured H460 cells resulted in cell cycle arrest at the G2/M phase, initial upregulation, followed by the downregulation of cell cycle regulator cyclin D and E, upregulation of Bax, Bad and FAS/CD95 and downregulation of Bcl-2, Bcl-xL, and XIAP protein expression, increase in ROS, intracellular Ca^{2+} and endoplasmic reticulum stress, which led to a loss of mitochondrial membrane potential ($\Delta\Psi_m$) and activation of caspase-3, release of growth arrest and DNA damage inducible gene 153 (*GADD153*) and glucose-regulated protein 78 (*GRP78*) from mitochondria to cytosol and nuclei, and decreased CDK1, CDK2, CDK4, and CDK6 protein expression and increased caspase 8 and *Endo G* mRNA expression [145]. Similar results elucidating the mechanism underlying the apoptotic activity of curcumin have been reported by other research groups using different tumor cell lines. For example, curcumin inhibited the proliferation of A549 cells through upregulation of Bax and downregulation of Bcl-2 expression, and activation of the mitochondrial apoptosis pathway, as manifested by the decreased mitochondrial membrane potential and increased release of cytochrome C from mitochondria to cytoplasm [146]. The effect of curcumin on inhibiting cell growth and inducing cell cycle arrest at the G1/S phase and apoptosis in PC-9 cells has been associated with the upregulation of the expression of *GADD45*, *GADD153*, CDK inhibitors *p21* and *p27* genes, and downregulation of the expression of *cyclin D1*, *CDK2*, *CDK4*, and *CDK6* genes [144]. A501, a synthetic analogue of curcumin with improved anticancer activities, induced cell cycle arrest at the G2/M phase by decreasing the expression of cyclin B1 and cdc-2, and promoted apoptosis by increasing the expression of p53 and Bax and decreasing the expression of Bcl-2 [153].

Although apoptosis induction appears to be the main mechanism underlying the antitumor activities of curcumin in lung cancer, there is evidence of other mechanisms being involved in the inhibitory effect of curcumin on lung tumor survival and progression. The anti-proliferative effect of curcumin has been associated with the inactivation of the PI3K/Akt/mTOR signaling pathway [148,149], upregulation of miR-192-5p [148], and induction of autophagy [149,150]. In a study by Liao et al., the ability of curcumin to suppress the proliferation, invasion, and metastasis of A549 cells was attributable to its inhibitory effect on the expression of GLUT1, MT1-MMP, and MMP2 in A549 cells [151]. Targeting GLUT1 has been sought as an attractive approach for cancer therapy, as upregulation of GLUT1 expression in malignant tumor cells is known to be responsible for the increased glucose uptake needed to drive ATP production through aerobic glycolysis, also known as the "Warburg effect" [204–206]. However, the overexpression of GLUT1 in A549 cells was found to attenuate the inhibitory effect of curcumin against tumor cell invasion in vitro and metastasis in vivo and increase the intracellular expression levels of MT1-MMP and MMP2, implicating that curcumin inhibits lung tumor growth and metastasis through its modulatory effect on the GLUT1/MT1-MMP/MMP2 pathway, but not by targeting GLUT1. In addition, it is suggested that GLUT1 overexpression might potentially confer resistance to curcumin treatment in lung cancer [151]. In another study by Tsai et al., the anti-migratory and anti-invasive effect of curcumin was attributable to the inhibited adiponectin expression via blockage of the adiponectin receptor 1 expression, the inactivated p38 and ERK pathways, and the downregulated expression levels of p65, MMP-2, -9, -3, -13, and -14 [152]. Given the additional evidence indicating that adiponectin regulated NF-κB expression through the Akt pathway, it was concluded that curcumin inhibited lung cancer metastasis through the adiponectin/NF-κB/MMP signaling pathway [152].

The potential of curcumin in combination with other anticancer drugs for lung cancer treatment has been documented. Curcumin potentiated the anti-proliferative effect of gefitinib in three gefitinib-resistant NSCLC cell lines, including CL1-5 ($EGFR^{wt}$), A549 ($EGFR^{wt}$), and H1975 ($EGFR^{L858R + T790M}$) cell lines through blockage of EGFR activation and induction of EGFR degradation [154]. Moreover, curcumin enhanced the antitumor effect of gefitinib in CL1-5, A549, and H1975 xenografts in vivo. Notably, curcumin alone, and in combination with gefitinib, decreased the protein expression of EGFR and Akt in CL1-5 xenografts, which was not affected by gefitinib treatment alone. In addition, co-treatment with curcumin reduced the gefitinib-induced villi damage and apoptosis in mouse intestines possibly through the modulatory effect of curcumin on gefitinib-induced p38 activation [154]. Combined treatment with curcumin and carboplatin resulted in synergistic effect on cell proliferation, apoptosis, invasion, and migration [155]. This synergism appeared to be mediated by multiple mechanisms, including efficient downregulation of MMP-2 and MMP-9, substantial suppression of NF-kB via the inhibition of the Akt/IKKa pathway and enhanced ERK1/2 activity, augmented apoptosis induction through increased upregulation of p53 and p21, and downregulation of Bcl-2 protein expression [155].

4.4. *Quercetin*

Quercetin, a plant pigment and the most abundant dietary flavonol, is known to possess anti-proliferative and proapoptotic effects against many human cancers, including lung cancer [207]. It has been demonstrated that quercetin induces cytotoxicity and apoptosis in human NSCLC cells through multiple mechanisms. The mechanisms by which quercetin induces cell growth inhibition, cell cycle arrest at the G2/M phase and apoptosis involve the increase in the expression levels of survivin, cyclin B1, phospho-cdc2 (threonine 161), total p53 (DO-1), phospho-p53 (serine 15) and p21 proteins, and the induction of abnormal chromosome segregation [156]. Besides inactivation of Akt, quercetin-induced cleavage of caspase-3, caspase-7 and PARP has been found to be accompanied by the increased phosphorylation of MEK, ERK, c-Jun, and JNK, which suggests that the activation of the MEK-ERK pathway plays an important role in quercetin-induced apoptosis [157]. The results of the microarray analysis of quercetin-regulated genes in H460 cells revealed that quercetin upregulated genes that are associated with cell cycle arrest ($p21^{Cip1}$, GADD45), the death pathway (including TRAILR, FAS, TNFR1), the JNK pathway (MEKK1, MKK4, JNK), the IL1 receptor pathway (IL1, IL1R, IRAK), the caspase cascade (caspase-10, DFF45), and the NF-κB pathway (IκBα), while it downregulated genes that are involved in cell survival (NF-κB, IKK, AKT) and proliferation (SCF, SKP2, CDKs, cyclins) [158].

Quercetin has been demonstrated to exert anti-invasive and anti-metastatic activities in lung tumor cells through the downregulation of monocarboxylate transporter 1 (MCT1) [159], inhibition of aurora B kinase activity and histone 3 phosphorylation [160], disassembly of microfilaments, microtubules, and vimentin filaments along with the inhibition of vimentin and N-cadherin expression [161]. Quercetin treatment effectively suppressed the in vitro migration/invasion and in vivo bone metastasis of NSCLC cells by increasing the expression of the epithelial marker, E-cadherin, and decreasing the expressions of the mesenchymal markers, N-cadherin, and vimentin [162]. The mechanism that is associated with quercetin inhibited cell motility involved F-actin-containing microfilament bundle rearrangement and the suppression of EMT through both Snail-dependent Akt activation and Snail-independent ADAM9 pathway [162]. A recent study on the effect of five phytochemicals, including quercetin, curcumin, chrysin, apigenin, and luteolin on $NiCl_2$ (Ni)-induced the migration and invasion of cultured lung cancer cells revealed that the most efficient phytochemical compound inhibiting cell migration and invasion was quercetin, followed by chrysin and apigenin [163]. Further investigation demonstrated that quercetin and chrysin at 2 and 5 μM significantly suppressed Ni-induced rise in Toll-like receptor 4 (TLR4) expression, nuclear p65 level, and relative phospho-IKK-β and phospho-IKK-α levels, which suggests that the anti-invasive effect of quercetin is associated with the downregulation of TLR4/NF-κB signaling pathway [163].

Quercetin treatment in combination with Trichostatin A, a histone deacetylase inhibitor, significantly increased growth arrest and apoptosis through the mitochondrial pathway in A549 cells expressing wild-type p53, but not in H1299 cells harboring a p53 null mutation [164]. Moreover, quercetin treatment enhances TSA-induced acetylation of histones H3 and H4 through the p53-independent mechanism [164]. Cotreatment of quercetin with gemcitabine, a pyrimidine nucleoside analogue that inhibits DNA synthesis, promoted apoptosis via the inhibition of heat shock protein 70 (HSP70) expression [165]. It is evident that quercetin-induced HSP70 inhibition is associated with the caspase-dependent apoptosis through intrinsic apoptotic pathway, given the fact that quercetin-induced HSP70 inhibition significantly increased the caspase-3 activity, while the combination of quercetin and gemcitabine significantly increased caspase-9 activity [165]. HSP70 is known to control proteostasis and anti-stress responses in rapidly proliferating tumor cells and thus reduce the sensitivity of tumors to conventional anti-cancer drugs [208]. The mild toxicity profile of quercetin and its potential to act as a HSP70 inhibitor render it an attractive agent for use as part of a combination regimen to improve tumor response to chemotherapy with less severe side effects.

4.5. Other Naturally Occurring Polyphenols

Thymoquinone (TQ), the predominant bioactive constituent that is present in black seed oil (Nigella sativa), and Caffeic acid phenethyl ester (CAPE), a phenolic compound that is isolated from propolis, have been shown to induce G2/M cell cycle arrest and apoptosis through mechanisms similar to those of resveratrol [95]. Notably, all three agents (i.e., CAPE, TQ, and resveratrol) decreased the expression of cyclin D and increased the expression of TRAIL receptor 1 and 2, and p21 with the highest increase in p21 expression being observed in TQ-treated A549 cells. Moreover, CAPE and TQ upregulated Bax expression, while TQ and resveratrol downregulated Bcl-2, NF-κB, and IKK1 expression in A549 cells [95]. Based on those findings, further studies are warranted to evaluate the potential benefit of using TQ and CAPE in combination with other therapeutic agents for the treatment of lung cancer.

Pterostilbene (*trans*-3,5-dimethoxy-4′-hydroxystilbene), a naturally derived phytoalexin and a demethylated analog of resveratrol, was shown to inhibit A549 cell proliferation and induce S-phase cell cycle arrest by activating the ATM/ATR-CHK1/2-p53 signaling pathway [166]. Moreover, in two precancerous human bronchial epithelial cell lines, HBECR and HBECR/p53i, which have normal and reduced p53 expression levels, respectively, low-dose pterostilbene (at 1 and 5 μM) inhibited cell growth and induced cell cycle arrest in S phase and senescence in HBECR cells more efficiently than in HBECR/p53i cells, which suggests that the chemopreventive activity of pterostilbene is p53-dependent. This finding implicates that the use of pterostilbene as a chemopreventive agent for squamous lung carcinogenesis should be initiated at the early stage before p53 mutation occurs. Another analogue of resveratrol, bakuchiol (1-(4-hydroxyphenyl)-3,7-dimethyl-3-vinyl-1,6-octadiene) that was isolated from the seeds of *Psoralea corylifolia* L. (Leguminosae), exhibits a more significant cytotoxic effect in A549 cell line than in EA.hy926 endothelial cells, HUVECs, and primary cultured mouse embryo fibroblasts. It induces apoptosis and cell cycle arrest in S phase by increasing ROS production, interrupting mitochondrial homeostasis, increasing Bax/Bcl-2 ratio, upregulating p53, and activating Caspase 9/3, which suggests that the apoptotic effect of bakuchiol is p53-dependent and involves a mitochondrial-mediated pathway [167].

Chlorogenic acid (CGA) is the ester of caffeic acid and (−)-quinic acid, one of the most abundant phenolic acid compounds found in coffee and tea [209]. A substantial body of evidence has indicated that CGA exerts antioxidant [210,211], anti-inflammatory [212], antidiabetic [209], antimicrobial [213,214], and anticancer [215,216] activities. Different mechanisms that are associated with the antitumor properties of CGA have been proposed, including enhancing the activity of aryl hydrocarbon hydroxylase, suppressing the oxidative formation of 8-hydroxy-2′-deoxyguanosine (8-OH-dG) in DNA, reducing the production of ROS, and regulating the immune system [217–219]. A study by Part et al. demonstrated that CGA significantly decreased the HIF-1α protein level without changing its mRNA level in A549 cells under hypoxic conditions and subsequently suppressed the transcriptional activity of HIF-1α, leading to decreased expression of its downstream target VEGF [168]. Moreover, CGA inhibited hypoxia-stimulated HUVEC migration, invasion, and tumor formation in vitro and VEGF-stimulated angiogenesis in Matrigel plugs in vivo through the mechanism of inhibiting the HIF-1α/AKT signaling pathway [168]. The observed antiangiogenic potential of CGA suggests that CGA could be a novel therapeutic option for the treatment of lung cancer.

Fisetin (3,3′,4′,7-tetrahydroxyflavone), a naturally occurring diet-based flavonoid, exerts anticancer activity against different cancer cell lines, including NSCLC cell lines, when used alone or in combination with other chemotherapeutic agents [169–171,220–223]. The inhibitory effect of fisetin on lung tumor cell growth is attributable to dual suppression of PI3K/Akt and mTOR signaling, as evidenced by the activation of PTEN, phospho-AMPKα, and TSC2, and the inhibition of PI3K, phospho-Akt, phospho-mTOR, and several downstream targets of mTOR [169]. Fisetin was shown not only to inhibit the growth and induce the apoptosis of A549 cells with acquired cisplatin resistant, but also enhance the cisplatin cytotoxicity in cisplatin-resistant cells through the modulation of the MAPK/survivin/caspase pathway [170]. Fisetin showed a synergistic effect with paclitaxel on growth inhibition and mitotic catastrophe induction [171]. The fisetin-enhanced paclitaxel-induced mitotic catastrophe triggered cytoprotective autophagy, subsequently changing to autophagic cell death, which led to enhanced cytotoxicity [171].

Treatment with the ethyl acetate fraction of Glycyrrhiza uralensis extract that contains liquiritin, isoliquiritin, and isoliquirigenin decreased the viability of A549 cells, induced cell cycle arrest at G2/M phase, and apoptosis [172]. The ethyl acetate fraction significantly decreased the protein expression of PCNA, MDM2, phospho-GSK-3β, phospho-Akt, phospho-c-Raf, p-PTEN, caspase-3, pro-caspase-8, pro-caspase-9, PARP, and Bcl-2, and increased the expression of p53, p21, and Bax in a concentration-dependent manner, which suggested that the antitumor effects of liquiritin, isoliquiritin, and isoliquirigenin are orchestrated by the crosstalk among p53, Bcl-2 family, caspase cascades, and the Akt pathway [172].

Experimental evidence for the protective effects of several beverages and plant extracts against lung cancer through different mechanisms has been documented [15,173–175,177–179]. For example, the decoction extract of *Eucalyptus globulus* Labill. decreased the viability of H460 cells in a concentration-dependent manner, which was correlated with cell cycle arrest at the G0/G1 phase, decrease in cell proliferation, and increase in the expression of p53, p21, and cyclin D1 proteins [173].

Polyphenol compounds that were isolated from Selaginella tamariscina suppressed the migration of A549 cells by targeting matrix metalloproteinases (MMPs) [174]. The antitumor activity of the polyphenol-containing rosemary extract was associated with the inactivation of the Akt/mTOR signaling pathway [175]. The inhibitory effect of red wine on the proliferation and lonogenic survival of A549 cells was associated with the inhibition of basal and EGF-stimulated Akt and Erk phosphorylation and increased total and phosphorylated p53 levels [15]. Magnolol and polyphenol mixture derived from Magnolia officinali significantly suppressed the expression levels and function of class I histone deacetylases (HDACs) and enriched the histone acetyl mark (H3K27ac) in the promoter region of DR5, which is a key protein in the death receptor signaling pathway [177]. Pomegranate concentrate that was administered via drinking bottle to cigarette smoking (CS)-exposed mice prevented the formation of CS-induced lung nodules by reducing the mitotic activity and HIF-1αexpression in CS-exposed animals [178]. Oral administration of Achyranthes aspera (PCA) extract to urethane primed lung cancerous mice increased the expression and activities of antioxidant enzymes GST, GR, CAT, and SOD, decreased the expression and activity of LDH, downregulated the expression of pro-inflammatory cytokines IL-1β, IL-6, and TNF-α, along with TFs, NF-κB, and Stat3, and increased expression of Bax and p53 [179]. In addition, PCA was found to counteract urethane-mediated conformational changes of DNA evident by the shift in guanine and thymine bands in Fourier Trans-form Infrared (FTIR) spectroscopy, which suggests that the anticancer activity of PCA is associated with its immunomodulatory role and DNA conformation restoring effect [179].

5. Conclusions and Future Perspectives

Taken together, many years of research on the mechanisms of anticancer action of natural polyphenols have yielded an amazing amount of information. Strong lines of evidence have confirmed that certain natural polyphenols possess potential antitumor activities against lung cancer, which is the leading cause of cancer death in the United States and worldwide. Encouraging data from preclinical studies that were conducted in cell cultures and tumor models have provided much insight into a broad spectrum of molecular mechanisms underlying the anti-proliferative, anti-migratory, anti-metastasis, anti-angiogenic, and pro-apoptotic effects of various bioactive natural polyphenols in lung cancer. However, given that current chemotherapies for lung cancer have not advanced dramatically despite our increased knowledge base, much research is still needed to pave the way for the optimal integration of bioactive polyphenols with traditional chemotherapeutic regimens for lung cancer treatment, and for a full exploration of the polyphenol compounds that have the potential to form the basis for novel anticancer drugs of the future. In addition to continually refining and expanding our knowledge of the molecular mechanisms by which natural polyphenols exert their antiproliferative and proapoptotic activities against lung cancer, future research endeavors should also focus on the mechanistic understanding of bioavailability and the biodistribution process of natural polyphenols, which has been considered to be a challenging research field [224,225]. With the enhanced insight into the factors controlling tumor uptake of phenolic compounds and the advent of innovative drug delivery technologies, it is anticipated that new exploitable avenues will be opened for improved delivery of bioactive natural polyphenols to the site of action, thereby advancing their therapeutic utility in the treatment of lung cancer.

References

1. Jemal, A.; Siegel, R.; Ward, E.; Hao, Y.; Xu, J.; Murray, T.; Thun, M.J. Cancer statistics, 2008. *CA A Cancer J. Clin.* **2008**, *58*, 71–96. [CrossRef] [PubMed]
2. Herbst, R.S.; Heymach, J.V.; Lippman, S.M. Lung cancer. *N. Engl. J. Med.* **2008**, *359*, 1367–1380. [CrossRef] [PubMed]

3. Pesch, B.; Kendzia, B.; Gustavsson, P.; Jockel, K.H.; Johnen, G.; Pohlabeln, H.; Olsson, A.; Ahrens, W.; Gross, I.M.; Bruske, I.; et al. Cigarette smoking and lung cancer—Relative risk estimates for the major histological types from a pooled analysis of case-control studies. *Int. J. Cancer* **2012**, *131*, 1210–1219. [CrossRef]
4. Taylor, R.; Najafi, F.; Dobson, A. Meta-analysis of studies of passive smoking and lung cancer: Effects of study type and continent. *Int. J. Epidemiol.* **2007**, *36*, 1048–1059. [CrossRef]
5. Field, R.W.; Withers, B.L. Occupational and environmental causes of lung cancer. *Clin. Chest Med.* **2012**, *33*, 681–703. [CrossRef]
6. Hosgood, H.D.; Boffetta, P.; Greenland, S.; Lee, Y.C.; McLaughlin, J.; Seow, A.; Duell, E.J.; Andrew, A.S.; Zaridze, D.; Szeszenia-Dabrowska, N.; et al. In-home coal and wood use and lung cancer risk: A pooled analysis of the International Lung Cancer Consortium. *Environ. Health Perspect.* **2010**, *118*, 1743–1747. [CrossRef]
7. Chen, C.L.; Chiou, H.Y.; Hsu, L.I.; Hsueh, Y.M.; Wu, M.M.; Chen, C.J. Ingested arsenic, characteristics of well water consumption and risk of different histological types of lung cancer in northeastern Taiwan. *Environ. Res.* **2010**, *110*, 455–462. [CrossRef]
8. Brenner, D.R.; Boffetta, P.; Duell, E.J.; Bickeboller, H.; Rosenberger, A.; McCormack, V.; Muscat, J.E.; Yang, P.; Wichmann, H.E.; Brueske-Hohlfeld, I.; et al. Previous lung diseases and lung cancer risk: A pooled analysis from the International Lung Cancer Consortium. *Am. J. Epidemiol.* **2012**, *176*, 573–585. [CrossRef]
9. Littman, A.J.; Thornquist, M.D.; White, E.; Jackson, L.A.; Goodman, G.E.; Vaughan, T.L. Prior lung disease and risk of lung cancer in a large prospective study. *Cancer Causes Control* **2004**, *15*, 819–827. [CrossRef]
10. Feskanich, D.; Ziegler, R.G.; Michaud, D.S.; Giovannucci, E.L.; Speizer, F.E.; Willett, W.C.; Colditz, G.A. Prospective study of fruit and vegetable consumption and risk of lung cancer among men and women. *J. Natl. Cancer Inst.* **2000**, *92*, 1812–1823. [CrossRef]
11. Middleton, E.; Kandaswami, C.; Theoharides, T.C. The effects of plant flavonoids on mammalian cells: Implications for inflammation, heart disease, and cancer. *Pharmacol. Rev.* **2000**, *52*, 673–751. [PubMed]
12. Smith-Warner, S.A.; Spiegelman, D.; Yaun, S.S.; Albanes, D.; Beeson, W.L.; van den Brandt, P.A.; Feskanich, D.; Folsom, A.R.; Fraser, G.E.; Freudenheim, J.L.; et al. Fruits, vegetables and lung cancer: A pooled analysis of cohort studies. *Int. J. Cancer* **2003**, *107*, 1001–1011. [CrossRef] [PubMed]
13. Wright, M.E.; Park, Y.; Subar, A.F.; Freedman, N.D.; Albanes, D.; Hollenbeck, A.; Leitzmann, M.F.; Schatzkin, A. Intakes of fruit, vegetables, and specific botanical groups in relation to lung cancer risk in the NIH-AARP Diet and Health Study. *Am. J. Epidemiol.* **2008**, *168*, 1024–1034. [CrossRef] [PubMed]
14. Amararathna, M.; Johnston, M.R.; Rupasinghe, H.P. Plant Polyphenols as Chemopreventive Agents for Lung Cancer. *Int. J. Mol. Sci.* **2016**, *17*, 1352. [CrossRef]
15. Barron, C.C.; Moore, J.; Tsakiridis, T.; Pickering, G.; Tsiani, E. Inhibition of human lung cancer cell proliferation and survival by wine. *Cancer Cell Int.* **2014**, *14*, 6. [CrossRef]
16. Lim, S.L.; Goh, Y.M.; Noordin, M.M.; Rahman, H.S.; Othman, H.H.; Abu Bakar, N.A.; Mohamed, S. Morinda citrifolia edible leaf extract enhanced immune response against lung cancer. *Food Funct.* **2016**, *7*, 741–751. [CrossRef]
17. Christensen, K.Y.; Naidu, A.; Parent, M.E.; Pintos, J.; Abrahamowicz, M.; Siemiatycki, J.; Koushik, A. The risk of lung cancer related to dietary intake of flavonoids. *Nutr. Cancer* **2012**, *64*, 964–974. [CrossRef]
18. Grosso, G.; Godos, J.; Lamuela-Raventos, R.; Ray, S.; Micek, A.; Pajak, A.; Sciacca, S.; D'Orazio, N.; Del Rio, D.; Galvano, F. A comprehensive meta-analysis on dietary flavonoid and lignan intake and cancer risk: Level of evidence and limitations. *Mol. Nutr. Food Res.* **2017**, *61*, 1600930. [CrossRef]
19. Wessner, B.; Strasser, E.M.; Koitz, N.; Schmuckenschlager, C.; Unger-Manhart, N.; Roth, E. Green tea polyphenol administration partly ameliorates chemotherapy-induced side effects in the small intestine of mice. *J. Nutr.* **2007**, *137*, 634–640. [CrossRef]
20. Yao, Q.; Ye, X.; Wang, L.; Gu, J.; Fu, T.; Wang, Y.; Lai, Y.; Wang, Y.; Wang, X.; Jin, H.; et al. Protective effect of curcumin on chemotherapy-induced intestinal dysfunction. *Int. J. Clin. Exp. Pathol.* **2013**, *6*, 2342–2349.
21. Khan, R.; Khan, A.Q.; Qamar, W.; Lateef, A.; Tahir, M.; Rehman, M.U.; Ali, F.; Sultana, S. Chrysin protects against cisplatin-induced colon. toxicity via amelioration of oxidative stress and apoptosis: Probable role of p38MAPK and p53. *Toxicol. Appl. Pharmacol.* **2012**, *258*, 315–329. [CrossRef] [PubMed]
22. Lissoni, P.; Tancini, G.; Barni, S.; Paolorossi, F.; Ardizzoia, A.; Conti, A.; Maestroni, G. Treatment of cancer chemotherapy-induced toxicity with the pineal hormone melatonin. *Support Care Cancer* **1997**, *5*, 126–129. [CrossRef]

23. Ghielmini, M.; Pagani, O.; de Jong, J.; Pampallona, S.; Conti, A.; Maestroni, G.; Sessa, C.; Cavalli, F. Double-blind randomized study on the myeloprotective effect of melatonin in combination with carboplatin and etoposide in advanced lung cancer. *Br. J. Cancer* **1999**, *80*, 1058–1061. [CrossRef] [PubMed]
24. Jaakkola, K.; Lahteenmaki, P.; Laakso, J.; Harju, E.; Tykka, H.; Mahlberg, K. Treatment with antioxidant and other nutrients in combination with chemotherapy and irradiation in patients with small-cell lung cancer. *Anticancer Res.* **1992**, *12*, 599–606. [PubMed]
25. Pace, A.; Savarese, A.; Picardo, M.; Maresca, V.; Pacetti, U.; Del Monte, G.; Biroccio, A.; Leonetti, C.; Jandolo, B.; Cognetti, F.; et al. Neuroprotective effect of vitamin E supplementation in patients treated with cisplatin chemotherapy. *J. Clin. Oncol.* **2003**, *21*, 927–931. [CrossRef] [PubMed]
26. Schmidinger, M.; Budinsky, A.C.; Wenzel, C.; Piribauer, M.; Brix, R.; Kautzky, M.; Oder, W.; Locker, G.J.; Zielinski, C.C.; Steger, G.G. Glutathione in the prevention of cisplatin induced toxicities. A prospectively randomized pilot trial in patients with head and neck cancer and non small cell lung cancer. *Wien. Klin. Wochenschr.* **2000**, *112*, 617–623.
27. Ferry, D.R.; Smith, A.; Malkhandi, J.; Fyfe, D.W.; deTakats, P.G.; Anderson, D.; Baker, J.; Kerr, D.J. Phase I clinical trial of the flavonoid quercetin: Pharmacokinetics and evidence for in vivo tyrosine kinase inhibition. *Clin. Cancer Res.* **1996**, *2*, 659–668.
28. Albanes, D.; Heinonen, O.P.; Taylor, P.R.; Virtamo, J.; Edwards, B.K.; Rautalahti, M.; Hartman, A.M.; Palmgren, J.; Freedman, L.S.; Haapakoski, J.; et al. Alpha-Tocopherol and beta-carotene supplements and lung cancer incidence in the alpha-tocopherol, beta-carotene cancer prevention study: Effects of base-line characteristics and study compliance. *J. Natl. Cancer Inst.* **1996**, *88*, 1560–1570. [CrossRef]
29. Pisters, K.M.; Newman, R.A.; Coldman, B.; Shin, D.M.; Khuri, F.R.; Hong, W.K.; Glisson, B.S.; Lee, J.S. Phase I trial of oral green tea extract in adult patients with solid tumors. *J. Clin. Oncol.* **2001**, *19*, 1830–1838. [CrossRef]
30. Hakim, I.A.; Harris, R.B.; Brown, S.; Chow, H.H.; Wiseman, S.; Agarwal, S.; Talbot, W. Effect of increased tea consumption on oxidative DNA damage among smokers: A randomized controlled study. *J. Nutr.* **2003**, *133*, 3303–3309. [CrossRef]
31. Goodman, G.E.; Thornquist, M.D.; Balmes, J.; Cullen, M.R.; Meyskens, F.L.; Omenn, G.S.; Valanis, B.; Williams, J.H. The Beta-Carotene and Retinol Efficacy Trial: Incidence of lung cancer and cardiovascular disease mortality during 6-year follow-up after stopping beta-carotene and retinol supplements. *J. Natl. Cancer Inst.* **2004**, *96*, 1743–1750. [CrossRef] [PubMed]
32. Laurie, S.A.; Miller, V.A.; Grant, S.C.; Kris, M.G.; Ng, K.K. Phase I study of green tea extract in patients with advanced lung cancer. *Cancer Chemother. Pharmacol.* **2005**, *55*, 33–38. [CrossRef] [PubMed]
33. Pathak, A.K.; Bhutani, M.; Guleria, R.; Bal, S.; Mohan, A.; Mohanti, B.K.; Sharma, A.; Pathak, R.; Bhardwaj, N.K.; Prasad, K.N.; et al. Chemotherapy alone vs. chemotherapy plus high dose multiple antioxidants in patients with advanced non small cell lung cancer. *J. Am. Coll. Nutr.* **2005**, *24*, 16–21. [CrossRef]
34. Osada, H.; Takahashi, T. Genetic alterations of multiple tumor suppressors and oncogenes in the carcinogenesis and progression of lung cancer. *Oncogene* **2002**, *21*, 7421–7434. [CrossRef]
35. Blanco, D.; Vicent, S.; Fraga, M.F.; Fernandez-Garcia, I.; Freire, J.; Lujambio, A.; Esteller, M.; Ortiz-de-Solorzano, C.; Pio, R.; Lecanda, F.; et al. Molecular analysis of a multistep lung cancer model induced by chronic inflammation reveals epigenetic regulation of p16 and activation of the DNA damage response pathway. *Neoplasia* **2007**, *9*, 840–852. [CrossRef]
36. Bettio, D.; Venci, A.; Achille, V.; Alloisio, M.; Santoro, A. Lung cancer in which the hypothesis of multi-step progression is confirmed by array-CGH results: A case report. *Exp. Ther. Med.* **2016**, *11*, 98–100. [CrossRef]
37. Gazdar, A.F.; Minna, J.D. Angiogenesis and the multistage development of lung cancers. *Clin. Cancer Res.* **2000**, *6*, 1611–1612.
38. McClelland, M.R.; Carskadon, S.L.; Zhao, L.; White, E.S.; Beer, D.G.; Orringer, M.B.; Pickens, A.; Chang, A.C.; Arenberg, D.A. Diversity of the angiogenic phenotype in non-small cell lung cancer. *Am. J. Respir. Cell Mol. Biol.* **2007**, *36*, 343–350. [CrossRef]
39. Hilbe, W.; Manegold, C.; Pircher, A. Targeting angiogenesis in lung cancer—Pitfalls in drug development. *Transl. Lung Cancer Res.* **2012**, *1*, 122–128. [CrossRef]

40. Lambert, A.W.; Wong, C.K.; Ozturk, S.; Papageorgis, P.; Raghunathan, R.; Alekseyev, Y.; Gower, A.C.; Reinhard, B.M.; Abdolmaleky, H.M.; Thiagalingam, S. Tumor Cell-Derived Periostin Regulates Cytokines That Maintain Breast Cancer Stem Cells. *Mol. Cancer Res.* **2016**, *14*, 103–113. [CrossRef]
41. Popper, H.H. Progression and metastasis of lung cancer. *Cancer Metastasis Rev.* **2016**, *35*, 75–91. [CrossRef] [PubMed]
42. Vogelstein, B.; Papadopoulos, N.; Velculescu, V.E.; Zhou, S.; Diaz, L.A.; Kinzler, K.W. Cancer genome landscapes. *Science* **2013**, *339*, 1546–1558. [CrossRef] [PubMed]
43. Pao, W.; Girard, N. New driver mutations in non-small-cell lung cancer. *Lancet Oncol.* **2011**, *12*, 175–180. [CrossRef]
44. Chan, B.A.; Hughes, B.G. Targeted therapy for non-small cell lung cancer: Current standards and the promise of the future. *Transl. Lung Cancer Res.* **2015**, *4*, 36–54. [CrossRef] [PubMed]
45. Vecchiarelli, S.; Bennati, C. Oncogene addicted non-small-cell lung cancer: Current standard and hot topics. *Future Oncol.* **2018**, *14*, 3–17. [CrossRef] [PubMed]
46. Facchinetti, F.; Rossi, G.; Bria, E.; Soria, J.C.; Besse, B.; Minari, R.; Friboulet, L.; Tiseo, M. Oncogene addiction in non-small cell lung cancer: Focus on ROS1 inhibition. *Cancer Treat. Rev.* **2017**, *55*, 83–95. [CrossRef] [PubMed]
47. Tsakonas, G.; Ekman, S. Oncogene-addicted non-small cell lung cancer and immunotherapy. *J. Thorac. Dis.* **2018**, *10*, 1547–1555. [CrossRef] [PubMed]
48. Peifer, M.; Fernandez-Cuesta, L.; Sos, M.L.; George, J.; Seidel, D.; Kasper, L.H.; Plenker, D.; Leenders, F.; Sun, R.; Zander, T.; et al. Integrative genome analyses identify key somatic driver mutations of small-cell lung cancer. *Nat. Genet.* **2012**, *44*, 1104–1110. [CrossRef] [PubMed]
49. George, J.; Lim, J.S.; Jang, S.J.; Cun, Y.; Ozretic, L.; Kong, G.; Leenders, F.; Lu, X.; Fernandez-Cuesta, L.; Bosco, G.; et al. Comprehensive genomic profiles of small cell lung cancer. *Nature* **2015**, *524*, 47–53. [CrossRef]
50. Brambilla, E.; Gazdar, A. Pathogenesis of lung cancer signalling pathways: Roadmap for therapies. *Eur. Respir. J.* **2009**, *33*, 1485–1497. [CrossRef]
51. Ciuffreda, L.; Incani, U.C.; Steelman, L.S.; Abrams, S.L.; Falcone, I.; Curatolo, A.D.; Chappell, W.H.; Franklin, R.A.; Vari, S.; Cognetti, F.; et al. Signaling intermediates (MAPK and PI3K) as therapeutic targets in NSCLC. *Curr. Pharm. Des.* **2014**, *20*, 3944–3957. [CrossRef] [PubMed]
52. Giaccia, A.J.; Kastan, M.B. The complexity of p53 modulation: Emerging patterns from divergent signals. *Genes Dev.* **1998**, *12*, 2973–2983. [CrossRef] [PubMed]
53. Lohrum, M.A.; Vousden, K.H. Regulation and activation of p53 and its family members. *Cell Death Differ.* **1999**, *6*, 1162–1168. [CrossRef]
54. Lee, J.S.; Yoon, A.; Kalapurakal, S.K.; Ro, J.Y.; Lee, J.J.; Tu, N.; Hittelman, W.N.; Hong, W.K. Expression of p53 oncoprotein in non-small-cell lung cancer: A favorable prognostic factor. *J. Clin. Oncol. Off. J. Am. Soc. Clin. Oncol.* **1995**, *13*, 1893–1903. [CrossRef]
55. Canale, M.; Petracci, E.; Delmonte, A.; Chiadini, E.; Dazzi, C.; Papi, M.; Capelli, L.; Casanova, C.; De Luigi, N.; Mariotti, M.; et al. Impact of TP53 Mutations on Outcome in EGFR-Mutated Patients Treated with First-Line Tyrosine Kinase Inhibitors. *Clin. Cancer Res.* **2017**, *23*, 2195–2202. [CrossRef]
56. Shivapurkar, N.; Reddy, J.; Chaudhary, P.M.; Gazdar, A.F. Apoptosis and lung cancer: A review. *J. Cell. Biochem.* **2003**, *88*, 885–898. [CrossRef]
57. Liu, G.; Pei, F.; Yang, F.; Li, L.; Amin, A.D.; Liu, S.; Buchan, J.R.; Cho, W.C. Role of Autophagy and Apoptosis in Non-Small-Cell Lung Cancer. *Int. J. Mol. Sci.* **2017**, *18*, 367. [CrossRef]
58. Ouyang, L.; Shi, Z.; Zhao, S.; Wang, F.T.; Zhou, T.T.; Liu, B.; Bao, J.K. Programmed cell death pathways in cancer: A review of apoptosis, autophagy and programmed necrosis. *Cell Prolif.* **2012**, *45*, 487–498. [CrossRef]
59. Li, H.; Zhu, H.; Xu, C.J.; Yuan, J. Cleavage of BID by caspase 8 mediates the mitochondrial damage in the Fas pathway of apoptosis. *Cell* **1998**, *94*, 491–501. [CrossRef]
60. Zou, H.; Li, Y.; Liu, X.; Wang, X. An APAF-1.cytochrome c multimeric complex is a functional apoptosome that activates procaspase-9. *J. Biol. Chem.* **1999**, *274*, 11549–11556. [CrossRef]
61. Hata, A.N.; Engelman, J.A.; Faber, A.C. The BCL2 Family: Key Mediators of the Apoptotic Response to Targeted Anticancer Therapeutics. *Cancer Discov.* **2015**, *5*, 475–487. [CrossRef] [PubMed]
62. Luthi, A.U.; Martin, S.J. The CASBAH: A searchable database of caspase substrates. *Cell Death Differ.* **2007**, *14*, 641–650. [CrossRef] [PubMed]
63. Hanahan, D.; Weinberg, R.A. Hallmarks of cancer: The next generation. *Cell* **2011**, *144*, 646–674. [CrossRef] [PubMed]

64. Fennell, D.A. Caspase regulation in non-small cell lung cancer and its potential for therapeutic exploitation. *Clin. Cancer Res.* **2005**, *11*, 2097–2105. [CrossRef] [PubMed]
65. Choi, H.S.; Cho, M.C.; Lee, H.G.; Yoon, D.Y. Indole-3-carbinol induces apoptosis through p53 and activation of caspase-8 pathway in lung cancer A549 cells. *Food Chem. Toxicol. Int. J. Publ. Br. Ind. Biol. Res. Assoc.* **2010**, *48*, 883–890. [CrossRef]
66. Chirumbolo, S. Dietary assumption of plant polyphenols and prevention of allergy. *Curr. Pharm. Des.* **2014**, *20*, 811–839. [CrossRef]
67. Pandey, K.B.; Rizvi, S.I. Plant polyphenols as dietary antioxidants in human health and disease. *Oxid. Med. Cell Longev.* **2009**, *2*, 270–278. [CrossRef]
68. Tsao, R. Chemistry and biochemistry of dietary polyphenols. *Nutrients* **2010**, *2*, 1231–1246. [CrossRef]
69. Manach, C.; Scalbert, A.; Morand, C.; Remesy, C.; Jimenez, L. Polyphenols: Food sources and bioavailability. *Am. J. Clin. Nutr.* **2004**, *79*, 727–747. [CrossRef]
70. Panche, A.N.; Diwan, A.D.; Chandra, S.R. Flavonoids: An overview. *J. Nutr. Sci.* **2016**, *5*, e47. [CrossRef]
71. Shen, T.; Wang, X.N.; Lou, H.X. Natural stilbenes: An overview. *Nat. Prod. Rep.* **2009**, *26*, 916–935. [CrossRef]
72. Teponno, R.B.; Kusari, S.; Spiteller, M. Recent advances in research on lignans and neolignans. *Nat. Prod. Rep.* **2016**, *33*, 1044–1092. [CrossRef] [PubMed]
73. Haslam, E. Polyphenol-protein interactions. *Biochem. J.* **1974**, *139*, 285–288. [CrossRef] [PubMed]
74. Hansch, C.; Gao, H. Comparative QSAR: Radical Reactions of Benzene Derivatives in Chemistry and Biology. *Chem. Rev.* **1997**, *97*, 2995–3060. [CrossRef]
75. Nandi, S.; Vracko, M.; Bagchi, M.C. Anticancer activity of selected phenolic compounds: QSAR studies using ridge regression and neural networks. *Chem. Biol. Drug Des.* **2007**, *70*, 424–436. [CrossRef]
76. Scotti, L.; Bezerra, M.F.J.; Magalhaes, M.D.R.; da Silva, M.S.; Pitta, I.R.; Scotti, M.T. SAR, QSAR and docking of anticancer flavonoids and variants: A review. *Curr. Top. Med. Chem.* **2012**, *12*, 2785–2809. [CrossRef]
77. Selassie, C.; Shusterman, A.; Kapur, S.P.; Verma, R.; Zhang, L.; Hansch, C. On the toxicity of phenols to fast growing cells. A QSAR model for a radical-based toxicity. *J. Chem. Soc. Perkin Trans.* **1999**, *2*, 2729–2733. [CrossRef]
78. Verma, R.P.; Kapur, S.; Barberena, O.; Shusterman, A.; Hansch, C.H.; Selassie, C.D. Synthesis, cytotoxicity, and QSAR analysis of X-thiophenols in rapidly dividing cells. *Chem. Res. Toxicol.* **2003**, *16*, 276–284. [CrossRef]
79. Oliver, C.L.; Miranda, M.B.; Shangary, S.; Land, S.; Wang, S.; Johnson, D.E. (-)-Gossypol acts directly on the mitochondria to overcome Bcl-2- and Bcl-X(L)-mediated apoptosis resistance. *Mol. Cancer Ther.* **2005**, *4*, 23–31.
80. Bruncko, M.; Oost, T.K.; Belli, B.A.; Ding, H.; Joseph, M.K.; Kunzer, A.; Martineau, D.; McClellan, W.J.; Mitten, M.; Ng, S.C.; et al. Studies leading to potent, dual inhibitors of Bcl-2 and Bcl-xL. *J. Med. Chem.* **2007**, *50*, 641–662. [CrossRef]
81. Kitada, S.; Leone, M.; Sareth, S.; Zhai, D.; Reed, J.C.; Pellecchia, M. Discovery, characterization, and structure-activity relationships studies of proapoptotic polyphenols targeting B-cell lymphocyte/leukemia-2 proteins. *J. Med. Chem.* **2003**, *46*, 4259–4264. [CrossRef] [PubMed]
82. Kitada, S.; Kress, C.L.; Krajewska, M.; Jia, L.; Pellecchia, M.; Reed, J.C. Bcl-2 antagonist apogossypol (NSC736630) displays single-agent activity in Bcl-2-transgenic mice and has superior efficacy with less toxicity compared with gossypol (NSC19048). *Blood* **2008**, *111*, 3211–3219. [CrossRef] [PubMed]
83. Wang, G.; Nikolovska-Coleska, Z.; Yang, C.Y.; Wang, R.; Tang, G.; Guo, J.; Shangary, S.; Qiu, S.; Gao, W.; Yang, D.; et al. Structure-based design of potent small-molecule inhibitors of anti-apoptotic Bcl-2 proteins. *J. Med. Chem.* **2006**, *49*, 6139–6142. [CrossRef] [PubMed]
84. Tang, G.; Yang, C.Y.; Nikolovska-Coleska, Z.; Guo, J.; Qiu, S.; Wang, R.; Gao, W.; Wang, G.; Stuckey, J.; Krajewski, K.; et al. Pyrogallol-based molecules as potent inhibitors of the antiapoptotic Bcl-2 proteins. *J. Med. Chem.* **2007**, *50*, 1723–1726. [CrossRef]
85. Tang, G.; Nikolovska-Coleska, Z.; Qiu, S.; Yang, C.Y.; Guo, J.; Wang, S. Acylpyrogallols as inhibitors of antiapoptotic Bcl-2 proteins. *J. Med. Chem.* **2008**, *51*, 717–720. [CrossRef]
86. Larsen, C.A.; Bisson, W.H.; Dashwood, R.H. Tea catechins inhibit hepatocyte growth factor receptor (MET kinase) activity in human colon cancer cells: Kinetic and molecular docking studies. *J. Med. Chem.* **2009**, *52*, 6543–6545. [CrossRef]
87. Ciechanover, A.; Orian, A.; Schwartz, A.L. Ubiquitin-mediated proteolysis: Biological regulation via destruction. *Bioessays* **2000**, *22*, 442–451. [CrossRef]

88. Nam, S.; Smith, D.M.; Dou, Q.P. Ester bond-containing tea polyphenols potently inhibit proteasome activity in vitro and in vivo. *J. Biol. Chem.* **2001**, *276*, 13322–13330. [CrossRef]
89. Kazi, A.; Wang, Z.; Kumar, N.; Falsetti, S.C.; Chan, T.H.; Dou, Q.P. Structure-activity relationships of synthetic analogs of (-)-epigallocatechin-3-gallate as proteasome inhibitors. *Anticancer Res.* **2004**, *24*, 943–954.
90. Whyte, L.; Huang, Y.Y.; Torres, K.; Mehta, R.G. Molecular mechanisms of resveratrol action in lung cancer cells using dual protein and microarray analyses. *Cancer Res.* **2007**, *67*, 12007–12017. [CrossRef]
91. Li, W.; Shi, Y.; Wang, R.; Pan, L.; Ma, L.; Jin, F. Resveratrol promotes the sensitivity of small-cell lung cancer H446 cells to cisplatin by regulating intrinsic apoptosis. *Int. J. Oncol.* **2018**, *53*, 2123–2130. [CrossRef] [PubMed]
92. Rasheduzzaman, M.; Jeong, J.K.; Park, S.Y. Resveratrol sensitizes lung cancer cell to TRAIL by p53 independent and suppression of Akt/NF-kappaB signaling. *Life Sci.* **2018**, *208*, 208–220. [CrossRef] [PubMed]
93. Sun, L.; Chen, B.; Jiang, R.; Li, J.; Wang, B. Resveratrol inhibits lung cancer growth by suppressing M2-like polarization of tumor associated macrophages. *Cell Immunol.* **2017**, *311*, 86–93. [CrossRef]
94. Ma, L.; Li, W.; Wang, R.; Nan, Y.; Wang, Q.; Liu, W.; Jin, F. Resveratrol enhanced anticancer effects of cisplatin on non-small cell lung cancer cell lines by inducing mitochondrial dysfunction and cell apoptosis. *Int. J. Oncol.* **2015**, *47*, 1460–1468. [CrossRef]
95. Ulasli, S.S.; Celik, S.; Gunay, E.; Ozdemir, M.; Hazman, O.; Ozyurek, A.; Koyuncu, T.; Unlu, M. Anticancer effects of thymoquinone, caffeic acid phenethyl ester and resveratrol on A549 non-small cell lung cancer cells exposed to benzo (a) pyrene. *Asian Pac. J. Cancer Prev.* **2013**, *14*, 6159–6164. [CrossRef]
96. Wright, C.; Iyer, A.K.V.; Yakisich, J.S.; Azad, N. Anti-Tumorigenic Effects of Resveratrol in Lung Cancer Cells Through Modulation of c-FLIP. *Curr. Cancer Drug Targets* **2017**, *17*, 669–680. [CrossRef]
97. Luo, H.; Yang, A.; Schulte, B.A.; Wargovich, M.J.; Wang, G.Y. Resveratrol induces premature senescence in lung cancer cells via ROS-mediated DNA damage. *PLoS ONE* **2013**, *8*, e60065. [CrossRef]
98. Luo, H.; Wang, L.; Schulte, B.A.; Yang, A.; Tang, S.; Wang, G.Y. Resveratrol enhances ionizing radiation-induced premature senescence in lung cancer cells. *Int. J. Oncol.* **2013**, *43*, 1999–2006. [CrossRef]
99. Zhu, Y.; He, W.; Gao, X.; Li, B.; Mei, C.; Xu, R.; Chen, H. Resveratrol overcomes gefitinib resistance by increasing the intracellular gefitinib concentration and triggering apoptosis, autophagy and senescence in PC9/G NSCLC cells. *Sci. Rep.* **2015**, *5*, 17730. [CrossRef]
100. Nie, P.; Hu, W.; Zhang, T.; Yang, Y.; Hou, B.; Zou, Z. Synergistic Induction of Erlotinib-Mediated Apoptosis by Resveratrol in Human Non-Small-Cell Lung Cancer Cells by Down-Regulating Survivin and Up-Regulating PUMA. *Cell Physiol. Biochem.* **2015**, *35*, 2255–2271. [CrossRef]
101. Ko, J.C.; Syu, J.J.; Chen, J.C.; Wang, T.J.; Chang, P.Y.; Chen, C.Y.; Jian, Y.T.; Jian, Y.J.; Lin, Y.W. Resveratrol Enhances Etoposide-Induced Cytotoxicity through Down-Regulating ERK1/2 and AKT-Mediated X-ray Repair Cross-Complement Group 1 (XRCC1) Protein Expression in Human Non-Small-Cell Lung Cancer Cells. *Basic Clin. Pharm. Toxicol.* **2015**, *117*, 383–391. [CrossRef] [PubMed]
102. Bae, S.; Lee, E.M.; Cha, H.J.; Kim, K.; Yoon, Y.; Lee, H.; Kim, J.; Kim, Y.J.; Lee, H.G.; Jeung, H.K.; et al. Resveratrol alters microRNA expression profiles in A549 human non-small cell lung cancer cells. *Mol. Cells* **2011**, *32*, 243–249. [CrossRef] [PubMed]
103. Han, Z.; Yang, Q.; Liu, B.; Wu, J.; Li, Y.; Yang, C.; Jiang, Y. MicroRNA-622 functions as a tumor suppressor by targeting K-Ras and enhancing the anticarcinogenic effect of resveratrol. *Carcinogenesis* **2012**, *33*, 131–139. [CrossRef]
104. Yu, Y.H.; Chen, H.A.; Chen, P.S.; Cheng, Y.J.; Hsu, W.H.; Chang, Y.W.; Chen, Y.H.; Jan, Y.; Hsiao, M.; Chang, T.Y.; et al. MiR-520h-mediated FOXC2 regulation is critical for inhibition of lung cancer progression by resveratrol. *Oncogene* **2013**, *32*, 431–443. [CrossRef]
105. Lee, E.J.; Min, H.Y.; Joo Park, H.; Chung, H.J.; Kim, S.; Nam Han, Y.; Lee, S.K. G2/M cell cycle arrest and induction of apoptosis by a stilbenoid, 3,4,5-trimethoxy-4′-bromo-cis-stilbene, in human lung cancer cells. *Life Sci.* **2004**, *75*, 2829–2839. [CrossRef]
106. Wang, X.; Wang, D.; Zhao, Y. Effect and Mechanism of Resveratrol on the Apoptosis of Lung Adenocarcinoma Cell Line A549. *Cell Biochem. Biophys.* **2015**, *73*, 527–531. [CrossRef]
107. He, L.; Fan, F.; Hou, X.; Gao, C.; Meng, L.; Meng, S.; Huang, S.; Wu, H. Resveratrol suppresses pulmonary tumor metastasis by inhibiting platelet-mediated angiogenic responses. *J. Surg. Res.* **2017**, *217*, 113–122. [CrossRef]

108. Li, X.; Wang, D.; Zhao, Q.C.; Shi, T.; Chen, J. Resveratrol Inhibited Non-small Cell Lung Cancer Through Inhibiting STAT-3 Signaling. *Am. J. Med. Sci.* **2016**, *352*, 524–530. [CrossRef]
109. Li, W.; Ma, X.; Li, N.; Liu, H.; Dong, Q.; Zhang, J.; Yang, C.; Liu, Y.; Liang, Q.; Zhang, S.; et al. Resveratrol inhibits Hexokinases II mediated glycolysis in non-small cell lung cancer via targeting Akt signaling pathway. *Exp. Cell Res.* **2016**, *349*, 320–327. [CrossRef]
110. Lee, Y.S.; Doonan, B.B.; Wu, J.M.; Hsieh, T.C. Combined metformin and resveratrol confers protection against UVC-induced DNA damage in A549 lung cancer cells via modulation of cell cycle checkpoints and DNA repair. *Oncol. Rep.* **2016**, *35*, 3735–3741. [CrossRef]
111. Sahin, E.; Baycu, C.; Koparal, A.T.; Burukoglu Donmez, D.; Bektur, E. Resveratrol reduces IL-6 and VEGF secretion from co-cultured A549 lung cancer cells and adipose-derived mesenchymal stem cells. *Tumour Biol. J. Int. Soc. Oncodev. Biol. Med.* **2016**, *37*, 7573–7582. [CrossRef] [PubMed]
112. Yuan, L.; Zhang, Y.; Xia, J.; Liu, B.; Zhang, Q.; Liu, J.; Luo, L.; Peng, Z.; Song, Z.; Zhu, R. Resveratrol induces cell cycle arrest via a p53-independent pathway in A549 cells. *Mol. Med. Rep.* **2015**, *11*, 2459–2464. [CrossRef] [PubMed]
113. Bai, T.; Dong, D.S.; Pei, L. Synergistic antitumor activity of resveratrol and miR-200c in human lung cancer. *Oncol. Rep.* **2014**, *31*, 2293–2297. [CrossRef] [PubMed]
114. Wang, H.; Zhang, H.; Tang, L.; Chen, H.; Wu, C.; Zhao, M.; Yang, Y.; Chen, X.; Liu, G. Resveratrol inhibits TGF-beta1-induced epithelial-to-mesenchymal transition and suppresses lung cancer invasion and metastasis. *Toxicology* **2013**, *303*, 139–146. [CrossRef]
115. Liao, H.F.; Kuo, C.D.; Yang, Y.C.; Lin, C.P.; Tai, H.C.; Chen, Y.Y.; Chen, Y.J. Resveratrol enhances radiosensitivity of human non-small cell lung cancer NCI-H838 cells accompanied by inhibition of nuclear factor-kappa B activation. *J. Radiat. Res.* **2005**, *46*, 387–393. [CrossRef]
116. Liu, P.L.; Tsai, J.R.; Charles, A.L.; Hwang, J.J.; Chou, S.H.; Ping, Y.H.; Lin, F.Y.; Chen, Y.L.; Hung, C.Y.; Chen, W.C.; et al. Resveratrol inhibits human lung adenocarcinoma cell metastasis by suppressing heme oxygenase 1-mediated nuclear factor-kappaB pathway and subsequently downregulating expression of matrix met alloproteinases. *Mol. Nutr. Food Res.* **2010**, *54*, 196–204. [CrossRef]
117. Zhao, W.; Bao, P.; Qi, H.; You, H. Resveratrol down-regulates survivin and induces apoptosis in human multidrug-resistant SPC-A-1/CDDP cells. *Oncol. Rep.* **2010**, *23*, 279–286. [CrossRef]
118. Kim, Y.A.; Lee, W.H.; Choi, T.H.; Rhee, S.H.; Park, K.Y.; Choi, Y.H. Involvement of p21WAF1/CIP1, pRB, Bax and NF-kappaB in induction of growth arrest and apoptosis by resveratrol in human lung carcinoma A549 cells. *Int. J. Oncol.* **2003**, *23*, 1143–1149.
119. Karthikeyan, S.; Hoti, S.L.; Prasad, N.R. Resveratrol loaded gelatin nanoparticles synergistically inhibits cell cycle progression and constitutive NF-kappaB activation, and induces apoptosis in non-small cell lung cancer cells. *Biomed. Pharmacother.* **2015**, *70*, 274–282. [CrossRef]
120. Thomas, E.; Gopalakrishnan, V.; Hegde, M.; Kumar, S.; Karki, S.S.; Raghavan, S.C.; Choudhary, B. A Novel Resveratrol Based Tubulin Inhibitor Induces Mitotic Arrest and Activates Apoptosis in Cancer Cells. *Sci. Rep.* **2016**, *6*, 34653. [CrossRef]
121. Savio, M.; Ferraro, D.; Maccario, C.; Vaccarone, R.; Jensen, L.D.; Corana, F.; Mannucci, B.; Bianchi, L.; Cao, Y.; Stivala, L.A. Resveratrol analogue 4,4′-dihydroxy-trans-stilbene potently inhibits cancer invasion and metastasis. *Sci. Rep.* **2016**, *6*, 19973. [CrossRef] [PubMed]
122. Malhotra, A.; Nair, P.; Dhawan, D.K. Premature mitochondrial senescence and related ultrastructural changes during lung carcinogenesis modulation by curcumin and resveratrol. *Ultrastruct. Pathol.* **2012**, *36*, 179–184. [CrossRef] [PubMed]
123. Weng, C.J.; Yang, Y.T.; Ho, C.T.; Yen, G.C. Mechanisms of apoptotic effects induced by resveratrol, dibenzoylmethane, and their analogues on human lung carcinoma cells. *J. Agric. Food Chem.* **2009**, *57*, 5235–5243. [CrossRef] [PubMed]
124. Lee, E.O.; Lee, H.J.; Hwang, H.S.; Ahn, K.S.; Chae, C.; Kang, K.S.; Lu, J.; Kim, S.H. Potent inhibition of Lewis lung cancer growth by heyneanol A from the roots of Vitis amurensis through apoptotic and anti-angiogenic activities. *Carcinogenesis* **2006**, *27*, 2059–2069. [CrossRef] [PubMed]
125. Yamauchi, R.; Sasaki, K.; Yoshida, K. Identification of epigallocatechin-3-gallate in green tea polyphenols as a potent inducer of p53-dependent apoptosis in the human lung cancer cell line A549. *Toxicol. In Vitro* **2009**, *23*, 834–839. [CrossRef]

126. Okabe, S.; Suganuma, M.; Hayashi, M.; Sueoka, E.; Komori, A.; Fujiki, H. Mechanisms of growth inhibition of human lung cancer cell line, PC-9, by tea polyphenols. *Jpn. J. Cancer Res.* **1997**, *88*, 639–643. [CrossRef]
127. Honda, Y.; Takigawa, N.; Ichihara, E.; Ninomiya, T.; Kubo, T.; Ochi, N.; Yasugi, M.; Murakami, T.; Yamane, H.; Tanimoto, M.; et al. Effects of (-)-epigallocatechin-3-gallate on EGFR- or Fusion Gene-driven Lung Cancer Cells. *Acta Med. Okayama* **2017**, *71*, 505–512. [CrossRef]
128. Okabe, S.; Fujimoto, N.; Sueoka, N.; Suganuma, M.; Fujiki, H. Modulation of gene expression by (-)-epigallocatechin gallate in PC-9 cells using a cDNA expression array. *Biol. Pharm. Bull.* **2001**, *24*, 883–886. [CrossRef]
129. Zhou, H.; Chen, J.X.; Yang, C.S.; Yang, M.Q.; Deng, Y.; Wang, H. Gene regulation mediated by microRNAs in response to green tea polyphenol EGCG in mouse lung cancer. *BMC Genom.* **2014**, *15*, S3. [CrossRef]
130. Suganuma, M.; Kurusu, M.; Suzuki, K.; Tasaki, E.; Fujiki, H. Green tea polyphenol stimulates cancer preventive effects of celecoxib in human lung cancer cells by upregulation of GADD153 gene. *Int. J. Cancer* **2006**, *119*, 33–40. [CrossRef]
131. Zhang, Y.; Wang, X.; Han, L.; Zhou, Y.; Sun, S. Green tea polyphenol EGCG reverse cisplatin resistance of A549/DDP cell line through candidate genes demethylation. *Biomed. Pharmacother.* **2015**, *69*, 285–290. [CrossRef] [PubMed]
132. Amin, A.R.; Wang, D.; Zhang, H.; Peng, S.; Shin, H.J.; Brandes, J.C.; Tighiouart, M.; Khuri, F.R.; Chen, Z.G.; Shin, D.M. Enhanced anti-tumor activity by the combination of the natural compounds (-)-epigallocatechin-3-gallate and luteolin: Potential role of p53. *J. Biol. Chem.* **2010**, *285*, 34557–34565. [CrossRef] [PubMed]
133. Ganguly, C.; Saha, P.; Panda, C.K.; Das, S. Inhibition of growth, induction of apoptosis and alteration of gene expression by tea polyphenols in the highly metastatic human lung cancer cell line NCI-H460. *Asian Pac. J. Cancer Prev.* **2005**, *6*, 326–331. [PubMed]
134. Banerjee, S.; Manna, S.; Mukherjee, S.; Pal, D.; Panda, C.K.; Das, S. Black tea polyphenols restrict benzopyrene-induced mouse lung cancer progression through inhibition of Cox-2 and induction of caspase-3 expression. *Asian Pac. J. Cancer Prev.* **2006**, *7*, 661–666. [PubMed]
135. Banerjee, S.; Manna, S.; Saha, P.; Panda, C.K.; Das, S. Black tea polyphenols suppress cell proliferation and induce apoptosis during benzo(a)pyrene-induced lung carcinogenesis. *Eur. J. Cancer Prev.* **2005**, *14*, 215–221. [CrossRef]
136. Gu, Q.; Hu, C.; Chen, Q.; Xia, Y.; Feng, J.; Yang, H. Development of a rat model by 3,4-benzopyrene intra-pulmonary injection and evaluation of the effect of green tea drinking on p53 and bcl-2 expression in lung carcinoma. *Cancer Detect. Prev.* **2009**, *32*, 444–451. [CrossRef]
137. Gu, Q.; Hu, C.; Chen, Q.; Xia, Y. Tea polyphenols prevent lung from preneoplastic lesions and effect p53 and bcl-2 gene expression in rat lung tissues. *Int. J. Clin. Exp. Pathol.* **2013**, *6*, 1523–1531.
138. Roy, P.; Nigam, N.; Singh, M.; George, J.; Srivastava, S.; Naqvi, H.; Shukla, Y. Tea polyphenols inhibit cyclooxygenase-2 expression and block activation of nuclear factor-kappa B and Akt in diethylnitrosoamine induced lung tumors in Swiss mice. *Investig. New Drugs* **2010**, *28*, 466–471. [CrossRef]
139. Pan, J.; Zhang, Q.; Xiong, D.; Vedell, P.; Yan, Y.; Jiang, H.; Cui, P.; Ding, F.; Tichelaar, J.W.; Wang, Y.; et al. Transcriptomic analysis by RNA-seq reveals AP-1 pathway as key regulator that green tea may rely on to inhibit lung tumorigenesis. *Mol. Carcinog.* **2014**, *53*, 19–29. [CrossRef]
140. Lu, Q.Y.; Yang, Y.; Jin, Y.S.; Zhang, Z.F.; Heber, D.; Li, F.P.; Dubinett, S.M.; Sondej, M.A.; Loo, J.A.; Rao, J.Y. Effects of green tea extract on lung cancer A549 cells: Proteomic identification of proteins associated with cell migration. *Proteomics* **2009**, *9*, 757–767. [CrossRef]
141. Lu, G.; Xiao, H.; You, H.; Lin, Y.; Jin, H.; Snagaski, B.; Yang, C.S. Synergistic inhibition of lung tumorigenesis by a combination of green tea polyphenols and atorvastatin. *Clin. Cancer Res.* **2008**, *14*, 4981–4988. [CrossRef] [PubMed]
142. Izdebska, M.; Klimaszewska-Wisniewska, A.; Halas, M.; Gagat, M.; Grzanka, A. Green tea extract induces protective autophagy in A549 non-small lung cancer cell line. *Postepy. Hig. Med. Dosw.* **2015**, *69*, 1478–1484.
143. Radhakrishna, P.G.; Srivastava, A.S.; Hassanein, T.I.; Chauhan, D.P.; Carrier, E. Induction of apoptosis in human lung cancer cells by curcumin. *Cancer Lett.* **2004**, *208*, 163–170. [CrossRef] [PubMed]
144. Saha, A.; Kuzuhara, T.; Echigo, N.; Fujii, A.; Suganuma, M.; Fujiki, H. Apoptosis of human lung cancer cells by curcumin mediated through up-regulation of "growth arrest and DNA damage inducible genes 45 and 153". *Biol. Pharm. Bull.* **2010**, *33*, 1291–1299. [CrossRef]

145. Wu, S.H.; Hang, L.W.; Yang, J.S.; Chen, H.Y.; Lin, H.Y.; Chiang, J.H.; Lu, C.C.; Yang, J.L.; Lai, T.Y.; Ko, Y.C.; et al. Curcumin induces apoptosis in human non-small cell lung cancer NCI-H460 cells through ER stress and caspase cascade- and mitochondria-dependent pathways. *Anticancer Res.* **2010**, *30*, 2125–2133.
146. Li, Y.; Zhang, S.; Geng, J.X.; Hu, X.Y. Curcumin inhibits human non-small cell lung cancer A549 cell proliferation through regulation of Bcl-2/Bax and cytochrome C. *Asian Pac. J. Cancer Prev.* **2013**, *14*, 4599–4602. [CrossRef]
147. Yang, C.L.; Ma, Y.G.; Xue, Y.X.; Liu, Y.Y.; Xie, H.; Qiu, G.R. Curcumin induces small cell lung cancer NCI-H446 cell apoptosis via the reactive oxygen species-mediated mitochondrial pathway and not the cell death receptor pathway. *DNA Cell Biol.* **2012**, *31*, 139–150. [CrossRef]
148. Jin, H.; Qiao, F.; Wang, Y.; Xu, Y.; Shang, Y. Curcumin inhibits cell proliferation and induces apoptosis of human non-small cell lung cancer cells through the upregulation of miR-192-5p and suppression of PI3K/Akt signaling pathway. *Oncol. Rep.* **2015**, *34*, 2782–2789. [CrossRef]
149. Wang, A.; Wang, J.; Zhang, S.; Zhang, H.; Xu, Z.; Li, X. Curcumin inhibits the development of non-small cell lung cancer by inhibiting autophagy and apoptosis. *Exp. Ther. Med.* **2017**, *14*, 5075–5080. [CrossRef]
150. Liu, F.; Gao, S.; Yang, Y.; Zhao, X.; Fan, Y.; Ma, W.; Yang, D.; Yang, A.; Yu, Y. Curcumin induced autophagy anticancer effects on human lung adenocarcinoma cell line A549. *Oncol. Lett.* **2017**, *14*, 2775–2782. [CrossRef]
151. Liao, H.; Wang, Z.; Deng, Z.; Ren, H.; Li, X. Curcumin inhibits lung cancer invasion and metastasis by attenuating GLUT1/MT1-MMP/MMP2 pathway. *Int. J. Clin. Exp. Med.* **2015**, *8*, 8948–8957. [PubMed]
152. Tsai, J.R.; Liu, P.L.; Chen, Y.H.; Chou, S.H.; Cheng, Y.J.; Hwang, J.J.; Chong, I.W. Curcumin Inhibits Non-Small Cell Lung Cancer Cells Metastasis through the Adiponectin/NF-kappab/MMPs Signaling Pathway. *PLoS ONE* **2015**, *10*, e0144462. [CrossRef] [PubMed]
153. Xia, Y.Q.; Wei, X.Y.; Li, W.L.; Kanchana, K.; Xu, C.C.; Chen, D.H.; Chou, P.H.; Jin, R.; Wu, J.Z.; Liang, G. Curcumin analogue A501 induces G2/M arrest and apoptosis in non-small cell lung cancer cells. *Asian Pac. J. Cancer Prev.* **2014**, *15*, 6893–6898. [CrossRef] [PubMed]
154. Lee, J.Y.; Lee, Y.M.; Chang, G.C.; Yu, S.L.; Hsieh, W.Y.; Chen, J.J.; Chen, H.W.; Yang, P.C. Curcumin induces EGFR degradation in lung adenocarcinoma and modulates p38 activation in intestine: The versatile adjuvant for gefitinib therapy. *PLoS ONE* **2011**, *6*, e23756. [CrossRef] [PubMed]
155. Kang, J.H.; Kang, H.S.; Kim, I.K.; Lee, H.Y.; Ha, J.H.; Yeo, C.D.; Kang, H.H.; Moon, H.S.; Lee, S.H. Curcumin sensitizes human lung cancer cells to apoptosis and metastasis synergistically combined with carboplatin. *Exp. Biol. Med.* **2015**, *240*, 1416–1425. [CrossRef] [PubMed]
156. Kuo, P.C.; Liu, H.F.; Chao, J.I. Survivin and p53 modulate quercetin-induced cell growth inhibition and apoptosis in human lung carcinoma cells. *J. Biol. Chem.* **2004**, *279*, 55875–55885. [CrossRef] [PubMed]
157. Nguyen, T.T.; Tran, E.; Nguyen, T.H.; Do, P.T.; Huynh, T.H.; Huynh, H. The role of activated MEK-ERK pathway in quercetin-induced growth inhibition and apoptosis in A549 lung cancer cells. *Carcinogenesis* **2004**, *25*, 647–659. [CrossRef] [PubMed]
158. Youn, H.; Jeong, J.C.; Jeong, Y.S.; Kim, E.J.; Um, S.J. Quercetin potentiates apoptosis by inhibiting nuclear factor-kappaB signaling in H460 lung cancer cells. *Biol. Pharm. Bull.* **2013**, *36*, 944–951. [CrossRef]
159. Izumi, H.; Takahashi, M.; Uramoto, H.; Nakayama, Y.; Oyama, T.; Wang, K.Y.; Sasaguri, Y.; Nishizawa, S.; Kohno, K. Monocarboxylate transporters 1 and 4 are involved in the invasion activity of human lung cancer cells. *Cancer Sci.* **2011**, *102*, 1007–1013. [CrossRef]
160. Zhu, X.; Ma, P.; Peng, D.; Wang, Y.; Wang, D.; Chen, X.; Zhang, X.; Song, Y. Quercetin suppresses lung cancer growth by targeting Aurora B kinase. *Cancer Med.* **2016**, *5*, 3156–3165. [CrossRef]
161. Klimaszewska-Wisniewska, A.; Halas-Wisniewska, M.; Izdebska, M.; Gagat, M.; Grzanka, A.; Grzanka, D. Antiproliferative and antimetastatic action of quercetin on A549 non-small cell lung cancer cells through its effect on the cytoskeleton. *Acta Histochem.* **2017**, *119*, 99–112. [CrossRef] [PubMed]
162. Chang, J.H.; Lai, S.L.; Chen, W.S.; Hung, W.Y.; Chow, J.M.; Hsiao, M.; Lee, W.J.; Chien, M.H. Quercetin suppresses the metastatic ability of lung cancer through inhibiting Snail-dependent Akt activation and Snail-independent ADAM9 expression pathways. *Biochim. Biophys. Acta Mol. Cell Res.* **2017**, *1864*, 1746–1758. [CrossRef] [PubMed]
163. Wu, T.C.; Chan, S.T.; Chang, C.N.; Yu, P.S.; Chuang, C.H.; Yeh, S.L. Quercetin and chrysin inhibit nickel-induced invasion and migration by downregulation of TLR4/NF-kappaB signaling in A549cells. *Chem. Biol. Interact.* **2018**, *292*, 101–109. [CrossRef]

164. Chan, S.T.; Yang, N.C.; Huang, C.S.; Liao, J.W.; Yeh, S.L. Quercetin enhances the antitumor activity of trichostatin A through upregulation of p53 protein expression in vitro and in vivo. *PLoS ONE* **2013**, *8*, e54255. [CrossRef]
165. Lee, S.H.; Lee, E.J.; Min, K.H.; Hur, G.Y.; Lee, S.H.; Lee, S.Y.; Kim, J.H.; Shin, C.; Shim, J.J.; In, K.H.; et al. Quercetin Enhances Chemosensitivity to Gemcitabine in Lung Cancer Cells by Inhibiting Heat Shock Protein 70 Expression. *Clin. Lung Cancer* **2015**, *16*, 235–243. [CrossRef]
166. Lee, H.; Kim, Y.; Jeong, J.H.; Ryu, J.H.; Kim, W.Y. ATM/CHK/p53 Pathway Dependent Chemopreventive and Therapeutic Activity on Lung Cancer by Pterostilbene. *PLoS ONE* **2016**, *11*, e0162335. [CrossRef]
167. Chen, Z.; Jin, K.; Gao, L.; Lou, G.; Jin, Y.; Yu, Y.; Lou, Y. Anti-tumor effects of bakuchiol, an analogue of resveratrol, on human lung adenocarcinoma A549 cell line. *Eur. J. Pharmacol.* **2010**, *643*, 170–179. [CrossRef]
168. Park, J.J.; Hwang, S.J.; Park, J.H.; Lee, H.J. Chlorogenic acid inhibits hypoxia-induced angiogenesis via down-regulation of the HIF-1alpha/AKT pathway. *Cell. Oncol.* **2015**, *38*, 111–118. [CrossRef]
169. Khan, N.; Afaq, F.; Khusro, F.H.; Mustafa Adhami, V.; Suh, Y.; Mukhtar, H. Dual inhibition of phosphatidylinositol 3-kinase/Akt and mammalian target of rapamycin signaling in human nonsmall cell lung cancer cells by a dietary flavonoid fisetin. *Int. J. Cancer* **2012**, *130*, 1695–1705. [CrossRef]
170. Zhuo, W.; Zhang, L.; Zhu, Y.; Zhu, B.; Chen, Z. Fisetin, a dietary bioflavonoid, reverses acquired Cisplatin-resistance of lung adenocarcinoma cells through MAPK/Survivin/Caspase pathway. *Am. J. Transl. Res.* **2015**, *7*, 2045–2052.
171. Klimaszewska-Wisniewska, A.; Halas-Wisniewska, M.; Tadrowski, T.; Gagat, M.; Grzanka, D.; Grzanka, A. Paclitaxel and the dietary flavonoid fisetin: A synergistic combination that induces mitotic catastrophe and autophagic cell death in A549 non-small cell lung cancer cells. *Cancer Cell Int.* **2016**, *16*, 10. [CrossRef] [PubMed]
172. Zhou, Y.; Ho, W.S. Combination of liquiritin, isoliquiritin and isoliquirigenin induce apoptotic cell death through upregulating p53 and p21 in the A549 non-small cell lung cancer cells. *Oncol. Rep.* **2014**, *31*, 298–304. [CrossRef] [PubMed]
173. Teixeira, A.; DaCunha, D.C.; Barros, L.; Caires, H.R.; Xavier, C.P.R.; Ferreira, I.; Vasconcelos, M.H. Eucalyptus globulus Labill. decoction extract inhibits the growth of NCI-H460 cells by increasing the p53 levels and altering the cell cycle profile. *Food Funct.* **2019**, *6*. [CrossRef] [PubMed]
174. Wang, C.G.; Yao, W.N.; Zhang, B.; Hua, J.; Liang, D.; Wang, H.S. Lung cancer and matrix met alloproteinases inhibitors of polyphenols from Selaginella tamariscina with suppression activity of migration. *Bioorg. Med. Chem. Lett.* **2018**, *28*, 2413–2417. [CrossRef] [PubMed]
175. Moore, J.; Megaly, M.; MacNeil, A.J.; Klentrou, P.; Tsiani, E. Rosemary extract reduces Akt/mTOR/p70S6K activation and inhibits proliferation and survival of A549 human lung cancer cells. *Biomed. Pharmacother.* **2016**, *83*, 725–732. [CrossRef]
176. Tang, X.L.; Yan, L.; Zhu, L.; Jiao, D.M.; Chen, J.; Chen, Q.Y. Salvianolic acid A reverses cisplatin resistance in lung cancer A549 cells by targeting c-met and attenuating Akt/mTOR pathway. *J. Pharm. Sci.* **2017**, *135*, 1–7. [CrossRef]
177. Liu, Y.; Tong, Y.; Yang, X.; Li, F.; Zheng, L.; Liu, W.; Wu, J.; Ou, R.; Zhang, G.; Hu, M.; et al. Novel histone deacetylase inhibitors derived from Magnolia officinalis significantly enhance TRAIL-induced apoptosis in non-small cell lung cancer. *Pharmacol. Res.* **2016**, *111*, 113–125. [CrossRef]
178. Husari, A.; Hashem, Y.; Zaatari, G.; El Sabban, M. Pomegranate Juice Prevents the Formation of Lung Nodules Secondary to Chronic Cigarette Smoke Exposure in an Animal Model. *Oxid. Med. Cell Longev.* **2017**, *2017*, 6063201. [CrossRef]
179. Narayan, C.; Kumar, A. Antineoplastic and immunomodulatory effect of polyphenolic components of Achyranthes aspera (PCA) extract on urethane induced lung cancer in vivo. *Mol. Biol. Rep.* **2014**, *41*, 179–191. [CrossRef]
180. Aichinger, G.; Pahlke, G.; Nagel, L.J.; Berger, W.; Marko, D. Bilberry extract, its major polyphenolic compounds, and the soy isoflavone genistein antagonize the cytostatic drug erlotinib in human epithelial cells. *Food Funct.* **2016**, *7*, 3628–3636. [CrossRef]
181. Aggarwal, B.B.; Bhardwaj, A.; Aggarwal, R.S.; Seeram, N.P.; Shishodia, S.; Takada, Y. Role of resveratrol in prevention and therapy of cancer: Preclinical and clinical studies. *Anticancer Res.* **2004**, *24*, 2783–2840. [PubMed]

182. Salehi, B.; Mishra, A.P.; Nigam, M.; Sener, B.; Kilic, M.; Sharifi-Rad, M.; Fokou, P.V.T.; Martins, N.; Sharifi-Rad, J. Resveratrol: A Double-Edged Sword in Health Benefits. *Biomedicines* **2018**, *6*, 91. [CrossRef]
183. Poulose, S.M.; Thangthaeng, N.; Miller, M.G.; Shukitt-Hale, B. Effects of pterostilbene and resveratrol on brain and behavior. *Neurochem. Int.* **2015**, *89*, 227–233. [CrossRef] [PubMed]
184. Ko, J.H.; Sethi, G.; Um, J.Y.; Shanmugam, M.K.; Arfuso, F.; Kumar, A.P.; Bishayee, A.; Ahn, K.S. The Role of Resveratrol in Cancer Therapy. *Int. J. Mol. Sci.* **2017**, *18*, 2589. [CrossRef]
185. Whitlock, N.C.; Baek, S.J. The anticancer effects of resveratrol: Modulation of transcription factors. *Nutr. Cancer* **2012**, *64*, 493–502. [CrossRef]
186. Bergman, M.; Levin, G.S.; Bessler, H.; Djaldetti, M.; Salman, H. Resveratrol affects the cross talk between immune and colon cancer cells. *Biomed. Pharmacother.* **2013**, *67*, 43–47. [CrossRef]
187. Su, J.L.; Chen, P.B.; Chen, Y.H.; Chen, S.C.; Chang, Y.W.; Jan, Y.H.; Cheng, X.; Hsiao, M.; Hung, M.C. Downregulation of microRNA miR-520h by E1A contributes to anticancer activity. *Cancer Res.* **2010**, *70*, 5096–5108. [CrossRef]
188. Graham, H.N. Green tea composition, consumption, and polyphenol chemistry. *Prev. Med.* **1992**, *21*, 334–350. [CrossRef]
189. Balentine, D.A.; Wiseman, S.A.; Bouwens, L.C. The chemistry of tea flavonoids. *Crit. Rev. Food Sci. Nutr.* **1997**, *37*, 693–704. [CrossRef]
190. Colomer, R.; Sarrats, A.; Lupu, R.; Puig, T. Natural Polyphenols and their Synthetic Analogs as Emerging Anticancer Agents. *Curr. Drug Targets* **2017**, *18*, 147–159. [CrossRef]
191. Sekher Pannala, A.; Chan, T.S.; O'Brien, P.J.; Rice-Evans, C.A. Flavonoid B-ring chemistry and antioxidant activity: Fast reaction kinetics. *Biochem. Biophys. Res. Commun.* **2001**, *282*, 1161–1168. [CrossRef] [PubMed]
192. Burda, S.; Oleszek, W. Antioxidant and antiradical activities of flavonoids. *J. Agric. Food Chem.* **2001**, *49*, 2774–2779. [CrossRef] [PubMed]
193. Sang, S.; Lambert, J.D.; Ho, C.T.; Yang, C.S. The chemistry and biotransformation of tea constituents. *Pharmacol. Res.* **2011**, *64*, 87–99. [CrossRef] [PubMed]
194. Yang, C.S.; Wang, X.; Lu, G.; Picinich, S.C. Cancer prevention by tea: Animal studies, molecular mechanisms and human relevance. *Nat. Rev. Cancer* **2009**, *9*, 429–439. [CrossRef] [PubMed]
195. Yang, C.S.; Wang, H.; Li, G.X.; Yang, Z.; Guan, F.; Jin, H. Cancer prevention by tea: Evidence from laboratory studies. *Pharmacol. Res.* **2011**, *64*, 113–122. [CrossRef] [PubMed]
196. Yang, C.S.; Wang, H.; Chen, J.X.; Zhang, J. Effects of Tea Catechins on Cancer Signaling Pathways. *Enzymes* **2014**, *36*, 195–221. [CrossRef] [PubMed]
197. Miyata, Y.; Matsuo, T.; Araki, K.; Nakamura, Y.; Sagara, Y.; Ohba, K.; Sakai, H. Anticancer Effects of Green Tea and the Underlying Molecular Mechanisms in Bladder Cancer. *Medicines* **2018**, *5*, 87. [CrossRef]
198. Wu, X.; Yu, H.; Amos, C.I.; Hong, W.K.; Spitz, M.R. Joint effect of insulin-like growth factors and mutagen sensitivity in lung cancer risk. *J. Natl. Cancer Inst.* **2000**, *92*, 737–743. [CrossRef]
199. Wang, H.; Bian, S.; Yang, C.S. Green tea polyphenol EGCG suppresses lung cancer cell growth through upregulating miR-210 expression caused by stabilizing HIF-1alpha. *Carcinogenesis* **2011**, *32*, 1881–1889. [CrossRef]
200. Liu, F.; Cao, X.; Liu, Z.; Guo, H.; Ren, K.; Quan, M.; Zhou, Y.; Xiang, H.; Cao, J. Casticin suppresses self-renewal and invasion of lung cancer stem-like cells from A549 cells through down-regulation of pAkt. *Acta Biochim. Biophys. Sin.* **2014**, *46*, 15–21. [CrossRef]
201. Singh, B.N.; Shankar, S.; Srivastava, R.K. Green tea catechin, epigallocatechin-3-gallate (EGCG): Mechanisms, perspectives and clinical applications. *Biochem. Pharmacol.* **2011**, *82*, 1807–1821. [CrossRef] [PubMed]
202. Vallianou, N.G.; Evangelopoulos, A.; Schizas, N.; Kazazis, C. Potential anticancer properties and mechanisms of action of curcumin. *Anticancer Res.* **2015**, *35*, 645–651. [PubMed]
203. Tomeh, M.A.; Hadianamrei, R.; Zhao, X. A Review of Curcumin and Its Derivatives as Anticancer Agents. *Int. J. Mol. Sci.* **2019**, *20*, 1033. [CrossRef]
204. Adekola, K.; Rosen, S.T.; Shanmugam, M. Glucose transporters in cancer metabolism. *Curr. Opin. Oncol.* **2012**, *24*, 650–654. [CrossRef]
205. Liu, Y.; Cao, Y.; Zhang, W.; Bergmeier, S.; Qian, Y.; Akbar, H.; Colvin, R.; Ding, J.; Tong, L.; Wu, S.; et al. A small-molecule inhibitor of glucose transporter 1 downregulates glycolysis, induces cell-cycle arrest, and inhibits cancer cell growth in vitro and in vivo. *Mol. Cancer Ther.* **2012**, *11*, 1672–1682. [CrossRef]
206. Meng, Y.; Xu, X.; Luan, H.; Li, L.; Dai, W.; Li, Z.; Bian, J. The progress and development of GLUT1 inhibitors targeting cancer energy metabolism. *Future Med. Chem.* **2019**, *11*, 2333–2352. [CrossRef]

207. Rauf, A.; Imran, M.; Khan, I.A.; Ur-Rehman, M.; Gilani, S.A.; Mehmood, Z.; Mubarak, M.S. Anticancer potential of quercetin: A comprehensive review. *Phytother. Res.* **2018**, *32*, 2109–2130. [CrossRef]
208. Garrido, C.; Schmitt, E.; Cande, C.; Vahsen, N.; Parcellier, A.; Kroemer, G. HSP27 and HSP70: Potentially oncogenic apoptosis inhibitors. *Cell Cycle* **2003**, *2*, 579–584. [CrossRef]
209. Meng, S.; Cao, J.; Feng, Q.; Peng, J.; Hu, Y. Roles of chlorogenic Acid on regulating glucose and lipids metabolism: A review. *Evid. Based Complementary Altern. Med.* **2013**, *2013*, 801457. [CrossRef]
210. Santana-Galvez, J.; Cisneros-Zevallos, L.; Jacobo-Velazquez, D.A. Chlorogenic Acid: Recent Advances on Its Dual Role as a Food Additive and a Nutraceutical against Metabolic Syndrome. *Molecules* **2017**, *22*, 358. [CrossRef]
211. Naveed, M.; Hejazi, V.; Abbas, M.; Kamboh, A.A.; Khan, G.J.; Shumzaid, M.; Ahmad, F.; Babazadeh, D.; FangFang, X.; Modarresi-Ghazani, F.; et al. Chlorogenic acid (CGA): A pharmacological review and call for further research. *Biomed. Pharmacother.* **2018**, *97*, 67–74. [CrossRef] [PubMed]
212. Liu, C.C.; Zhang, Y.; Dai, B.L.; Ma, Y.J.; Zhang, Q.; Wang, Y.; Yang, H. Chlorogenic acid prevents inflammatory responses in IL1betastimulated human SW1353 chondrocytes, a model for osteoarthritis. *Mol. Med. Rep.* **2017**, *16*, 1369–1375. [CrossRef] [PubMed]
213. Karunanidhi, A.; Thomas, R.; van Belkum, A.; Neela, V. In vitro antibacterial and antibiofilm activities of chlorogenic acid against clinical isolates of Stenotrophomonas maltophilia including the trimethoprim/sulfamethoxazole resistant strain. *Biomed. Res. Int.* **2013**, *2013*, 392058. [CrossRef] [PubMed]
214. Sung, W.S.; Lee, D.G. Antifungal action of chlorogenic acid against pathogenic fungi, mediated by membrane disruption. *Pure Appl. Chem.* **2010**, *82*, 219–226. [CrossRef]
215. Shimizu, M.; Yoshimi, N.; Yamada, Y.; Matsunaga, K.; Kawabata, K.; Hara, A.; Moriwaki, H.; Mori, H. Suppressive effects of chlorogenic acid on N-methyl-N-nitrosourea-induced glandular stomach carcinogenesis in male F344 rats. *J. Toxicol. Sci.* **1999**, *24*, 433–439. [CrossRef]
216. Matsunaga, K.; Katayama, M.; Sakata, K.; Kuno, T.; Yoshida, K.; Yamada, Y.; Hirose, Y.; Yoshimi, N.; Mori, H. Inhibitory Effects of Chlorogenic Acid on Azoxymethane-induced Colon Carcinogenesis in Male F344 Rats. *Asian Pac. J. Cancer Prev.* **2002**, *3*, 163–166.
217. Kasai, H.; Fukada, S.; Yamaizumi, Z.; Sugie, S.; Mori, H. Action of chlorogenic acid in vegetables and fruits as an inhibitor of 8-hydroxydeoxyguanosine formation in vitro and in a rat carcinogenesis model. *Food Chem. Toxicol. Int. J. Publ. Br. Ind. Biol. Res. Assoc.* **2000**, *38*, 467–471. [CrossRef]
218. Ignatowicz, E.; Balana, B.; Vulimiri, S.V.; Szaefer, H.; Baer-Dubowska, W. The effect of plant phenolics on the formation of 7,12-dimethylbenz[a]anthracene-DNA adducts and TPA-stimulated polymorphonuclear neutrophils chemiluminescence in vitro. *Toxicology* **2003**, *189*, 199–209. [CrossRef]
219. Kang, T.Y.; Yang, H.R.; Zhang, J.; Li, D.; Lin, J.; Wang, L.; Xu, X. The studies of chlorogenic Acid antitumor mechanism by gene chip detection: The immune pathway gene expression. *J. Anal. Methods Chem.* **2013**, *2013*, 617243. [CrossRef]
220. Khan, N.; Afaq, F.; Syed, D.N.; Mukhtar, H. Fisetin, a novel dietary flavonoid, causes apoptosis and cell cycle arrest in human prostate cancer LNCaP cells. *Carcinogenesis* **2008**, *29*, 1049–1056. [CrossRef]
221. Syed, D.N.; Adhami, V.M.; Khan, M.I.; Mukhtar, H. Inhibition of Akt/mTOR signaling by the dietary flavonoid fisetin. *Anticancer Agents Med. Chem.* **2013**, *13*, 995–1001. [CrossRef] [PubMed]
222. Yang, P.M.; Tseng, H.H.; Peng, C.W.; Chen, W.S.; Chiu, S.J. Dietary flavonoid fisetin targets caspase-3-deficient human breast cancer MCF-7 cells by induction of caspase-7-associated apoptosis and inhibition of autophagy. *Int. J. Oncol.* **2012**, *40*, 469–478. [CrossRef] [PubMed]
223. Kashyap, D.; Garg, V.K.; Tuli, H.S.; Yerer, M.B.; Sak, K.; Sharma, A.K.; Kumar, M.; Aggarwal, V.; Sandhu, S.S. Fisetin and Quercetin: Promising Flavonoids with Chemopreventive Potential. *Biomolecules* **2019**, *9*, 174. [CrossRef]
224. D'Archivio, M.; Filesi, C.; Vari, R.; Scazzocchio, B.; Masella, R. Bioavailability of the polyphenols: Status and controversies. *Int. J. Mol. Sci.* **2010**, *11*, 1321–1342. [CrossRef]
225. Teng, H.; Chen, L. Polyphenols and bioavailability: An update. *Crit. Rev. Food Sci. Nutr.* **2019**, *59*, 2040–2051. [CrossRef]

8

The Chalcone Lonchocarpin Inhibits Wnt/β-Catenin Signaling and Suppresses Colorectal Cancer Proliferation

Danilo Predes [1,†], Luiz F. S. Oliveira [1,†], Laís S. S. Ferreira [1,†], Lorena A. Maia [1,†], João M. A. Delou [1], Anderson Faletti [1], Igor Oliveira [1], Nathalia G. Amado [1], Alice H. Reis [1], Carlos A. M. Fraga [1], Ricardo Kuster [2], Fabio A. Mendes [1], Helena L. Borges [1] and Jose G. Abreu [1,*]

[1] Program of Cell and Developmental Biology, Institute of Biomedical Sciences, Federal University of Rio de Janeiro, Rio de Janeiro 21941-902, Brazil; danilopredes@gmail.com (D.P.); oliveira.lfs2@gmail.com (L.F.S.O.); ssflais@gmail.com (L.S.S.F.); agostini.maia@gmail.com (L.A.M.); jmdelou@gmail.com (J.M.A.D.); 7andersonfaletti7@gmail.com (A.F.); igor.oliveira93@outlook.com (I.O.); ngamado@gmail.com (N.G.A.); alicehreis@gmail.com (A.H.R.); cmfraga@ccsdecania.ufrj.br (C.A.M.F.); famendes@gmail.com (F.A.M.); hborges@icb.ufrj.br (H.L.B.)

[2] Department of Chemistry, Federal University of Espírito Santo, Espírito Santo 29075-910, Brazil; kusterrm@gmail.com

* Correspondence: garciajr@icb.ufrj.br

† These authors contributed equally.

Abstract: The deregulation of the Wnt/β-catenin signaling pathway is a central event in colorectal cancer progression, thus a promising target for drug development. Many natural compounds, such as flavonoids, have been described as Wnt/β-catenin inhibitors and consequently modulate important biological processes like inflammation, redox balance, cancer promotion and progress, as well as cancer cell death. In this context, we identified the chalcone lonchocarpin isolated from *Lonchocarpus sericeus* as a Wnt/β-catenin pathway inhibitor, both in vitro and in vivo. Lonchocarpin impairs β-catenin nuclear localization and also inhibits the constitutively active form of TCF4, dnTCF4-VP16. *Xenopus laevis* embryology assays suggest that lonchocarpin acts at the transcriptional level. Additionally, we described lonchocarpin inhibitory effects on cell migration and cell proliferation on HCT116, SW480, and DLD-1 colorectal cancer cell lines, without any detectable effects on the non-tumoral intestinal cell line IEC-6. Moreover, lonchocarpin reduces tumor proliferation on the colorectal cancer AOM/DSS mice model. Taken together, our results support lonchocarpin as a novel Wnt/β-catenin inhibitor compound that impairs colorectal cancer cell growth in vitro and in vivo.

Keywords: anticancer drugs; flavonoids; natural compounds; *Xenopus laevis*; AOM/DSS model

---

1. Introduction

Colorectal cancer (CRC) is the third most commonly diagnosed cancer and the second most common cause of cancer death. According to World Health Organization (WHO), it is expected that there were 1.8 million cases and 862,000 deaths in 2018 [1]. Sporadic CRC initiation, promotion, and progression is mostly driven by a sequence of known genetic mutations in key signaling pathways, frequently related to DNA damage response and sustained proliferation in the absence of growth factors. In CRC, 93% of the cases have at least one mutation of one Wnt/β-catenin pathway component [2]. The most frequently mutated gene in colorectal cancer is *APC* (adenomatous polyposis coli) that is a β-catenin destruction complex component. *APC* mutation occurs in 81% of non-hypermutated colorectal cancers cases and in 51% of hypermutated colorectal cancer cases, triggering tumorigenesis in intestinal polyps of patients with familial adenomatous polyposis [3]. The Wnt/β-catenin signaling pathway coordinates several cell behavior aspects, such as cell proliferation, differentiation, stemness, polarity, and migration [4,5]. In the absence of Wnt ligands, the destruction complex is active in the cytoplasm, phosphorylating β-catenin, a key component of the canonical Wnt pathway, leading to its degradation by the proteasome [6,7]. Wnt interaction with its receptors Frizzled (Fzd) and LDL receptor-related protein 5/6 (LRP5/6) disrupts the destruction complex assembly leading to β-catenin stabilization, cytoplasmic accumulation, translocation to the nucleus and binding to the T-cell factor/lymphoid enhancer factor (TCF/LEF), allowing Wnt target gene transcription [8]. Despite the crucial role of Wnt signaling on colorectal tumorigenesis, there is no Wnt/β-catenin inhibitor approved for clinical use [9]. Due to the importance of Wnt/β-catenin and its frequent mutations upstream to β-catenin translocation to the nucleus, it is crucial to find anticancer drugs that target the pathway downstream to this phenomenon [2].

Addressing normal and pathological Wnt/β-catenin signaling functioning requires multidisciplinary experiments combining in vitro and in vivo approaches. Among different models for studying Wnt/β-catenin signaling in vivo, *Xenopus laevis* stands out for its liability and efficiency. Wnt/β-catenin signaling plays a key role in two fundamental steps during the Xenopus early development that can be exploited for the screening of new drug candidates: the dorso-ventral and the antero-posterior axis patterning [10–12]. Indeed, the Xenopus model system has been explored to discover Pyrvinium, an FDA approved compound, as a Wnt signaling inhibitor that acts downstream of β-catenin. Pyrvinium impaired Xenopus embryo secondary axis induction in a dose-dependent manner and decreased colon cancer cells viability [13].

In addition, the AOM/DSS mouse model stands as a relevant preclinical inflammation-associated CRC model with histologic and phenotypic features that recapitulates the aberrant crypt foci-adenoma-carcinoma found in the human CRC [14]. Consistent with CRC development, in the AOM/DSS murine model, β-catenin nuclear translocation is observed in both flat and polypoid lesions likely due to β-catenin mutation [15]. In this context, the study of synthetic and natural compounds able to inhibit the Wnt/β-catenin signaling pathway have been explored as possible antitumor prototypes. Among the small natural molecules studied, the flavonoids, polyphenolic compounds found in many plants with a wide range of biological effects, stand out. Many flavonoids have been described as inhibitors of Wnt signaling and potential antitumor compounds, such as apigenin, EGCG, silibin, kaempferol, isorhamnetin, quercetin, isoquercitrin, derricin, and derricidin [16–25]. However, the specific mechanism by which some of these compounds affect Wnt/β-catenin signaling as well as its capacity to impair CRC growth is still not elucidated. Along the flavonoid biosynthesis pathway, the chalcones are well known as precursors of the flavonoids. Lonchocarpin is a chalcone first isolated from *Lonchocarpus sericeus* (as known as *Derris sericeu*) by Baudrenghien and colleagues in 1949 [26], and its correct structure was elucidated by the same researchers in 1953. The cytotoxic effects of the chalcone lonchocarpin have been previously described in neuroblastoma and leukemia cell lines [27], however, its role in CRC and the Wnt/β-catenin pathway is unknown.

In the present work, we describe lonchocarpin ability of inhibiting Wnt/β-catenin both in vitro, in colon cancer cell lines, and in vivo, with Wnt specific *Xenopus laevis* embryonic assays. In addition, acute administration of lonchocarpin in a preclinical CRC mouse model reduced cell proliferation in adenocarcinomas. Altogether, our data show lonchocarpin as a potent Wnt/β-catenin inhibitor that impairs cancer cell proliferation both in vitro and in vivo, and a promising compound for further antitumor clinical investigation and development.

2. Results

2.1. Lonchocarpin Inhibits Wnt/β-Catenin Pathway and Reduces Nuclear β-Catenin Levels

It has been shown that natural compounds, including chalcones, have growth-inhibitory properties in cancer cell lines by modulating Wnt/β-catenin signaling [17,18]. We employed an RKO pBAR/Renilla based screening of natural compounds and found lonchocarpin as a Wnt signaling modulator hit (data not shown). In this context, we evaluated whether lonchocarpin, a chalcone isolated from *Lonchocarpus sericeus*, is able to inhibit the Wnt signaling pathway in human colorectal cancer cell lines RKO pBAR/Renilla stimulated with Wnt3a CM (conditioned medium) for 24 h and non-stimulated SW480 pBAR/Renilla (Figure 1A). SW480 does not need Wnt stimulation, since it harbors an APC mutation that overactivates the canonical Wnt signaling. Cells were treated with lonchocarpin overnight, with or without the conditioned medium. Lonchocarpin decreased luciferase reporter activity in a concentration-dependent manner, starting at 3 μM in RKO pBAR/Renilla and 5 μM in SW480 pBAR/Renilla (Figure 1B,C), and presented the half maximal inhibitory concentration (IC50) of 4 μM in SW480 pBAR/Renilla (Figure 1D).

In order to validate the Wnt/β-catenin reporter gene assay inhibition, we performed immunocytochemistry on SW480 cells. In order to activate the pathway, we treated RKO cells with Wnt3a CM for 24 h and performed immunocytochemistry to assess nuclear β-catenin cell count. These cells were cotreated with DMSO (vehicle), 10 or 20 μM lonchocarpin. L-cell CM treated cells displayed 34% β-catenin positive nuclei (Figure 1E–E"), while Wnt3a CM treatment increased the mean to 86% (Figure 1F–F"). RKO cells cotreated with 10 μM (Figure 1G–G") or 20 μM Figure 1H–H") lonchocarpin showed 54% and 30% nuclear β-catenin positive cells, respectively (Figure 1J). This data show that lonchocarpin treatment decreased β-catenin nuclear translocation in a concentration-dependent manner (Figure 1E–H"). To assess whether lonchocarpin affects total β-catenin protein level, we performed immunoblotting assay of RKO cells stimulated overnight with Wnt3a CM or 1 μM BIO, cotreated with DMSO or 20 μM lonchocarpin (Figure 1K). Immunoblot assay showed that lonchocarpin did not expressively reduced β-catenin total levels (Figure 1K), suggesting that β-catenin degradation, or β-catenin stabilization impairment might not be a lonchocarpin mechanism of action. In order to further validate our immunocytochemistry analysis, we performed immunoblotting of RKO cytosolic and nuclear fractions (Figure 1L). These cells were treated accordingly to previous assay. Immunoblotting showed that lonchocarpin reduces β-catenin nuclear level, suggesting an inhibition of nuclear translocation, or, possibly, an inhibition of β-catenin nuclear interaction with other proteins or DNA. Thus, this data suggests that lonchocarpin inhibits Wnt/β-catenin signaling pathway and impairs β-catenin nuclear localization.

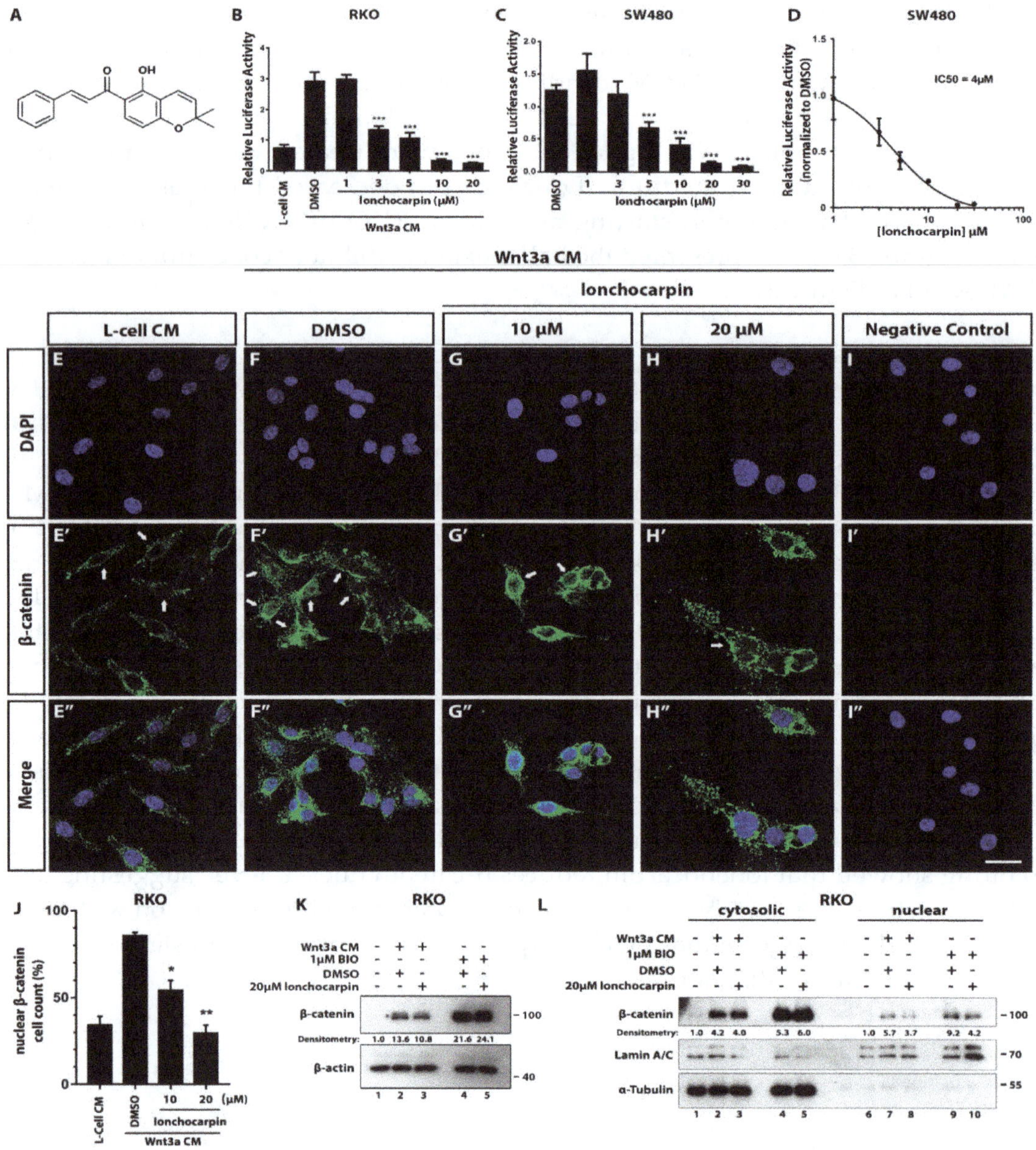

Figure 1. Lonchocarpin inhibits the Wnt/β-catenin pathway. Treatment with lonchocarpin inhibits Wnt reporter activity. (**A**) Lonchocarpin chemical structure, (**B**) RKO-pBAR/Renilla, and (**C**) SW480-pBAR/Renila gene reporter luciferase assay. (**D**) Lonchocarpin half maximal inhibitory concentration is 4 μM in the SW480-pBAR/Renilla cell lineage. Graph bars represent mean and SD. (**E–I**) SW480 β-catenin and DAPI immunocytochemistry staining showed that lonchocarpin decreases β-catenin translocation after lonchocarpin treatment. RKO cells were treated with (**E–E"**) L-cell control conditioned medium or Wnt3a conditioned medium with (**F–F"**) DMSO, (**G–G"**) 10 μM or (**H–H"**) 20 μM lonchocarpin. (**I–I"**) Immunocytochemistry negative control. (**J**) Quantification of nuclear β-catenin positive cell count ratio. Graph bars represent mean and SEM. (**K**) Immunoblotting depicting β-catenin and β-actin total levels of RKO cells treated with Wnt3a CM (conditioned medium) for 7 h. Densitometry is shown as the ratio of β-catenin/β-actin. (**K**) Immunoblot of cell lysate of RKO cells treated with 1-L-cell CM, 2-Wnt3a CM + DMSO, 3-Wnt3a CM + lonchocarpin 20 μM, 4-BIO 1 μM + DMSO, 5-BIO 1 μM + lonchocarpin 20 μM. (**L**) Immunoblot of cytosolic and nuclear fractions of RKO cells treated with 1,6-L-cell CM, 2,7-Wnt3a CM + DMSO, 3,8-Wnt3a CM + lonchocarpin 20 μM, 4,9-BIO 1 μM + DMSO, 5,10-BIO 1 μM + lonchocarpin 20 μM. Cytosolic densitometry was calculated considering α-Tubulin as the loading control, while nuclear densitometry considered Lamin A/C as the loading control. * $p < 0.05$, ** $p < 0.01$, *** $p < 0.001$. Scale bar represents 20 μm.

2.2. Lonchocarpin Inhibits the Canonical Wnt Pathway Downstream of the Destruction Complex

SW480 harbors a mutation in APC that deletes its carboxyl-terminus domain, preventing the destruction complex assembly [28,29]. Considering that lonchocarpin inhibited the Wnt reporter gene in SW480 pBAR/Renilla (Figure 1C,D), and also prevented β-catenin nuclear localization (Figure 1L), we speculated that the flavonoid could act downstream of the destruction complex. To test this hypothesis, we performed epistasis assay using Wnt/β-catenin-specific reporter (Super TOPFLASH) transfected cells induced by Wnt3a CM (Figure 2A), or co-transfected with wild type β-catenin (Figure 2B), constitutively active β-catenin S33A (Figure 2C), or dnTCF4 VP16 (Figure 2D), a constitutive active TCF4 form that does not rely on β-catenin for inducing the pathway.

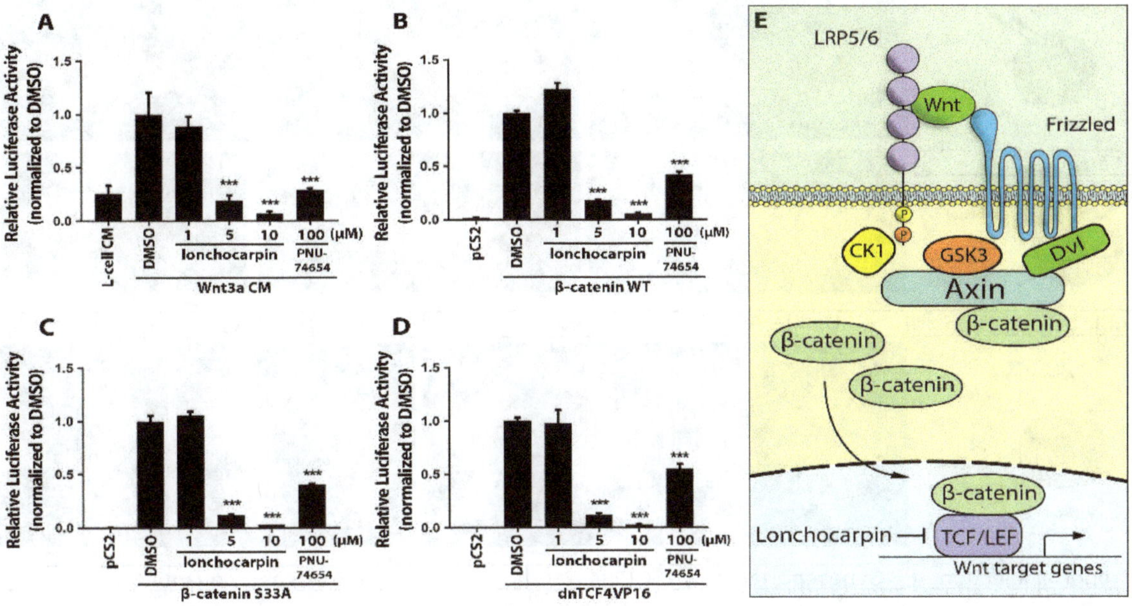

Figure 2. Lonchocarpin inhibits Wnt/β-catenin pathway downstream to TCF4. Lonchocarpin suppresses Wnt/β-catenin pathway induced by Wnt3a CM treatment (**A**) or by transfection with (**B**) β-catenin, (**C**) β-catenin S33A, or (**D**) dnTCF4VP16 in HEK293T cells. (**E**) Proposed lonchocarpin mechanism of action. Graph bars represent mean and SD. *** $p < 0.001$.

Our results showed that lonchocarpin inhibits Wnt/β-catenin signaling activation when pathway activation is triggered by wild-type β-catenin, β-catenin S33A, or dnTCF4 VP16 overexpression (Figure 2A–D). Interestingly, lonchocarpin showed a more potent and efficient inhibitory effect than the previously published compound PNU-74654 (Figure 2A–D) [30]. In this scenario, we propose that lonchocarpin acts downstream of the destruction complex and impairs TCF4 mediated transcription.

Together, these data suggest that lonchocarpin inhibits Wnt/β-catenin signaling by impairing β-catenin nuclear localization while also hindering TCF activity.

2.3. Lonchocarpin Treatment Disturbs Xenopus laevis Embryos Axial Patterning and Rescues Wnt Overactivation Phenotypes

Our in vitro data suggest that lonchocarpin inhibits Wnt/β-catenin by impairing β-catenin nuclear localization (Figure 1E–L) while also suppressing TCF mediated transcription (Figure 2D). Next, we investigated if this inhibitory effect is also observed in vivo. Manipulation of *Xenopus laevis* embryonic development has been successfully used to validate compounds targeting Wnt/β-catenin signaling through the interpretation of embryonic phenotypes and Wnt signaling overactivation [11]. In this context, injection of 1.6 pmol lonchocarpin in the embryo animal dorsal blastomeres (Figure 3A) induced head defects, characterized by reduction of anterior structures in 23% of injected embryos, such as the cement gland and diminished eyes (Figure 3D) while uninjected or DMSO-injected embryos developed normally (Figure 3B,C). Considering that Wnt/β-catenin is active in the dorsal side of the Xenopus embryo, which will organize the anterior-posterior axis, this result suggests an inhibition of the pathway by lonchocarpin. In order to confirm this result, we injected 10 pmol of lonchocarpin into the blastocoele space of stage 9 embryos (Figure 3E). Lonchocarpin injection induced anterior structures enlargement, such as the head and cement gland in 48% of the embryos (Figure 3H), while uninjected and DMSO injected embryos developed normally (Figure 3F,G). This lonchocarpin effect is consistent with Wnt/β-catenin inhibition in the embryo anterior region, since the signaling at this embryonic stage induces posterior structures.

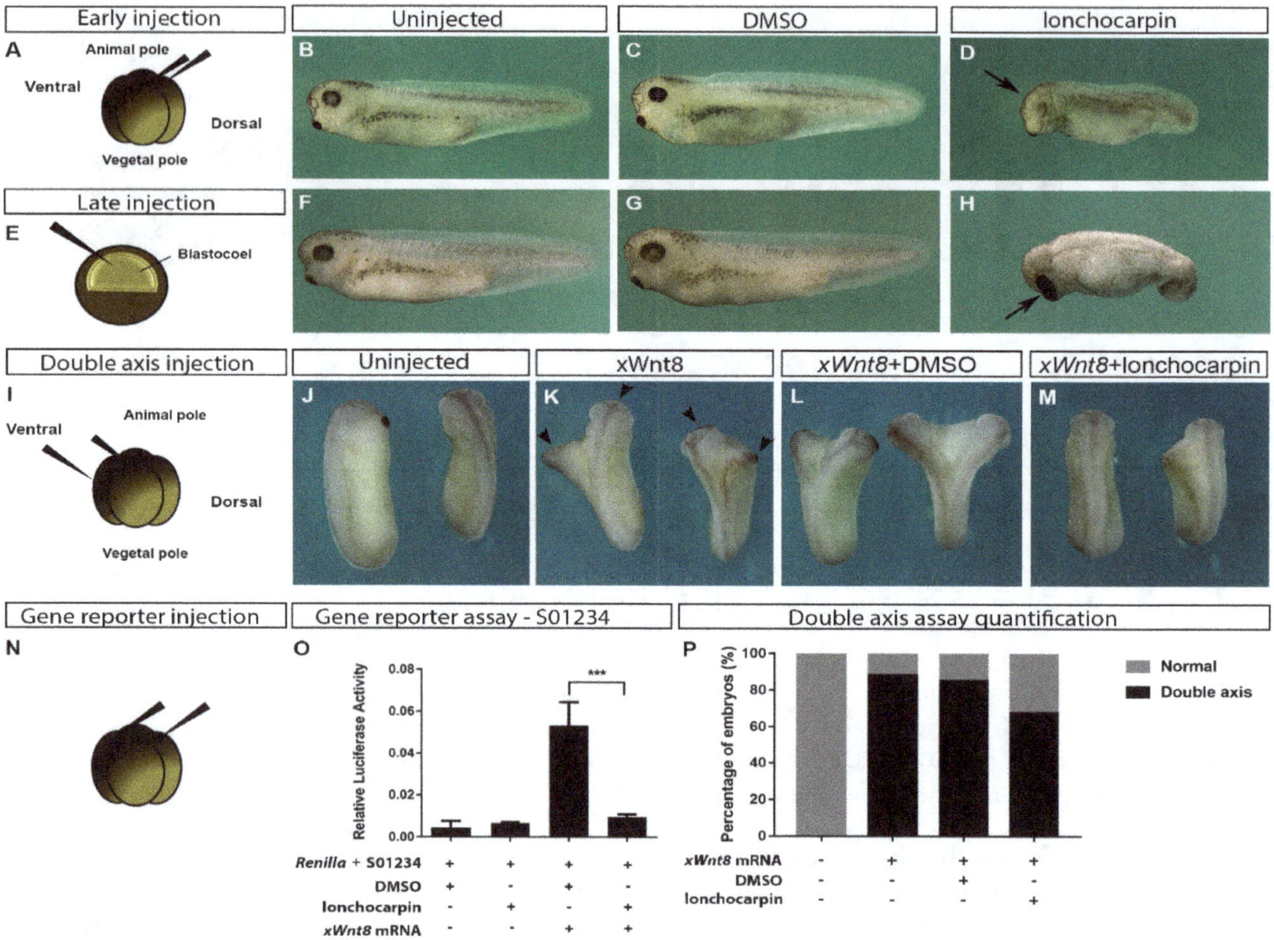

Figure 3. Lonchocarpin alters axial patterning in *Xenopus laevis* embryos and inhibits Wnt-8 induced axis and S01234-luciferase reporter. The 4-cell stage injected embryos display a smaller head compared uninjected and DMSO-injected embryos (**A**–**D**). Stage 9 blastulae injected embryos display a larger head (arrow) and cement gland (arrow) compared to uninjected or DMSO-injected embryos (**E**–**H**). Injection of xWnt8 mRNA into ventral blastomere induced ectopic axis (arrowhead) compared to uninjected embryos (**I**–**K**,**P**). Lonchocarpin inhibited Wnt8-induced secondary axis (**M**,**P**), but not DMSO (**L**,**P**). Lonchocarpin injection inhibits Wnt8-induced S01234-luciferase specific reporter activation in *Xenopus laevis* embryo (**N**,**O**) *** $p < 0.001$. Graph bars represent mean and SD (see also Figure S1).

It is well established that Wnt/β-catenin signaling overactivation in the Xenopus embryo 4-cell stage ventral side induces ectopic axis containing head and dorsal structures [10,12,31]. We injected 10 pg of xWnt8 mRNA combined or not with 10 pmol lonchocarpin or DMSO into two ventral blastomeres at 4-cell stage embryo (Figure 3I). xWnt8 or xWnt8 + DMSO-injected embryos developed a secondary axis in 90% of the embryos, while only 60% of the lonchocarpin-injected embryos developed a secondary axis (Figure 3K–M,P).

Thus, these results strongly suggest lonchocarpin induces phenotypes consistent with Wnt/β-catenin inhibition in Xenopus embryos (see also Figure S1 for quantification). To confirm whether lonchocarpin inhibits Wnt signaling in Xenopus, we coinjected a Wnt/β-catenin specific gene reporter S01234-luciferase with xWnt8 mRNA and 2.4 pmol lonchocarpin or DMSO into 4-cell *stage Xenopus laevis* embryos (Figure 3N). Lonchocarpin suppressed 82% of Wnt/β-catenin signaling gene reporter activation (Figure 3O).

These data support that lonchocarpin inhibits Wnt/β-catenin signaling pathway activation both in vivo and in vitro.

2.4. Lonchocarpin Reduces HCT116, SW480, and DLD-1 Cell Proliferation

Since lonchocarpin inhibited Wnt/β-catenin downstream to the destruction complex both in vitro and in vivo, we asked whether lonchocarpin has antitumor effects on colorectal cancer cell lines where Wnt/β-catenin signaling has a critical role on tumorigenesis. Canonical Wnt signaling activation leads to proliferation in many cell types, including colorectal cancer cells, thus we asked whether lonchocarpin inhibits colon cancer cell proliferation. We treated HCT116, SW480, DLD-1, and IEC-6 cell lines with 5, 10, or 20 μM lonchocarpin for 24 h and performed the Click-it EdU proliferation assay.

Lonchocarpin inhibited 33% of HCT116 EdU positive cell count at 5 and 10 μM and reduced 75% of EdU positive cell count at 30 μM (Figure 4B–E). Lonchocarpin inhibited 50% and 85% of SW480 EdU positive cell count at 10 and 20 μM, respectively (Figure 4H–J). Lonchocarpin inhibited 40% and 75% of DLD-1 proliferative cells ratio at 10 and 20 μM, respectively (Figure 4M–O). However, lonchocarpin did not affect the non-tumoral intestinal cell line IEC-6 proliferating cells ratio (Figure 4Q–T). These data show that lonchocarpin suppresses colorectal cancer cell lines proliferation while not affecting the non-tumoral cell line IEC-6 proliferation. Next, we asked whether lonchocarpin suppresses proliferation through cell toxicity. In order to assess cellular viability, we performed MTT assay after treatment with 10, 20, 30, 40, and 50 μM lonchocarpin for 24, 48, or 72 h (Figure 4). We noticed that 20 to 50 μM lonchocarpin at all treatment intervals reduced relative 570 nm absorbance of HCT116, SW480, and DLD-1 colorectal cancer cell lines but 10 μM had no effect (Figure 4U–W). Curiously, 20 μM lonchocarpin did not decrease relative 570 nm absorbance, but maintained the same reading throughout the experiment, suggesting a proliferation inhibition.

However, in the non-tumoral intestinal cell line IEC-6, lonchocarpin decreased relative 570 nm absorbance only at 50 μM. Exclusively at 72 h of treatment there was noticeable absorbance reduction in 40 μM lonchocarpin (Figure 4X). These data show that lonchocarpin inhibits cell proliferation and viability preferentially in the colorectal cancer cell lines.

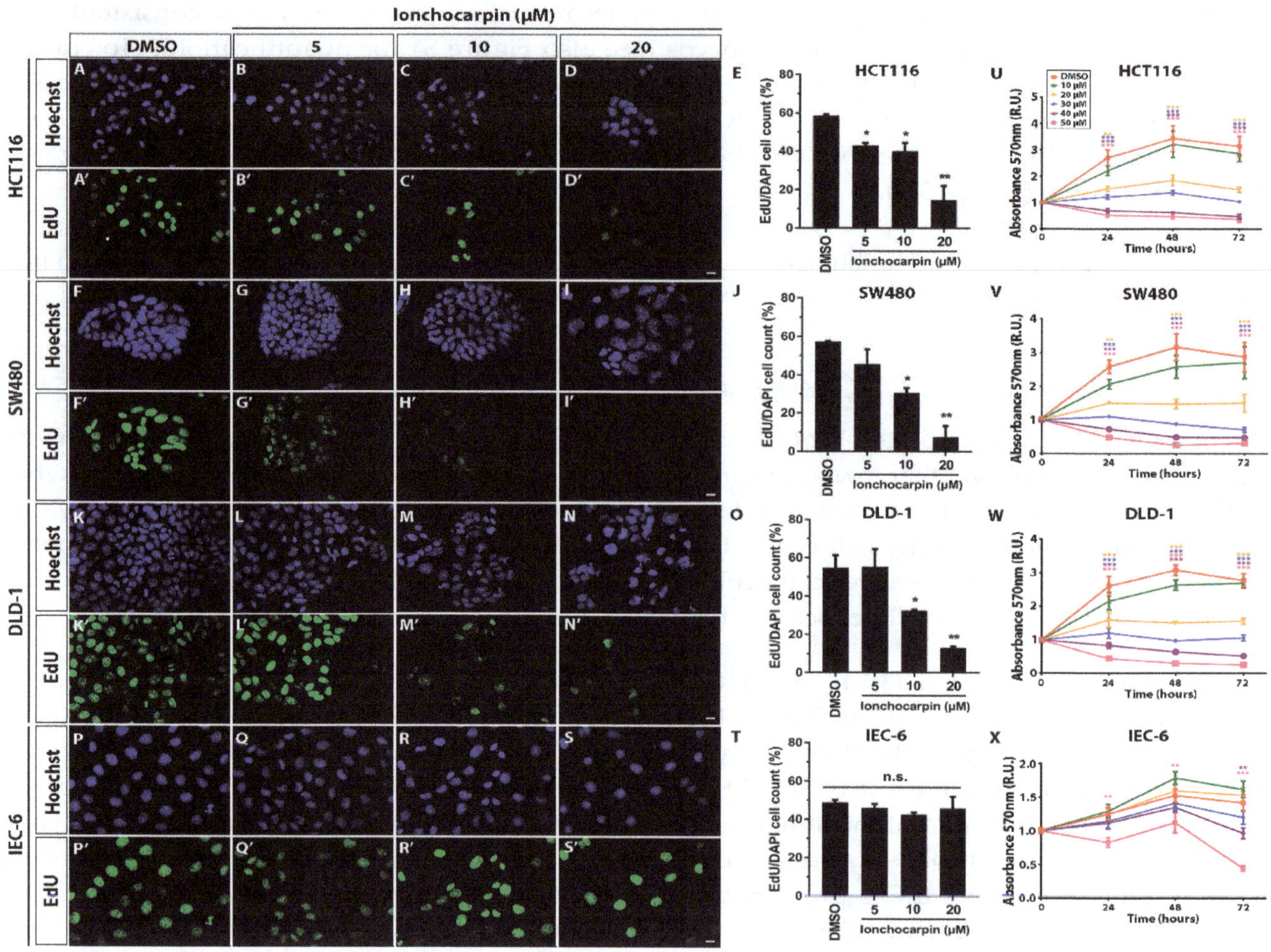

Figure 4. Lonchocarpin inhibits HCT116, SW480, and DLD-1 colorectal cancer cell lines proliferation. Proliferation assay shows that lonchocarpin suppresses proliferation of HCT116, SW480, and DLD-1 colorectal cancer cell lines, while not affecting IEC-6 non-tumor small intestine cell line proliferation. DAPI and EdU stained cells micrographs acquired 24 h post 5, 10, and 20 μM lonchocarpin treatment. (**A–E**) HCT116, (**F–J**) SW480, (**K–O**) DLD-1, (**P–T**) IEC-6. Graphs show the percentage of EdU positive cells. Scale bar represents 10 μm. Graph bars represent mean and SD. MTT assay shows that lower lonchocarpin concentrations are less cytotoxic to the non-tumor cell line IEC-6 compared to the tumor cell lines. MTT assay performed after treatment with 10, 20, 30, 40, and 50 μM lonchocarpin of (**U**) HCT116, (**V**) SW480, (**W**) DLD-1, and (**X**) IEC-6 cells during 24, 48, and 72 h. R.U. (Relative Units). * $p < 0.1$, ** $p < 0.01$. Graphs show mean and SEM.

2.5. Lonchocarpin Reduces Cell Migration in HCT116, SW480, and DLD-1 Colorectal Cancer Cell Lines

Canonical Wnt signaling key protein β-catenin interacts with adhesion proteins in the membrane that may affect cell adhesion and migration. We evaluated whether lonchocarpin affects HCT116, SW480 and DLD-1 colorectal cancer cell lines and IEC-6 non-tumoral intestinal cell line migration by performing scratch assay. HCT116 lonchocarpin treatment reduced 55% of scratch closure at 20 μM (Figure 5A–E). Lonchocarpin treatment of SW480 reduced 40% and 55% of scratch closure at 10 and 20 μM, respectively (Figure 5F–J). Likewise, DLD-1 lonchocarpin treatment reduced 45% of scratch closure at 20 μM (Figure 5K–O). However, lonchocarpin treatment did not affect cell migration of the non-tumoral cell line IEC-6 (Figure 5P–T). These data show that lonchocarpin treatment impairs cell migration of colorectal cell lines, while not affecting the migration of the non-tumoral cell line.

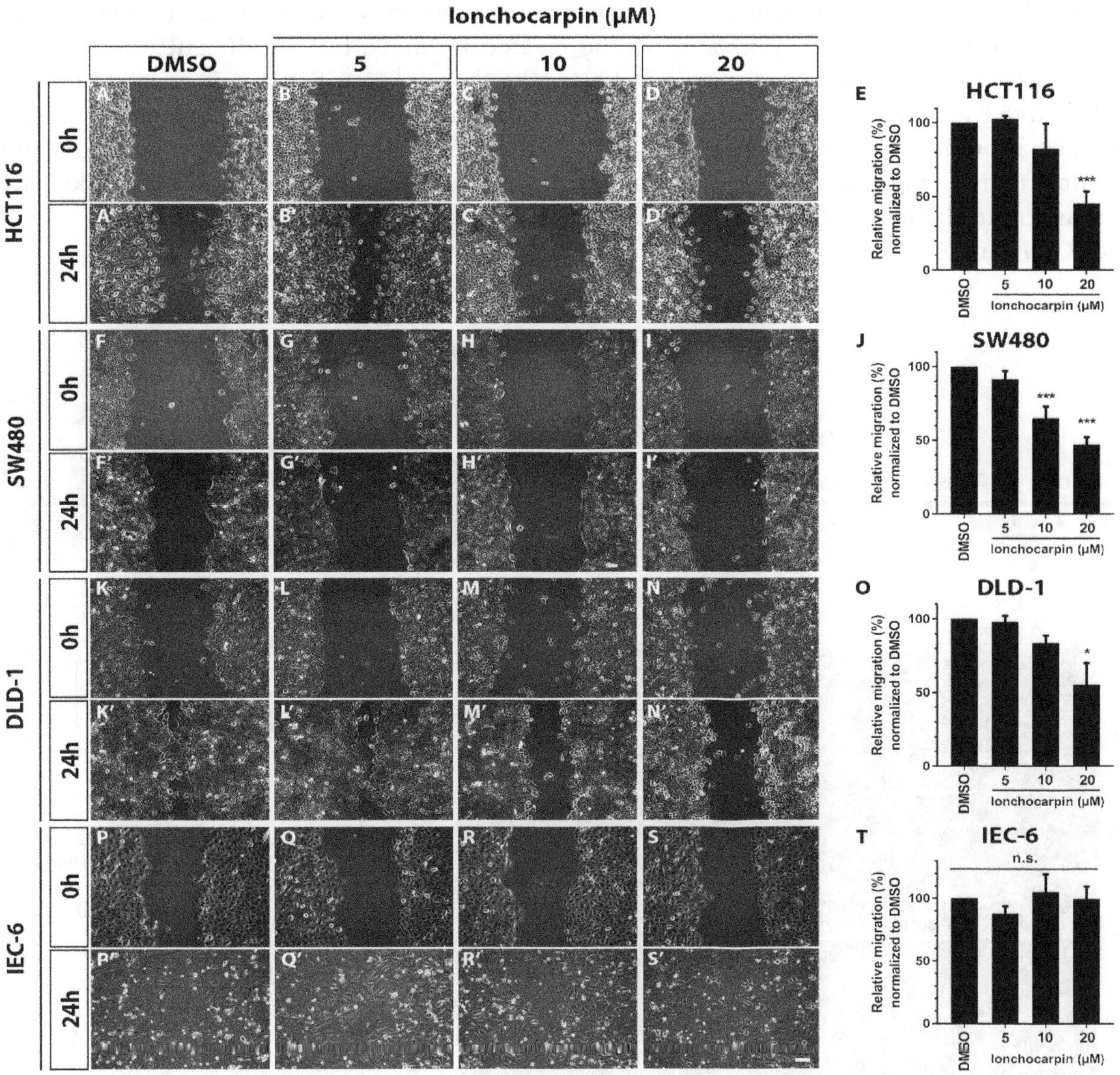

Figure 5. Lonchocarpin inhibits cell migration in HCT116, SW480, and DLD-1 colorectal cancer cell lines. Scratch assay shows that lonchocarpin impairs migration of HCT116, SW480, and DLD-1 colorectal cancer cell lines while not interfering with the IEC-6 non-tumor intestine cell line migration. Images show cell migration through the scratch healing 24 h post treatment with 5, 10, and 20 μM lonchocarpin (**A–E**) HCT116, (**F–J**) SW480, (**K–O**) DLD-1, (**P–T**) IEC-6. Graph shows relative wound area closure relative to time 0 h. All conditions were normalized to DMSO. * $p < 0.1$, *** $p < 0.001$. Scale bar represents 100 μm. Graph bars represent mean and SD.

2.6. Lonchocarpin Decreases Cell Proliferation in Azoxymethane (AOM)/Dextran Sulfate Sodium (DSS) Induced Adenocarcinomas

Lonchocarpin inhibits Wnt/β-catenin in vitro and in vivo, while also presenting antitumor effects in vitro. We asked whether lonchocarpin also has antitumor effects in vivo. We assessed the efficacy of lonchocarpin therapeutic administration in an azoxymethane (AOM)/dextran sulfate sodium (DSS)-induced model of colon cancer. After three cycles of DSS, when colon tumors were expected in most animals, lonchocarpin (50 or 100 mg·kg^{-1}·day^{-1}) was injected intraperitoneally for four days, and the mice were assessed 3 h after the last injection (Figure 6A). Colon tumors were macroscopically observed in almost all mice submitted to the protocol (77%), and histopathological analyses revealed several changes in the intestinal mucosa (Figure S2). The most frequent alterations included no presence of mononuclear and polymorphonuclear leukocyte infiltrates in the lamina propria and submucosa, hyperplastic epithelium, in addition several adenomas and adenocarcinomas (Figure 6B). Lonchocarpin did not show any toxicity to the treated animals, but significantly reduced tumor proliferation (Figure 6C–F″). Lonchocarpin at 100 mg·kg^{-1}·day^{-1} significantly decreased 31% and 38% of proliferative Ki-67 and BrdU positive cells in adenocarcinomas of the treated mice compared either with vehicle groups, respectively (Figure 6G,H, Tables S1 and S2). However, lonchocarpin showed a more efficient antiproliferative effect when administered at the highest dosage (100 mg·kg^{-1}·day^{-1}) in comparison to the lower dosage (50 mg·kg^{-1}·day^{-1}), in which no statistical relevance was found (Figure 6G,H, Tables S1 and S2).

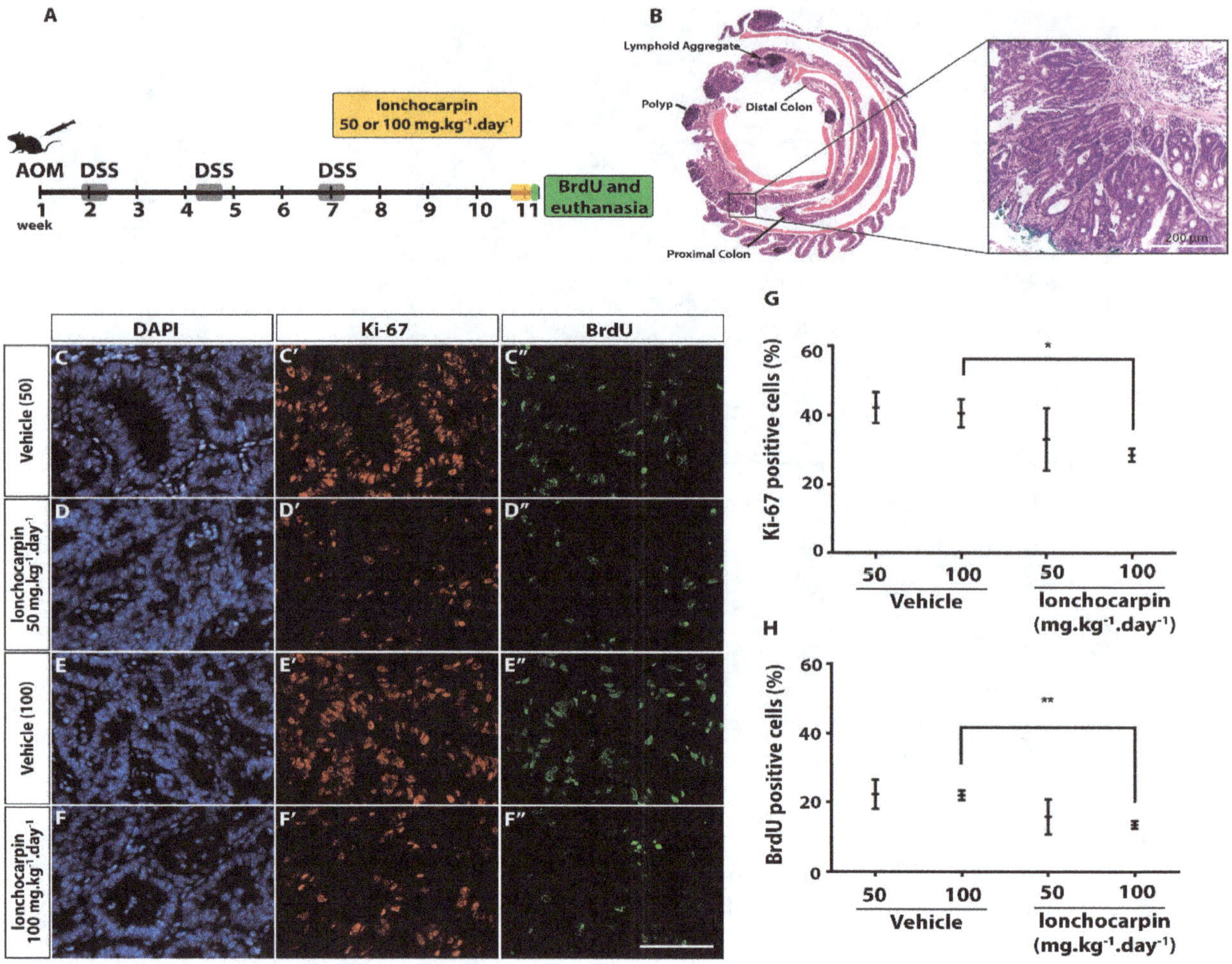

Figure 6. Lonchocarpin decreases cell proliferation in adenocarcinomas. (**A**) Timeline of inflammation-driven colon cancer tumorigenesis model (azoxymethane (AOM)/dextran sulfate sodium (DSS)) protocol in adult mice. Groups were divided as follows, vehicle 50 or 100: i.p. vehicle corresponding to volume for the respective dose in the treated group; treated groups: i.p. injections of 2.5 mg/mL lonchocarpin 50 or 100 mg·kg^{-1}·day^{-1} for four days. Vehicle: PEG400 30% in sterile NaCl 0.9%. BrdU i.p. injection (100 µg/kg) 1 h before euthanasia. (**B**) Representative H&E swiss-roll image of a colon section from a mouse subjected to AOM/DSS protocol. The zoom picture shows the corresponding area of an adenocarcinoma. Scale bar represents 200 µm. (**C**) Representative immunofluorescence photomicrographs of adenocarcinoma areas from colon sections stained for proliferation markers (**C′–F′**) Ki-67 (red, Cy3) and (**C″–F″**) BrdU (green, Alexa 488). (**C–F**) Nuclei stained with DAPI (blue). (**D,E**) Quantification of the percentage of (**G**) Ki-67 (**H**) or BrdU positive cells per indicated group. Scale bar represents 100 µm. Graphs represent mean and SEM. * $p < 0.05$ ** $p < 0.01$ Student *t*-test of lonchocarpin treatment condition in comparison to vehicle.

Taken together, our data demonstrate that lonchocarpin suppress the colorectal cancer cell growth in vitro and in vivo.

3. Discussion

The Wnt/β-catenin pathway plays a key role in colorectal tumorigenesis Integrated analysis of 195 colorectal tumors revealed that Wnt signaling pathway components were mutated in 94% of all tumors, and these mutations occurred mostly downstream to APC[10]. Hence, describing the novel canonical Wnt signaling pathway inhibiting small molecules that act downstream to APC is a recurrent strategy to improve colorectal cancer treatability.

Several studies show the antitumor effect of natural compounds that act as inhibitors of multiple components of the Wnt/β-catenin pathway [17]. Quercetin has been described to disrupt TCF/β-catenin interaction [23,32]. Epigallocatechin-3-gallate (EGCG) has been shown as a Wnt/β-catenin inhibitor by promoting β-catenin degradation [33]. Isoquercitrin has been described as an inhibitor of the Wnt signaling both in vitro and in vivo, and impairing tumor growth in vitro [34]. The chalcones derricin and derricidin have also been reported as canonical Wnt signaling inhibitors impairing tumor growth in vitro [18].

The present work is the first to identify lonchocarpin as a negative modulator of the Wnt/β-catenin pathway in RKO and SW480 colon tumor cell lines and in the HEK293T embryonic kidney cell line. We further elucidate that lonchocarpin acts downstream to β-catenin stabilization, probably at the TCF level, since it inhibits the overactivation of the Wnt/β-catenin pathway induced by the transfection of wild-type β-catenin, constitutively active β-catenin S33A or the constitutively active dnTCF4 VP16 in the HEK293T epistasis assay, while also inhibiting the Wnt/β-catenin pathway reporter in SW480 pBAR/Renilla cells, which harbors an APC truncation. We also show that lonchocarpin inhibits proliferation, migration, and cell viability in most of the three colorectal cancer cell lines, HCT116, SW480, and DLD-1, while not altering any of these aspects of the non-tumoral intestinal rat cell line IEC-6.

Recent work has identified that 24 h treatment with 50 μM lonchocarpin of SK-N-SH neuroblastoma line induces AMPK phosphorylation, which results in increased glucose uptake and inhibits protein synthesis [27]. Although our data shows effects at lower concentrations, this work corroborates our findings that lonchocarpin decreases cell viability. Thus, the antitumor effects that we described may be also a consequence of modulation of other signaling pathways besides Wnt/β-catenin.

Previous work has also measured cell viability following lonchocarpin treatment through MTT assay, indicating that the IC_{50} for cell growth in the CEM leukemia cell line is 10.4 μg/mL, the same as 3.4 μM of lonchocarpin [35]. Although not explored by the authors, leukemia cell lines are known to have Wnt signaling activating mutations, and lonchocarpin growth inhibiting effect could be due to Wnt signaling inhibition [36]. In this same study, authors show that derricin also inhibits leukemia cell growth [35], a chalcone also described as a canonical Wnt signaling inhibitor [18]. Comparatively, our cell viability data in HCT116, SW480, and DLD-1 colorectal cancer cell lines show that lonchocarpin reduces cell viability starting at 20 μM. This disparity may be due to the different origin of the cell lines. Lonchocarpin has also been shown as inhibiting lung cancer cells H292 growth in vitro and murine sarcoma S180 graft growth in vivo by inducing Caspase-3 mediated cell death [37]. Curiously, increased cleaved Caspase-3 levels were found at 48 h [37], but not at 24 h, suggesting that canonical Wnt signaling is inhibited prior apoptosis induction. Thus, previous lonchocarpin biological effect descriptions confirm that the antitumor effect of this chalcone is not exclusive to colorectal cancer.

Additionally, we show that lonchocarpin inhibits Wnt/β-catenin signaling in vivo in the *Xenopus laevis* embryo model. Xenopus embryo is a robust and reliable system to approach Wnt/β-catenin signaling in vivo since it is critical for axis patterning [10]. In that sense, Wnt signaling plays two major roles in early Xenopus development: a prior role that is composed by maternal Wnt components, and a latter role that is regulated by genes transcribed by the embryo itself. We show that injection of lonchocarpin at 4-cell stage, a stage where the embryo has no functioning transcription machinery, induced microcephaly and impaired Wnt8-induced axis, although a not very strong effect, most likely due to low lonchocarpin concentration into the embryo blastomere (Figure 3). Consistently, lonchocarpin injection into the blastocoele as well as co-injection with Wnt8-specific reporter (S01234), both addressing a moment where the embryo transcribes genes by itself, induced head enlargement and suppressed 82% of Wnt/β-catenin signaling gene reporter activation (Figure 3). These results are consistent with previous epistasis assay showing that lonchocarpin inhibits Wnt pathway downstream to β-catenin stabilization level, by impairing TCF mediated transcription (Figure 2).

Considering the relevance of the lonchocarpin Wnt/β-catenin inhibition and its functional effects on CRC cell lines as well as in Xenopus embryo, we tested lonchocarpin therapeutic administration in an inflammation-associated CRC mouse model. The AOM/DSS model has been widely used for CRC studies since it is highly reproducible, and recapitulates human cancer histological features and the major driven mutations. Indeed, it has become a powerful platform for chemopreventive and anticancer drug discovery studies. AOM is a procarcinogen metabolized into alkylating agent methylazocymethanol (MAM) in the liver. After excretion into the bile, it induces mutagenesis of the colonic epithelium. Colonic tumors are accelerated by a heparin-like polysaccharide DSS, which causes colonic epithelial damage, mirroring some of the features of inflammatory bowel disease [38]. Acute lonchocarpin i.p. administration in mice containing fully developed carcinomas reduced Ki-67 positive and BrdU positive cell count (Figure 6). Therefore, indicating lonchocarpin as an acute anti-proliferative agent in AOM/DSS induced adenocarcinoma. Although very promising, only the lonchocarpin highest dose produced anti-proliferative effects suggesting that its biological activity should be further enhanced through the synthesis of novel optimized analogues, or by using alternative administration approaches. In the middle of the 1950s, it was first isolated from the stem wood of *Camptotheca acuminata* the precursor of one of the most used chemotherapeutic agents for colorectal cancer treatment, the alkaloid camptothecin [39]. First described as showing antileukemic and antitumor activities, for the following three decades many camptothecin analogues have been described in order to enhance its antitumor properties. One of these analogues was CPT-11, currently known as Irinotecan, that is widely used to treat colorectal cancer [40]. Together with Irinotecan, 5-FU is also widely used clinically. Intriguingly, Wnt signaling inhibition has been shown to decrease resistance of colorectal cells to these chemotherapy drugs' treatment [41]. Interestingly, MEK signaling inhibitors have been shown to increase canonical Wnt signaling in CRC [42], and the co-treatment of MEK inhibitors and Wnt signaling inhibitors resulted in a reduction of tumor growth [42]. Thus, MEK inhibitors should also be addressed as a cotreatment with lonchocarpin.

There are currently 55 clinical trials aiming to inhibit Wnt signaling pathway in cancers, in which 21 are CRC studies (clinicaltrials.gov). Among the 21 CRC clinical trials, only two tested compounds inhibit canonical Wnt signaling at the transcriptional level, PRI-724 and resveratrol. In this context, in comparison with these compounds, the in vitro IC50 of lonchocarpin Wnt signaling inhibition is noticeable. PRI-724 inhibited the Wnt signaling pathway at 25 μM in vitro [43] (authors used cyclin D1 Western blot to check Wnt signaling modulation), resveratrol inhibited at 20 μM [44] (authors used a Wnt signaling specific gene reporter assay), whereas 4 uM lonchocarpin reached the IC50. The PRI-724 clinical trial has been withdrawn due to supply issues (NCT02413853) and resveratrol results have not been published yet (NCT00256334). We believe that lonchocarpin anticancer effects should be further addressed in preclinical studies, so it can be a possible clinical trial candidate.

The use of natural compounds as drug candidates has been improved by the use of alternative delivery approaches such as controlled delivery systems. Indeed, nanostructuration has been used to circumvent solubility issues [45–47]. These strategies can solve instability and poor water solubility issues [48,49] and improve a drug candidate pharmacokinetic profile. These systems could be used to further enhance lonchocarpin anticancer properties in vivo.

At last, the similarity of lonchocarpin and derricin chemical structure deserves to be noticed. These two natural compounds inhibit Wnt signaling through similar mechanisms, while derricidin has a different one [18]. This comparison paves a new way for structure-function studies, and the quest for new Wnt signaling inhibitor pharmacophores.

4. Materials and Methods

4.1. Cell Lines and Chemical Compounds

HEK293T, SW480, HCT116, DLD-1, and IEC-6 cell lines were purchased from ATCC and RKO-pBAR/Renilla and SW480-pBAR/Renilla were a gift from Professor Xi He (Harvard Medical School). All cell lines were maintained in DMEM-F-12 (Gibco, Life Technologies Limited, Paisley, UK) enriched with 10% fetal bovine serum (Gibco). The chalcone lonchocarpin was purified by Nascimento and Mors, 1972 [50] and kindly donated for this study by professor Ricardo Kuster (Federal University of Espirito Santo). PNU-74654 was synthesized at the Laboratory of Evaluation and Synthesis of Bioactives substances (Biomedical Sciences Institute, UFRJ). Both compounds were diluted in DMSO (Sigma-Aldrich, Saint Louis, MO, USA) at the concentration of 10 mM. PNU-74654 has been previously described as an inhibitor of Wnt/β-catenin pathway by blocking the interaction between β-catenin and TCF [30]. L-cell conditioned medium (CM) and Wnt3a CM were obtained according to the ATCC protocol. L-cells and L-Wnt3a cells were plated into 75 cm^2 flasks at 50% confluence with 10 mL DMEM medium containing 10% FBS. After 4 days, the first batch of medium was obtained and kept at 4 °C. Three days later, the last batch of medium was obtained and combined with the first one. Finally, L-cell CM and Wnt3a CM were passed through a 0.22 μm filter, and kept at 20 °C.

4.2. Wnt/β-Catenin Luciferase Reporter Assay

First, 1.2×10^4 cells/well RKO-pBAR/Renilla and SW480-pBAR/Renilla cells were cultured on 96-well plates in DMEM/F-12 containing 10% fetal bovine serum (Gibco). Then, 24 h later, cells were treated with lonchocarpin at the concentrations of 1, 3, 5, 10, 20, and 30 μM in the presence of Wnt3a conditioned medium for an additional 24 h. L-cell CM was used as negative control, and 0.3% DMSO was used as vehicle control. After 24 h of treatment, Firefly and Renilla luciferase activities were detected according to the manufacturer's protocol (Dual Luciferase Reporter Assay System, Promega, Madison, WI, USA).

The 1.2×10^4 cells/well HEK293T cells were cultured on 96-well plates in DMEM/F-12 containing 10% fetal bovine serum (Gibco). At 70% confluence, each well was transfected with 100 ng TOP-Flash plasmid, 10 ng Renilla-luciferase plasmid, and 100 ng wild type β-catenin or 100 ng β-catenin S33A using Lipofectamine 3000 (Invitrogen, Life Technologies Corporation, Carlsbad, CA, USA). Then, 18 h after transfection, cells were treated with 1, 5, and 10 μM of lonchocarpin. After 24 h, Firefly and Renilla luciferase activities were detected according to the manufacturer's protocol (Dual Luciferase Reporter Assay System, Promega).

4.3. Immunocytochemistry

SW480 cells were cultured in 24-well plates with 4.0×10^4 cells/well in DMEM-F12 media (Gibco) containing 10% fetal bovine serum (Gibco). Cells were fixed in 4% paraformaldehyde, washed with phosphate buffered saline, and permeabilized with 0.3% Triton X-100. Then, each well was blocked for 1 h with 5% bovine serum albumin. The rabbit anti-β-catenin primary antibody (Sigma Aldrich) was diluted in PBS containing 1% bovine serum albumin (1:200) and incubated overnight. The secondary antibody anti-rabbit Alexa Fluor 546 (Sigma Aldrich) was diluted (1:500) with 1% bovine serum albumin (1:500) and incubated for 2 h at room temperature. 4,6-diamidino-2-phenylindole staining (Cell Signaling) was performed for 15 min, and then slides were mounted with Fluoromount (Sigma Aldrich). Images were captured using the confocal microscope Leica TCS SP5.

4.4. Immunoblotting and Cell Fractionation

First, 2×10^5 cells/well RKO-pBAR/Renilla cells were cultured on 12-well plates and treated with 20 μM lonchocarpin for 24 h. Then, the cells were harvested in ice-cold PBS 1X, followed by cytosolic lysis in digitonin buffer with protease inhibitors (150 mM NaCl, 50 mM Tris, 25 μg/mL digitonin, pH 7.4) for 5 min. Then, the lysate was centrifugated for 10 min at 2000 G at 4 °C and the supernatant was collected and considered as the cytosolic fraction. Following digitonin extraction, the remaining cell pellets were washed in ice-cold PBS 1X and lysed in NP-40 buffer (150 mM NaCl, 50 mM Tris, 1%NP-40, pH 7.4) with protease inhibitors for 15 min and centrifuged for 10 min at 7000 G at 4 °C. The supernatant was collected and considered as the membrane fraction. After that, the cell pellets were washed again in ice-cold PBS 1X and lysed in RIPA buffer with protease inhibitors for 20 min and centrifugated after at 16,000 G at 4 °C. The supernatant was collected and considered as the nuclear fraction. Whole cell lysates were prepared using Triton buffer (150 mM NaCl, 50 mM Tris, 1% Triton X-100, 1 mM EDTA, 10% Glycerol, pH 7.5). Finally, cell lysates were denatured with Laemmli buffer at 95 for 5 min, and the protein samples were subjected to SDS-PAGE and transferred into PVDF membranes (Millipore, Merck KGaA, Darmstadt, Germany). The membrane was then blocked with 2% PVP (Sigma Aldrich) in TBS-Tween-20, incubated with primary monoclonal antibodies β-catenin (BD, 1:500), β-actin (SCBT, 1:2000); lamin A/C (CST, 1:500) and α-tubulin (Sigma, 1:2000) overnight at 4 °C. After three washes with TBS-T, the membranes were incubated for 1 h with HRP-conjugated secondary antibodies (CST). The immunoblots were visualized by chemiluminescence using SuperSignal West Pico and West Femto (ThermoFisher, Life Technologies Corporation, Carlsbad, CA, USA).

4.5. *Xenopus laevis* Embryo Manipulations

Frog experiments were carried out according to the guidelines granted by the Animal Care and Use Ethic Committee from the Federal University of Rio de Janeiro and were approved by this committee under the permission number 152/13. Female adult frogs (Nasco Inc., Fort Atkinson, WI, USA) were stimulated with 1000 IU human chorionic gonadotropin (Ferring Pharmaceuticals, Kiel, Germany). *Xenopus laevis* embryos were obtained through in vitro fertilization and staged according to Nieuwkoop and Farber [51]. All experiments were performed at 22 °C. For the Wnt/β-catenin signaling specific reporter assay, two transverse blastomeres of 4-cell stage embryos were injected with 4 nL containing 280 pg of S01234-luciferase plasmid, 50 pg of TK-Renilla plasmid, 1 pg of xWnt8 mRNA, and 1.2 pmol of lonchocarpin or DMSO each, for a total of 2.4 pmol of lonchocarpin per embryo. For synthetic xWnt8 mRNA, the plasmid was linearized with NotI and transcribed with SP6 RNA polymerase using the mMessage mMachine kit (Applied Biosystems, Austin, TX, USA). After microinjections, embryos were cultivated in 0.1× Barth (8.89 mM NaCl; 0.1 mM KCl; 0.24 mM $NaHCO_3$; 0.08 mM $MgSO_4{\cdot}7H_2O$; 1 mM Hepes; 0.03 mM $Ca(NO_3)_2{\cdot}4H_2O$; 0.04 mM $CaCl_2{\cdot}2H_2O$; pH 7.7) until sibling control embryos reached stage 10. Triplicates of four embryos were lysed using 50 μL of 1× Passive Lysis Buffer (Promega). Then, 10 μL of embryo lysate was used for gene reporter activity detection. Firefly and Renilla luciferase activities were detected according to the manufacturer's protocol (Dual Luciferase Reporter Assay System, Promega).

In order to modulate the maternal wave, 4-cell stage embryos dorsal blastomeres were injected in the animal pole with 4 nL containing 200 μM of lonchocarpin (0.8 pmol/embryo) or DMSO each, for a total of 1.6 pmol of lonchocarpin per embryo. In order to modulate the zygotic wave, stage 9 embryos were injected with 50 nL containing 200 μM of lonchocarpin (10 pmol/embryo) or DMSO into the blastocoel. After injection, embryos were maintained in 0.1X Barth, until stage 35, when the phenotypes were analyzed.

4.6. MTT Assay

3-(4,5-Dimethylthiazol-2-yl)-2,5-diphenyltetrazolium bromide (MTT) was used to assay mitochondrial activity in viable cells. Cells were plated at a concentration of 1.2×10^4 cells/well in

96-well tissue culture plates in DMEM/F-12 containing 10% fetal bovine serum (Gibco) and cultured for 24 h. Cells were treated for 24 h with 10, 20, 30, 40, or 50 μM of lonchocarpin and 0.5% DMSO was used as the vehicle control. MTT was added to each well at a final concentration of 0.25 mg/mL for 1 h. The formazan reaction product was dissolved with 100% DMSO and quantified spectrophotometrically at 570 nm (Modulus™ II Microplate Multimode Reader, Promega).

4.7. *Scratch Assay*

HCT116, SW480, DLD-1, and IEC-6 were cultured on 12-well plates in DMEM/F-12 containing 10% fetal bovine serum (Gibco). Confluent wells were scratched in the center of each well with a pipette tip and treated with the proliferation inhibitor Ara-C at 10 μM. After scratch, cells were treated with 5, 10, or 20 μM lonchocarpin for 24 h. Images were taken at 0 h and the wound areas were measured at 0 and 24 h after treatment. Each experiment was carried out in triplicate, and three fields were counted per well.

4.8. *Cell Proliferation Assay*

HCT116, SW480, DLD-1, and IEC-6 were cultured on 24-well plates with 4.0×10^4 cells/well in DMEM/F-12 containing 10% fetal bovine serum (Gibco). Then, 24 h later, cells were treated with 20 or 30 μM lonchocarpin. DMSO 0.3% was used as vehicle control. Then, 18 h later, we added EdU to the cells, and 6 h later cells were fixed with paraformaldehyde 4% and the experiment was conducted according to Click-iT EdU (Life Technologies Corporation, Carlsbad, CA, USA) manufacturer protocol.

4.9. *AOM/DSS Protocol*

Animal procedures were approved and carried out according to the guidelines by the Animal Care and Use Ethic Committee from the Federal University of Rio de Janeiro under register 85/15. Male and female 129SvJxC57BL6 mixed mice (8–12 weeks) were housed in microisolator cages and maintained at 23 °C with a 12/12-h light/dark cycle and free access to food and water. A total of 26 experimental mice were pre-treated with vermifuge (vetmax plus 0.04% and ivermectin 0.4%) in quarantine for 5 days. All mice were intraperitoneally injected with AOM (12.5 mg/kg; Sigma-Aldrich) once. Five days later, all animals received the first cycle of DSS treatment composed by 2% DSS (MP Biochemicals, Solon, OH, USA) in drinking water for five days, followed by a 2-week rest period without DSS. The 2% DSS treatment cycle was repeated once and followed by a last cycle of 1.5% DSS for 4 days. Mice were monitored every day. Any mouse that lost greater than 20% body weight, demonstrate hunched posture, or moved in a limited fashion was euthanized. Four weeks after the last DSS cycle the animals were randomized into five groups as follows: no treatment group (only AOM/DSS); i.p. injections of 50 or 100 $mg{\cdot}kg^{-1}{\cdot}day^{-1}$, of vehicle (30% polyethylene glycol 400 (PEG400) with 0.9% saline); and i.p. injections of 2.5 mg/mL lonchocarpin 50 or 100 $mg{\cdot}kg^{-1}{\cdot}day^{-1}$ for four days. Due to limitation of the lonchocarpin solubility, to reach 100 $mg{\cdot}kg^{-1}{\cdot}day^{-1}$ i.p was performed every 12 h with 50 mg/kg. Euthanasia was performed after the treatment and the animals received an i.p. BrdU injection (100 mg/kg) 1 h before euthanasia.

4.10. *Tissue Processing, Histopathology, H&E, and Immunofluorescence*

After euthanasia, the colons were removed, longitudinally opened, cleaned with phosphate-buffered saline (PBS) and fixed in 4% buffered paraformaldehyde for 24 h at 4 °C. The swiss-rolls were processed in sequential ethanol and xilol for paraplast inclusion and the tissues were sectioned in Leica RM2125 RTS microtome and stained with hematoxylin and eosin (H&E) for microscopic identification of lesions, adenomas, and adenocarcinomas. Indirect immunofluorescence was performed after serial deparaffinization in xilol and ethanol. Heat induced epitope retrieval was performed in sodium citrate buffer (10 mM Sodium citrate, 0.05% Tween 20, pH 6.0) in a steamer and nonspecific binding sites were blocked with bovine serum albumin 3% in PBS. The sections were incubated with monoclonal antibodies rat anti-Ki-67 (Invitrogen #14569882; 1:100) and mouse anti-BrdU (GE Healthcare #RPN202;

1:3) overnight at 4 °C. Anti-rat biotinylated and anti-mouse Alexa 488-conjugated secondary antibodies (Invitrogen) were used to visualize Ki-67 and BrdU, respectively and the nuclei were stained with DAPI. Images were captured using the Olympus Light Microscope BX53 with a LUCPLFLN 20XPH objective and a SC50 color camera (Olympus Life Science Solutions America, Waltham, MA, USA). Only the adenocarcinoma areas confirmed in H&E staining were considered in immunofluorescence analysis. All images were manually and independently counted by at least two authors (LFSO, JMAD and AF). The proportion of positive-stained nuclei in the epithelial crypt cells found in the adenocarcinoma area were calculated and compared between the groups.

4.11. Statistical Analysis

For MTT assays statistical analysis we used a two-way ANOVA following a Bonferroni post-test (GraphPad Prism version 6.0), error bars represent standard error. For all other results, we used a one-way ANOVA (GraphPad Prism version 6.0). Figures show the mean of three replicates performed three times; standard deviation and statistical significance was set at * $p < 0.05$ ** $p < 0.01$ *** $p < 0.001$.

5. Conclusions

In summary, our data describes lonchocarpin, a flavonoid from the chalcone class, as a potent inhibitor of the Wnt/β-catenin pathway that acts downstream to β-catenin stabilization level and impairs TCF mediated transcription. In addition, lonchocarpin presents anti-tumor growth properties in vitro and inhibits adenocarcinoma proliferation in an in vivo CRC model. Further studies should be conducted in order to improve its activity and perhaps propose lonchocarpin as an alternative in CRC treatment.

Author Contributions: Conceptualization: D.P., L.F.S.O., L.S.S.F., L.A.M., J.M.A.D., N.G.A., A.H.R., F.A.M., H.L.B. and J.G.A. Methodology: D.P., L.F.S.O., L.A.M., J.M.A.D., N.G.A., A.H.R., F.A.M, H.L.B. and J.G.A. Investigation: D.P., L.F.S.O., L.S.S.F., L.A.M., J.M.A.D., A.F., I.O. Resources: C.A.M.F, R.K., F.A.M., H.L.B. and J.G.A. Writing: D.P., L.F.S.O., L.S.S.F., L.A.M., J.M.A.D., F.A.M., H.L.B. and J.G.A. Review and editing: D.P., L.F.S.O., L.S.S.F., L.A.M., J.M.A.D., N.G.A., A.H.R., C.A.M.F., R.K., F.A.M., H.L.B. and J.G.A. Visualization: D.P., L.F.S.O., L.S.S.F., L.A.M., F.A.M. and J.G.A. Supervision: J.G.A. Project administration: J.G.A. Funding acquisition: F.A.M., H.L.B., and J.G.A.

Acknowledgments: We thank Walter B. Mors, in memoriam, one of the founders of the Research Institute of Natural Products at Federal University of Rio de Janeiro, for donation of lonchocapin purified compound. We thank Simone Rodrigues and Fabio Jorge da Silva for animal care. We thank Carolina Batista for providing technical assistance. This work was supported by the Conselho Nacional de Desenvolvimento Científico e Tecnológico (CNPq) and the Fundação Carlos Chagas Filho de Amparo à Pesquisa do Estado do Rio de Janeiro (FAPERJ).

References

1. Siegel, R.L.; Miller, K.D.; Jemal, A. Cancer statistics, 2018. *CA A Cancer J. Clin.* **2018**, *68*, 7–30. [CrossRef] [PubMed]
2. Network, C.G.A. Comprehensive molecular characterization of human colon and rectal cancer. *Nature* **2012**, *487*, 330–337. [CrossRef] [PubMed]
3. Kinzler, K.; Nilbert, M.; Vogelstein, B.; Bryan, T.; Levy, D.; Smith, K.; Preisinger, A.; Hedge, P.; Markham, A. Identification of a gene located at chromosome 5q21 that is mutated in colorectal cancers. *Science* **1991**, *251*, 1366–1370. [CrossRef] [PubMed]
4. Miki, T.; Yasuda, S.Y.; Kahn, M. Wnt/β-catenin Signaling in Embryonic Stem Cell Self-renewal and Somatic Cell Reprogramming. *Stem Cell Rev. Rep.* **2011**, *7*, 836–846. [CrossRef]
5. Van Amerongen, R.; Nusse, R. Towards an integrated view of Wnt signaling in development. *Development* **2009**, *136*, 3205–3214. [CrossRef]
6. Kim, S.-E.; Huang, H.; Zhao, M.; Zhang, X.; Zhang, A.; Semonov, M.V.; MacDonald, B.T.; Zhang, X.; Abreu, J.G.; Peng, L.; et al. Wnt stabilization of β-catenin reveals principles for morphogen receptor-scaffold assemblies. *Science* **2013**, *340*, 867–870. [CrossRef]

7. MacDonald, B.T.; Tamai, K.; He, X. Wnt/β-Catenin Signaling: Components, Mechanisms, and Diseases. *Dev. Cell* **2009**, *17*, 9–26. [CrossRef]
8. Tortelote, G.G.; Reis, R.R.; de Almeida Mendes, F.; Abreu, J.G. Complexity of the Wnt/β-catenin pathway: Searching for an activation model. *Cell. Signal.* **2017**, *40*, 30–43. [CrossRef]
9. Kahn, M. Can we safely target the WNT pathway? *Nat. Rev. Drug Discov.* **2014**, *13*, 513–532. [CrossRef]
10. Larabell, C.A.; Torres, M.; Rowning, B.A.; Yost, C.; Miller, J.R.; Wu, M.; Kimelman, D.; Moon, R.T. Establishment of the Dorso-ventral Axis in Xenopus Embryos Is Presaged by Early Asymmetries in β-Catenin That Are Modulated by the Wnt Signaling Pathway. *J. Cell Biol.* **1997**, *136*, 1123–1136. [CrossRef] [PubMed]
11. Maia, L.A.; Velloso, I.; Abreu, J.G. Advances in the use of Xenopus for successful drug screening. *Expert Opin. Drug Discov.* **2017**, *12*, 1153–1159. [CrossRef] [PubMed]
12. McMahon, A.P.; Moon, R.T. Ectopic expression of the proto-oncogene int-1 in Xenopus embryos leads to duplication of the embryonic axis. *Cell* **1989**, *58*, 1075–1084. [CrossRef]
13. Thorne, C.A.; Hanson, A.J.; Schneider, J.; Tahinci, E.; Orton, D.; Cselenyi, C.S.; Jernigan, K.K.; Meyers, K.C.; Hang, B.I.; Waterson, A.G.; et al. Small-molecule inhibition of Wnt signaling through activation of casein kinase 1α. *Nat. Chem. Biol.* **2010**, *6*, 829. [CrossRef] [PubMed]
14. Tanaka, T.; Kohno, H.; Suzuki, R.; Yamada, Y.; Sugie, S.; Mori, H. A novel inflammation-related mouse colon carcinogenesis model induced by azoxymethane and dextran sodium sulfate. *Cancer Sci.* **2003**, *94*, 965–973. [CrossRef]
15. Tanaka, T.; Suzuki, R.; Kohno, H.; Sugie, S.; Takahashi, M.; Wakabayashi, K. Colonic adenocarcinomas rapidly induced by the combined treatment with 2-amino-1-methyl-6-phenylimidazo[4,5-b]pyridine and dextran sodium sulfate in male ICR mice possess β-catenin gene mutations and increases immunoreactivity for β-catenin, cyclooxygenase-2 and inducible nitric oxide synthase. *Carcinogenesis* **2005**, *26*, 229–238.
16. Amado, N.G.; Cerqueira, D.M.; Menezes, F.S.; Da Silva, J.F.M.; Neto, V.M.; Abreu, J.G. Isoquercitrin isolated from Hyptis fasciculata reduces glioblastoma cell proliferation and changes β-catenin cellular localization. *Anti-Cancer Drugs* **2009**, *20*, 543–552. [CrossRef]
17. Amado, N.G.; Predes, D.; Moreno, M.M.; Carvalho, I.O.; Mendes, F.A.; Abreu, J.G. Flavonoids and Wnt/β-Catenin Signaling: Potential Role in Colorectal Cancer Therapies. *Int. J. Mol. Sci.* **2014**, *15*, 12094–12106. [CrossRef]
18. Fonseca, B.F.; Predes, D.; Cerqueira, D.M.; Reis, A.H.; Amado, N.G.; Cayres, M.C.L.; Kuster, R.M.; Oliveira, F.L.; Mendes, F.A.; Abreu, J.G. Derricin and Derricidin Inhibit Wnt/β-Catenin Signaling and Suppress Colon Cancer Cell Growth In Vitro. *PLoS ONE* **2015**, *10*, e0120919. [CrossRef]
19. Gao, Z.; Xu, Z.; Hung, M.S.; Lin, Y.C.; Wang, T.; Gong, M.; Zhi, X.; Jablon, D.M.; You, L. Promoter demethylation of WIF-1 by epigallocatechin-3-gallate in lung cancer cells. *Anticancer Res.* **2009**, *29*, 2025–2030.
20. Kaur, M.; Velmurugan, B.; Tyagi, A.; Agarwal, C.; Singh, R.P.; Agarwal, R. Silibinin Suppresses Growth of Human Colorectal Carcinoma SW480 Cells in Culture and Xenograft through Down-regulation of β-Catenin-Dependent Signaling. *Neoplasia* **2010**, *12*, 415–424. [CrossRef]
21. Landesman-Bollag, E.; Song, D.H.; Mourez, R.R.; Sussman, D.J.; Cardiff, R.D.; Sonenshein, G.E.; Seldin, D.C. Protein kinase CK2: Signaling and tumorigenesis in the mammary gland. *Mol. Cell. Biochem.* **2001**, *227*, 153–165. [CrossRef] [PubMed]
22. Li, Y.; Wang, Z.; Kong, D.; Li, R.; Sarkar, S.H.; Sarkar, F.H. Regulation of Akt/FOXO3a/GSK-3β/AR signaling network by isoflavone in prostate cancer cells. *J. Biol. Chem.* **2008**, *283*, 27707–27716. [CrossRef] [PubMed]
23. Park, C.H.; Chang, J.Y.; Hahm, E.R.; Park, S.; Kim, H.K.; Yang, C.H. Quercetin, a potent inhibitor against β-catenin/Tcf signaling in SW480 colon cancer cells. *Biochem. Biophys. Res. Commun.* **2005**, *328*, 227–234. [CrossRef] [PubMed]
24. Lee, J.; Lee, J.; Jung, E.; Hwang, W.; Kim, Y.S.; Park, D. Isorhamnetin-induced anti-adipogenesis is mediated by stabilization of β-catenin protein. *Life Sci.* **2010**, *86*, 416–423. [CrossRef]
25. Song, D.H.; Sussman, D.J.; Seldin, D.C. Endogenous Protein Kinase CK2 Participates in Wnt Signaling in Mammary Epithelial Cells. *J. Biol. Chem.* **2000**, *275*, 23790–23797. [CrossRef]
26. Baudrenghien, J.; Jadot, J.; Huis, R. Etablissement de la formule de structure de la lonchocarpine. *Bull. Soc. Roy. Sci. Liège* **1949**, *18*, 52.
27. Cursino, L.M.C.; Lima, N.M.; Murillo, R.; Nunez, C.V.; Merfort, I.; Humar, M. Isolation of Flavonoids from Deguelia duckeana and Their Effect on Cellular Viability, AMPK, eEF2, eIF2 and eIF4E. *Molecules* **2016**, *21*, 192. [CrossRef]

28. Korinek, V.; Barker, N.; Morin, P.J.; Van Wichen, D.; De Weger, R.; Kinzler, K.W.; Vogelstein, B.; Clevers, H. Constitutive transcriptional activation by a β-catenin-Tcf complex in APC−/− colon carcinoma. *Science* **1997**, *275*, 1784–1787. [CrossRef]
29. Munemitsu, S.; Albert, I.; Rubinfeld, B.; Polakis, P. Deletion of an amino-terminal sequence beta-catenin in vivo and promotes hyperphosporylation of the adenomatous polyposis coli tumor suppressor protein. *Mol. Cell. Biol.* **1996**, *16*, 4088–4094. [CrossRef]
30. Trosset, J.Y.; Dalvit, C.; Knapp, S.; Fasolini, M.; Veronesi, M.; Mantegani, S.; Gianellini, L.M.; Catana, C.; Sundström, M.; Stouten, P.F. Inhibition of protein–protein interactions: The discovery of druglike β-catenin inhibitors by combining virtual and biophysical screening. *Proteins Struct. Funct. Bioinform.* **2006**, *64*, 60–67. [CrossRef]
31. Zhang, X.; Abreu, J.G.; Yokota, C.; MacDonald, B.T.; Singh, S.; Coburn, K.L.A.; Cheong, S.-M.; Zhang, M.M.; Ye, Q.-Z.; Hang, H.C.; et al. Tiki1 is required for head formation via Wnt cleavage-oxidation and inactivation. *Cell* **2012**, *149*, 1565–1577. [CrossRef] [PubMed]
32. Amado, N.G.; Fonseca, B.F.; Cerqueira, D.M.; Reis, A.H.; Simas, A.B.C.; Kuster, R.M.; Mendes, F.A.; Abreu, J.G. Effects of natural compounds on Xenopus embryogenesis: A potential read out for functional drug discovery targeting Wnt/β-catenin signaling. *Curr. Top. Med. Chem.* **2012**, *12*, 2103–2113. [CrossRef] [PubMed]
33. Oh, S.; Gwak, J.; Park, S.; Yang, C.S. Green tea polyphenol EGCG suppresses Wnt/β-catenin signaling by promoting GSK-3β- and PP2A-independent β-catenin phosphorylation/degradation. *BioFactors* **2014**, *40*, 586–595. [CrossRef]
34. Amado, N.G.; Predes, D.; Fonseca, B.F.; Cerqueira, D.M.; Reis, A.H.; Dudenhoeffer, A.C.; Borges, H.L.; Mendes, F.A.; Abreu, J.G. Isoquercitrin suppresses colon cancer cell growth in vitro by targeting the Wnt/β-catenin signaling pathway. *J. Biol. Chem.* **2014**, *289*, 35456–35467. [CrossRef] [PubMed]
35. Cunha, G.M.D.; Fontenele, J.B.; Nobre Júnior, H.V.; de Sousa, F.C.; Silveira, E.R.; Nogueira, N.A.; de Moraes, M.O.; Viana, G.S.; Costa-Lotufo, L.V. Cytotoxic activity of chalcones isolated from *Lonchocarpus sericeus* (Pocr.) Kunth. *Phytother. Res.* **2003**, *17*, 155–159. [CrossRef] [PubMed]
36. Staal, F.; Famili, F.; Garcia Perez, L.; Pike-Overzet, K. Aberrant Wnt signaling in leukemia. *Cancers* **2016**, *8*, 78. [CrossRef]
37. Chen, G.; Zhou, D.; Li, X.Z.; Jiang, Z.; Tan, C.; Wei, X.Y.; Ling, J.; Jing, J.; Liu, F.; Li, N. A natural chalcone induces apoptosis in lung cancer cells: 3D-QSAR, docking and an in vivo/vitro assay. *Sci. Rep.* **2017**, *7*, 10729. [CrossRef]
38. De Robertis, M.; Massi, E.; Poeta, M.L.; Carotti, S.; Morini, S.; Cecchetelli, L.; Signori, E.; Fazio, V.M. The AOM/DSS murine model for the study of colon carcinogenesis: From pathways to diagnosis and therapy studies. *J. Carcinog.* **2011**, *10*. [CrossRef]
39. Wall, M.E.; Wani, M.C.; Cook, C.; Palmer, K.H.; McPhail, A.A.; Sim, G. Plant antitumor agents. I. The isolation and structure of camptothecin, a novel alkaloidal leukemia and tumor inhibitor from camptotheca acuminata. *J. Am. Chem. Soc.* **1966**, *88*, 3888–3890. [CrossRef]
40. Wall, M.E.; Wani, M.C. Discovery to clinic. *Ann. N. Y. Acad. Sci.* **1996**, *803*, 1–12. [CrossRef]
41. Chikazawa, N.; Tanaka, H.; Tasaka, T.; Nakamura, M.; Tanaka, M.; Onishi, H.; Katano, M. Inhibition of Wnt signaling pathway decreases chemotherapy-resistant side-population colon cancer cells. *Anticancer Res.* **2010**, *30*, 2041–2048.
42. Zhan, T.; Ambrosi, G.; Wandmacher, A.; Rauscher, B.; Betge, J.; Rindtorff, N.; Häussler, R.; Hinsenkamp, I.; Bamberg, L.; Hessling, B.; et al. MEK inhibitors activate Wnt signalling and induce stem cell plasticity in colorectal cancer. *Nat. Commun.* **2019**, *10*, 2197. [CrossRef] [PubMed]
43. Fang, F.; VanCleave, A.; Helmuth, R.; Torres, H.; Rickel, K.; Wollenzien, H.; Sun, H.; Zeng, E.; Zhao, J.; Tao, J. Targeting the Wnt/β-catenin pathway in human osteosarcoma cells. *Oncotarget* **2018**, *9*, 36780–36792. [CrossRef] [PubMed]
44. Chen, H.J.; Hsu, L.S.; Shia, Y.T.; Lin, M.W.; Lin, C.M. The β-catenin/TCF complex as a novel target of resveratrol in the Wnt/β-catenin signaling pathway. *Biochem. Pharmacol.* **2012**, *84*, 1143–1153. [CrossRef] [PubMed]
45. Arbain, N.H.; Salim, N.; Wui, W.T.; Basri, M.; Rahman, M.B.A. Optimization of Quercetin loaded Palm Oil Ester Based Nanoemulsion Formulation for Pulmonary Delivery. *J. Oleo Sci.* **2018**, *67*, 933–940. [CrossRef] [PubMed]

46. Kakran, M.; Shegokar, R.; Sahoo, N.G.; Al Shaal, L.; Li, L.; Müller, R.H. Fabrication of quercetin nanocrystals: Comparison of different methods. *Eur. J. Pharm. Biopharm.* **2012**, *80*, 113–121. [CrossRef]
47. Kumari, A.; Yadav, S.K.; Pakade, Y.B.; Singh, B.; Yadav, S.C. Development of biodegradable nanoparticles for delivery of quercetin. *Colloids Surf. B Biointerfaces* **2010**, *80*, 184–192. [CrossRef]
48. Ader, P. Bioavailability and metabolism of the flavonol quercetin in the pig. *Free Radic. Biol. Med.* **2000**, *28*, 1056–1067. [CrossRef]
49. Pool, H.; Quintanar, D.; Figueroa, J.D.D.; Mano, C.M.; Bechara, J.E.H.; Godínez, L.A.; Mendoza, S.; Godí Nez, L.A. Antioxidant Effects of Quercetin and Catechin Encapsulated into PLGA Nanoparticles. *J. Nanomater.* **2012**, *2012*, 86. [CrossRef]
50. Nascimento, M.C.D.; Mors, W. Chalcones of the root bark of Derris sericea. *Phytochemistry* **1972**, *11*, 3023–3028. [CrossRef]
51. Nieuwkoop, P.; Faber, J. *Normal Table of Xenopus Laevis*; North-Holland Publishing, Co.: Amsterdam, The Netherlands, 1967.

9

The Inhibitory Mechanisms of Tumor PD-L1 Expression by Natural Bioactive Gallic Acid in Non-Small-Cell Lung Cancer (NSCLC) Cells

Dong Young Kang [1,†], Nipin Sp [1,†], Eun Seong Jo [1], Alexis Rugamba [1], Dae Young Hong [2], Hong Ghi Lee [3], Ji-Seung Yoo [4], Qing Liu [5], Kyoung-Jin Jang [1,*] and Young Mok Yang [1,*]

1 Department of Pathology, School of Medicine, Institute of Biomedical Science and Technology, Konkuk University, Seoul 05029, Korea; kdy6459@naver.com (D.Y.K.); nipinsp@gmail.com (N.S.); eses0706@naver.com (E.S.J.); rugambalex@gmail.com (A.R.)
2 Department of Emergency Medicine, School of Medicine, Konkuk University, Seoul 05029, Korea; kuhemhdy@gmail.com
3 Division of Hematology-Oncology, Department of Internal Medicine, Konkuk University Medical Center, Seoul 05029, Korea; mlee@kuh.ac.kr
4 Department of Immunology, Hokkaido University Graduate School of Medicine, Sapporo 060-0808, Japan; jiseungy@pop.med.hokudai.ac.jp
5 Jilin Green Food Engineering Research Institute, Changchun 130000, Jilin, China; liuqing0523@hotmail.com
* Correspondence: jangkj@konkuk.ac.kr (K.-J.J.); ymyang@kku.ac.kr (Y.M.Y.)

† These authors contribute equally to this paper.

Abstract: Non-small-cell lung cancer (NSCLC) is the most common lung cancer subtype and accounts for more than 80% of all lung cancer cases. Epidermal growth factor receptor (EGFR) phosphorylation by binding growth factors such as EGF activates downstream prooncogenic signaling pathways including KRAS-ERK, JAK-STAT, and PI3K-AKT. These pathways promote the tumor progression of NSCLC by inducing uncontrolled cell cycle, proliferation, migration, and programmed death-ligand 1 (PD-L1) expression. New cytotoxic drugs have facilitated considerable progress in NSCLC treatment, but side effects are still a significant cause of mortality. Gallic acid (3,4,5-trihydroxybenzoic acid; GA) is a phenolic natural compound, isolated from plant derivatives, that has been reported to show anticancer effects. We demonstrated the tumor-suppressive effect of GA, which induced the decrease of PD-L1 expression through binding to EGFR in NSCLC. This binding inhibited the phosphorylation of EGFR, subsequently inducing the inhibition of PI3K and AKT phosphorylation, which triggered the activation of p53. The p53-dependent upregulation of miR-34a induced PD-L1 downregulation. Further, we revealed the combination effect of GA and anti-PD-1 monoclonal antibody in an NSCLC-cell and peripheral blood mononuclear–cell coculture system. We propose a novel therapeutic application of GA for immunotherapy and chemotherapy in NSCLC.

Keywords: natural bioactive compound; gallic acid; EGFR signaling; p53; PD-L1; immunotherapy

1. Introduction

Lung cancer, constituting 18% of all global cancer deaths, is one of the representative causes of death globally [1]. It is classified into two main groups: small-cell lung cancer (SCLC; 15% of all lung cancers) and non-SCLC (NSCLC; 85% of all lung cancers) [2,3]. NSCLC can be further subcategorized into three subtypes: adenocarcinoma, squamous cell carcinoma, and large cell carcinoma [4]. Despite many efforts to treat NSCLC, the overall survival rate is only 15.9% within five years [5]. Further, many patients receiving NSCLC chemotherapies struggle with adverse reactions, drug resistance, and the necessary target specificity of some types of drugs. Thus, unsatisfactory outcomes in NSCLC treatment have motivated researchers to identify novel agents such as natural compounds [6–8]. Moreover, the main advantage of such drugs having fewer side effects relative to non-natural drugs has spurred scientists to reveal their molecular mechanisms.

Gallic acid (3,4,5-trihydroxybenzoic acid; GA), a natural phenolic compound, is widely distributed in natural plants, fruits, and green tea [9,10]. Many studies have reported that GA exhibits anti oxidative, anti mutagenic, anti carcinogenic, antibacterial, antiviral, and anti-inflammatory effects [11–15]. However, the main interest in GA and its derivatives surrounds its anticancer activity. Previous studies have revealed that GA effectively induces selective apoptosis in various cancer cells, including HeLa, HCT-15, SH-SY5Y, and NSCLC cells [16–19] and inhibits proliferation and migration via regulating fatty acid synthase in TSGH-8301 cells [20]. Recent studies also revealed potential anticancer effects of GA is due to its ability to inhibit cell proliferation and to induce apoptosis *in vivo* [21,22].

Programmed cell death ligand-1 (PD-L1), also known as CD274 and B7-H1, is a transmembrane protein expressed on the surface of antigen-presenting cells such as dendritic cells, macrophages, and B-cells. It is also overexpressed and found in various types of cancer [23–26]. PD-L1 specifically binds to programmed cell death-1 (PD-1), which is an important inhibitory receptor expressed on the surface of immune-related lymphocytes like T-cells, B-cells, and myeloid cells [27]. The binding of PD-L1 to PD-1 inhibits the proliferation, cytokine generation and release, and cytotoxicity of T-cells. Thus, the binding leads to an immunosuppressive effect and allows cancer cells to escape immune eradication via assistance from tumor-specific T-cells [28]. PD-L1 overexpression in cancer cells promotes cancer progression and leads cancer cells to malignancy. Moreover, the intrinsic signal transduction by PD-L1 enhances the survival of cancer cells through increasing the resistance toward proapoptotic stimuli such as interferons [29]. PD-L1 expression at the transcriptional level is regulated individually or cooperatively by many oncogenic transcription factors such as MYC, AP-1, STAT, IRF1, HIF, and NF-κB. Some studies have demonstrated that there is a tendency toward higher PD-L1 expression in *TP53*-mutated and low p53-expression cancer cells, which imply that PD-L1 expression is considerably related to p53 status in cancer cells [30–33]. In addition, tumor suppressor gene *PTEN*, one of the most frequently mutated genes in human cancers, downregulates PD-L1 expression, which signifies that tumor suppressors play an important role in controlling PD-L1 expression [34–36].

Previous research has demonstrated that apigenin, a kind of flavonoid, induces growth-suppressive and proapoptotic effects in melanoma cells. Additionally, such significantly inhibits the expression of interferon (IFN)-γ-induced PD-L1, which may indicate the existence of an immunosuppressive effect shown by a natural compound [37]. In this study, we examined the anticancer and immunosuppressive activities of natural bioactive GA in NSCLC A549 and H292 cells (wild-type p53 and epidermal growth factor receptor (EGFR)), which are kinds of NSCLC cells. The binding of GA to EGFR inhibited the EGFR phosphorylation, leading to the promotion of p53 expression in both A549 and H292 cells. Furthermore, highly expressed p53 decreased PD-L1 protein expression through enhancing the miR-34a related to PD-L1 downregulation at the transcriptional level. As such, our results suggest an immunosuppressive effect of GA toward NSCLC cells, which might imply a potential possibility for clinical application in NSCLC treatment.

2. Results

2.1. GA Downregulates the PD-L1 Expression in NSCLC Cells

To determine whether GA inhibits the cell proliferation of A549 and H292 cell lines, GA-treated cells were compared with non-treated control cells. The results of MTT assay showed that the cell growth of GA-treated cells is significantly inhibited in a time- and concentration-dependent manner (Figure S1A). This result was confirmed with crystal violet assay by treating GA in A549 and H292 cells for 48 h (Figure S1B). From this data, we respectively identified an IC_{50} dosage of 400 μM in A549 and 100 μM in H292 cell lines at 48 hours, respectively, information which was used for further studies. We checked the same concentration in non-cancerous cells (HUVEC cell line) and found that

400 μM GA inducing around 8% cell death which indicated that this concentration does not make much toxicity in normal cells (Figure S2). Recently, cancer immunotherapy based on PD-1/PD-L1 blockade has shown clinical efficacy in the treatment of multiple cancers [26,28]. In addition, a study of the drug-induced inhibition of PD-L1 expression in cancer cells has been conducted [37]. To investigate whether GA influences PD-L1 expression, we assessed the expression levels of PD-L1 by the impact of GA in NSCLC cells. As shown in Figure 1A, results from western blotting suggested that GA strongly decreases the expression levels of PD-L1 protein in A549 and H292 NSCLC cells. In addition, GA showed a greater than 70% inhibitory effect as compared with in non-treated control cells among A549 cells (Figure 1B). Subsequently, we performed a real time PCR experiment to examine the influence of GA on the messenger RNA (mRNA) expression of PD-L1 in A549 and H292 cell lines. In accordance with data from real time PCR, GA also downregulated the expression of PD-L1 mRNA in a concentration-dependent manner in both A549 and H292 cells (Figure 1C). These results suggest that bioactive natural GA has a significant inhibitory effect on PD-L1 expression (both protein and mRNA) in A549 and H292 cell lines, which imply the potential of using it as an immune anticancer agent.

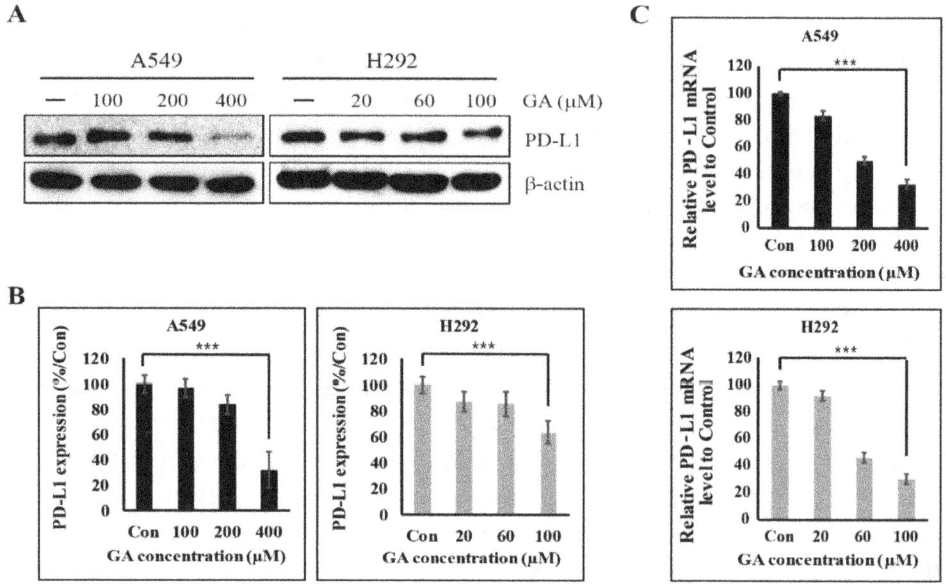

Figure 1. Gallic acid (GA) reduces the programmed death-ligand 1 (PD-L1) expression in non-small-cell lung cancer (NSCLC) cells. (**A**) The expression levels of PD-L1 protein in A549 and H292 cells were detected after GA treatment in concentrations indicated for 48 hours. (**B**) The relative expression levels of PD-L1 protein were determined by densitometry and normalized to β-actin. Data are representative of three independent experiments. *** $p < 0.001$ (t-test). (**C**) The expression levels of PD-L1 mRNA in A549 and H292 cells were detected after GA treatment in concentrations indicated for 48 hours. The relative expression levels of PD-L1 mRNA were determined by real time qPCR and normalized to GAPDH mRNA. Data are representative of three independent experiments. *** $p < 0.001$ (t-test).

2.2. GA Binds to EGFR and Then Inhibits its Phosphorylation

EGFR phosphorylation induces various oncogenic signaling pathways for cell proliferation, invasion, and metabolic reprogramming in many cancer cells [38]. Therefore, to inhibit EGFR phosphorylation in cancer cells, many clinical applications have been stimulated to develop EGFR tyrosine kinase inhibitors (TKIs) such as erlotinib, gefitinib, and lapatinib [39,40]. In previous studies, we found that the binding of natural compounds to EGFR, causing a decrease in EGFR phosphorylation, inhibited the proliferation, migration, invasion, and angiogenesis of human breast adenocarcinoma cells [41,42]. To understand the impact of GA for EGFR phosphorylation, we identified the binding ability of GA to EGFR. Molecular docking was performed with an AutoDock Vina platform (Oleg Trott, The Scripps Research Institute, La Jolla, CA, USA). We found that GA is docked in the ATP binding site of EGFR, and this result may imply the direct binding of GA to EGFR (Figure 2A). Subsequently, we further performed an immunoblot analysis for understanding whether the GA/EGFR binding influences the phosphorylation of EGFR and found that, GA significantly downregulated the phosphorylation of EGFR in both A549 and H292 cells (EGFR wild-type NSCLC cells) (Figure 2B,C). However, this treatment did not affect the expression levels of total EGFR mRNA (Figure 2D). These results may imply that GA could influence the inhibition of EGFR signal transduction in two NSCLC cells. Moreover, these results led us to investigate the binding specificity of GA to EGFR, where we conducted a competitive binding experiment of GA and EGF (25 ng/mL pre-treatment for 15 min) versus EGFR. Here, GA significantly inhibited EGF-induced EGFR phosphorylation in both A549 and H292 cells (Figure 2E,F). This result suggests that GA binds to EGFR as compared with the natural ligand (EGF) for EGFR, and this act of binding clearly induces the inhibition of EGFR phosphorylation.

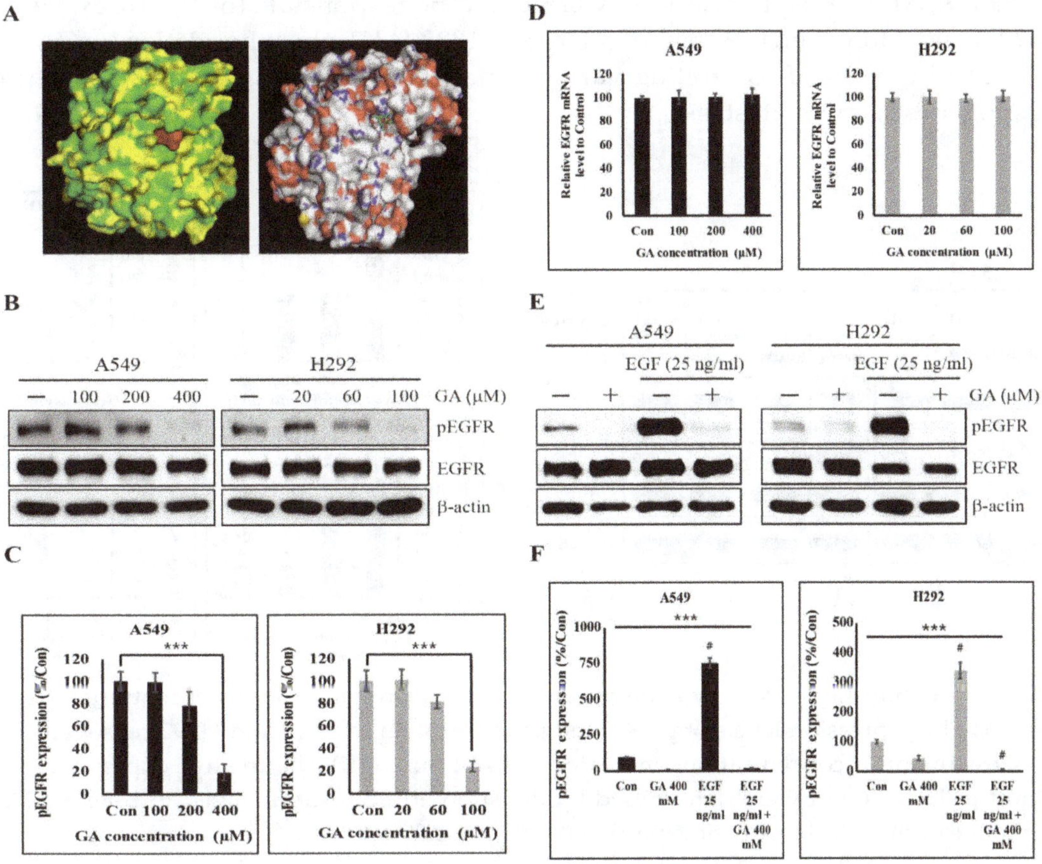

Figure 2. GA binding to epidermal growth factor receptor (EGFR) inhibits the phosphorylation of EGFR. (**A**) Binding of GA (PubChem CID: 370) to the ATP-binding domain of EGFR (Protein Data Bank ID: 4LQM) as determined by molecular docking using AutoDock Vina. (**B**) The expression levels of total EGFR and phosphorylated EGFR (pEGFR) protein in A549 and H292 cells were detected after GA treatment in concentrations indicated for 48 hours. (**C**) The relative levels of pEGFR protein were determined by densitometry and normalized to β-actin. Data are representative of three independent experiments. *** $p < 0.001$ (*t*-test). (**D**) The expression levels of EGFR mRNA in A549 and H292 cells were detected by real time PCR after GA treatment in concentrations indicated for 48 hours. The relative levels of EGFR mRNA were determined and normalized to GAPDH mRNA. Data are representative of three independent experiments. (**E**) A549 and H292 cells for detecting the expression levels of total EGFR and pEGFR protein were treated with or without 25 ng/mL EGF for 15 minutes and then further treated with GA (A549: 400 μM; H292: 100 μM) for 48 hours. (**F**) The relative levels of pEGFR protein were determined by densitometry and normalized to β-actin. Data are representative of three independent experiments. *** $p < 0.001$ (*t*-test). # $p < 0.001$ vs. control.

2.3. GA Reduces the Phosphorylation of PI3K/AKT That is One of the Downstream Targets of EGFR Signaling

EGF/EGFR signal transduction has been known to lead to the constitutive activation of downstream signaling pathways associated with MAPKs, STAT3, and PI3K for regulating PD-L1 expression in various cancer cells [43]. A previous study found that the PD-L1 expression of EGFR–mutated PC-9 cells was significantly higher than those of EGFR wild-type LU-99, A549, and PC-14 cells. In EGFR inhibitor experiments, the EGFR TKI gefitinib induced a lower expression of phosphorylated AKT and STAT3, which prompted the downregulation of PD-L1 expression [44]. To determine a key EGFR-downstream pathway associated with PD-L1 expression, we used an immunoblot analysis. As shown in Figure S3, GA treatment did not inhibit the phosphorylation of JAK2/STAT3, which is one of the main pathways. However, GA efficiently controlled the PI3K/AKT pathway by inhibiting their phosphorylation but not total protein level (Figure 3A,B). These results clearly show that the regulation of PI3K/AKT phosphorylation by GA could be responsible for PD-L1 expression in both A549 and H292 cells. Moreover, the downregulation of PI3K/AKT phosphorylation by GA may indicate a beneficial effect in terms of controlling various oncogenic signals, such as cellular proliferation, invasion, angiogenesis, and metastasis.

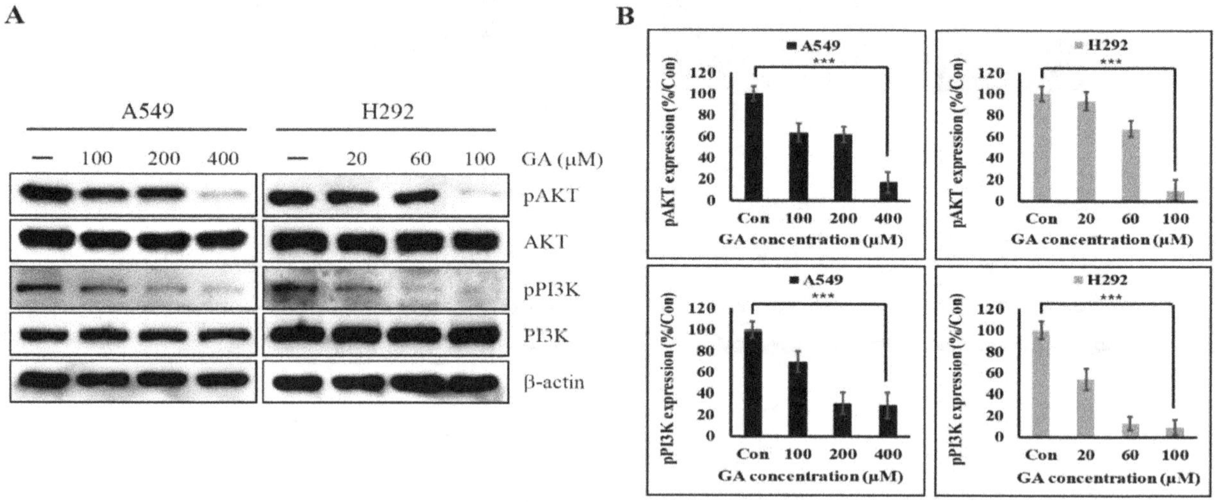

Figure 3. GA inhibits the phosphorylation of AKT and PI3K protein in a GA concentration-dependent manner. (**A**) The expression levels of pAKT and pPI3K protein in A549 and H292 cells were detected after GA treatment in concentrations indicated for 48 hours. (**B**) The relative expression levels of pAKT and pPI3K protein were determined by densitometry and normalized to β-actin. Data are representative of three independent experiments. *** $p < 0.001$ (t-test).

2.4. GA Activates the Expression of Tumor Suppressor Factor p53 for Inhibiting the Expression of PD-L1

The tumor suppressor factor p53 plays an important role in cell-cycle arrest and apoptosis induction in response to oncogenic or other stresses for the prevention of cancer development. However, it is downregulated or mutated in an inactive form in almost all human cancer cells. A previous study found that p53 is led into Mdm2-mediated ubiquitination and degradation by PI3K/AKT signal transduction in breast cancer MCF-7 cells but not p53 mRNA [45]. Furthermore, p53-regulated IFN-γ induced PD-L1 expression in melanoma cells [32]. To investigate the effect on p53 by GA, we checked the protein levels of p53 with or without GA treatment in A549 and H292 cells and found that GA upregulates the expression levels of p53 protein in a concentration-dependent manner (Figure 4A,B). In addition, the expression levels of p53 protein were nearly doubled in A549 cells. Further, the mRNA levels of p53 identified by real time PCR showed a significant increase in a GA concentration-dependent manner in H292 cells as well as in A549 cells (Figure 4C). From these data, although a previous study revealed that PI3K/AKT signaling induced by their phosphorylation regulates only p53 protein levels, the PI3K/AKT signaling controlled by GA plays a key role in regulating both protein and mRNA levels of p53. These results additional imply that GA regulates p53 from mRNA levels through the downregulation of PI3K/AKT phosphorylation. To further understand the role of p53 in PD-L1 regulation, we used GA with or without p53 siRNA and determined whether specific gene silencing influences PD-L1 expression in A549 and H292 cells. As shown in Figure 4D,E, the gene silencing of p53 significantly affected the increase in PD-L1 proteins compared to non-treated control, which was decreased by GA treatment. In contrast, the effect by GA regulated the protein levels of p53 and PD-L1 in two NSCLC cells. These results imply that the regulation of PD-L1 by GA is indirectly controlled by way of inducing an increase in p53 protein level. In addition, the upregulation of p53 by GA may induce various p53-mediated anti-oncogenic factors such as the regulation of miRNA.

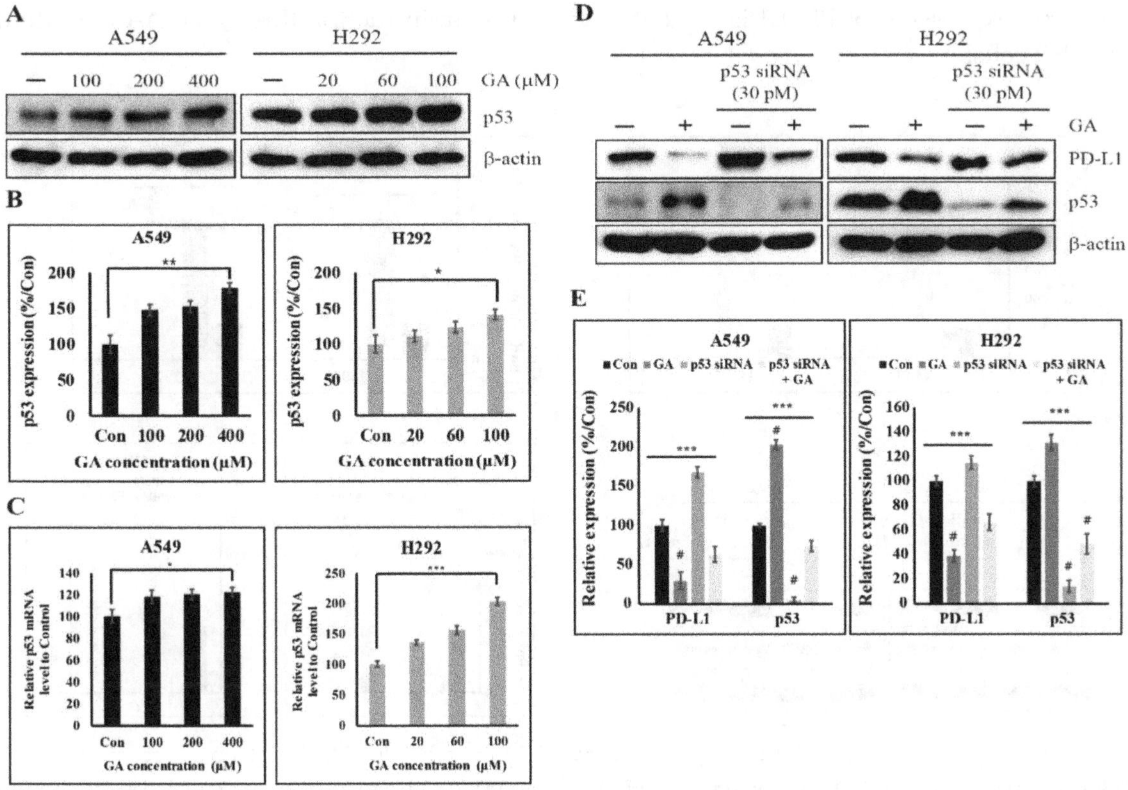

Figure 4. GA increased p53 expression. (**A**) The expression levels of p53 protein in A549 and H292 cells were detected after GA treatment in concentrations indicated for 48 hours. (**B**) The relative expression levels of p53 protein were determined by densitometry and normalized to β-actin. Data are representative of three independent experiments. * $p < 0.05$ and ** $p < 0.01$ (t-test). (**C**) The expression levels of p53 mRNA in A549 and H292 cells were detected by real time qPCR after GA treatment in concentrations indicated for 48 hours. The relative expression levels of p53 mRNA were determined and normalized to GAPDH mRNA. Data are representative of three independent experiments. * $p < 0.05$ and *** $p < 0.001$ (t-test). (**D**) The expression levels of p53 and PD-L1 protein in A549 and H292 cells, treated with GA (A549: 400 μM; H292: 100 μM) or 30 pM p53 siRNA, were detected by western blotting at 48 hours. (**E**) The relative expression levels of p53 and PD-L1 protein were determined using densitometry and normalized to β-actin. Data are representative of three independent experiments. *** $p < 0.001$ (ANOVA); # $p < 0.001$ vs. control.

2.5. GA Upregulates p53-Dependent MiR-34a for Inhibiting the Expression of PD-L1

miRNAs, a family of small noncoding RNAs, regulate wide biological processes including carcinogenesis, which severely is dysregulated in many cancer cells. Some miRNAs such as miR-513 and miR-570 directly target PD-L1 [46,47]. However, p53 indirectly regulates the expression levels of PD-L1 through inducing miR-34a in cancer cells [33]. Although many studies have shown results for the regulation of PD-L1 expression directly by miRNA, detailed studies of the actions brought on indirectly by p53 via drugs including natural compounds is poorly understood. To understand the expression level of miR-34a by GA, we performed a real time PCR experiment because miR-34a is a well-known molecule transcriptionally induced by p53. As shown in Figure 5A, we found that it was significantly increased in a time- and GA concentration-dependent manner in both A549 and H292 cells. To further investigate miR-34a regulation by GA via p53, we additionally used p53 siRNA. The expression levels of miR-34a were decreased by p53 siRNA, but their expression levels were slightly increased by additional GA (Figure 5B). These results clearly suggest that miR-34a expression is regulated by GA-dependent p53. Additionally, we used a miR-34a inhibitor with or without GA to determine a more detailed interrelation analysis in the regulation of PD-L1 expression. In this experiment, we demonstrated that the inhibition of miR-34a function by its inhibitor is induced into an increase of PD-L1 protein which reversed by GA, but not p53 (Figure 5C,D). These results support that the expression of PD-L1 is regulated via miR-34a-induction through GA-dependent p53 in A549 and H292 cells.

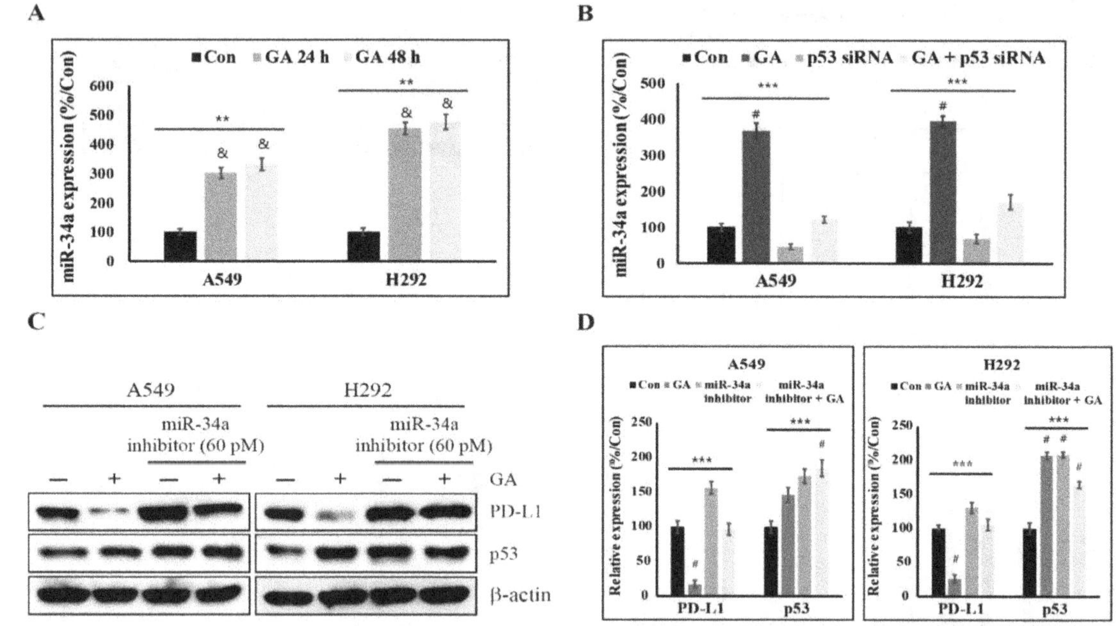

Figure 5. GA upregulates the PD-L1 expression by p53 via miR-34a. (**A**) Relative expression levels of miR34a after treatment of GA (A549: 400 μM; H292: 100 μM) for 24 and 48 hours. Data are representative of three independent experiments. ** $p < 0.01$ (ANOVA); & $p < 0.01$ vs. control. (**B**) The expression levels of miR-34a in A549 and H292 cells, treated with GA (A549: 400 μM; H292: 100 μM), p53 siRNA (60 pM) or GA plus p53 siRNA were detected by RT-PCR at 48 hours. The relative expression levels of miR-34a were determined using densitometry and normalized to U6. Data are representative of three independent experiments. *** $p < 0.001$ (ANOVA); # $p < 0.001$ vs. control. (**C**) The expression levels of p53 and PD-L1 protein in A549 and H292 cells, treated with GA (A549: 400 μM; H292: 100 μM) or 30 pM miR-34a inhibitor, were detected by western blotting at 48 hours. (**D**) The relative expression levels of p53 and PD-L1 protein were determined by densitometry and normalized to β-actin. Data are representative of three independent experiments. *** $p < 0.001$ (ANOVA); # $p < 0.001$ vs. control.

2.6. The Downregulation of PD-L1 Expression by GA Induces the Combination Effect with PD-1 Blockade

To test the combination effect of PD-1 blockade and GA on antitumor activity, we evaluated cytotoxicity in an NSCLC-cell and peripheral blood mononuclear-cell (PBMC) coculture system in the presence of the anti-PD-1 monoclonal antibody (mAb) nivolumab, GA, or both. We observed a considerable apoptotic effect in the presence of both PD-1 mAb and GA in A549 and H292 cells (Figure 6A). Further, GA reduced the viability of cancer cells more effectively in comparison with a single blockade of PD-1 with PD-1 mAb. These results may indicate that the decrease of PD-L1 expression by GA regulates not only reducing survival signals of PD-L1 downstream but also activates the T-cell-mediated immune response. To further investigate the combination effect on PBMC cytokine expression, we performed an IFN-γ analysis by enzyme-linked immunosorbent assay (ELISA). As shown in Figure 6B, GA treatment was observed to slightly increase the IFN-γ level more so than a single blockade of PD-1 with PD-1 mAb. In addition, treatment with both GA and PD-1 mAb considerably enhanced the IFN-γ production in the supernatant of the NSCLC-cell and PBMC coculture system. These results suggest that the decrease in PD-L1 expression brought about by GA enhances the effect observed with PD-1 mAb in the production of IFN-γ. Figure 7 is a graphical abstract which gave the conclusion of all these results. We checked the effect of this combination in a non-cancerous cell (HUVEC cell line) and found that these combination does not induce much cell toxicity in non-cancerous cells (Figure S3).

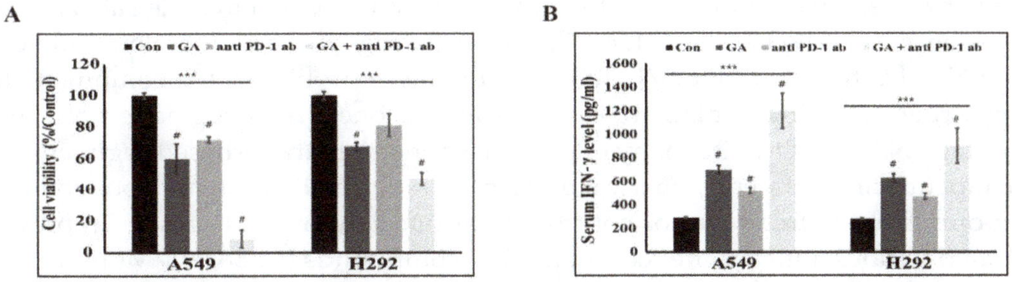

Figure 6. GA enhances the combination effect with anti-PD-1 mAb in an NSCLC-cell and peripheral blood mononuclear-cell (PBMC) coculture system. (**A**) The cell survival rates of NSCLC cells cocultured with PBMCs were examined after treatment with mock, GA (A549: 200 μM; H292: 50 μM), anti-PD-1 mAb (5 μg/mL), or both GA and anti-PD-1 mAb for 48 hours. *** $p < 0.001$ (ANOVA); # $p < 0.001$ vs. control. (**B**) The levels of interferon (IFN)-γ from the supernatants of the coculture system were measured by ELISA also following treatment with mock, GA (A549: 200 μM; H292: 50 μM), anti-PD-1 mAb (5 μg/mL), or both GA and anti-PD-1 mAb for 48 hours. *** $p < 0.001$ (ANOVA); # $p < 0.001$ vs. control.

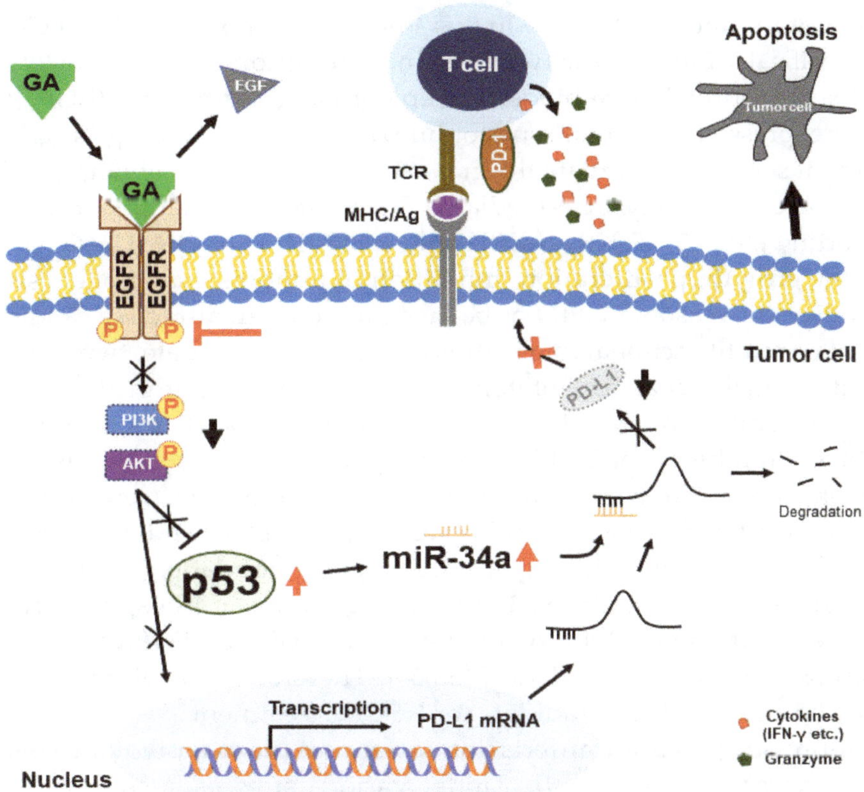

Figure 7. Molecular regulatory mechanism of programmed death-ligand 1 (PD-L1) by natural bioactive gallic acid in NSCLC cells and proposed combination effect for NSCLC immunotherapy.

3. Discussion

An important concept in cancer treatment is that the cancerous cells should ideally be removed without influencing normal cells. Chemotherapy is the most common type of treatment, where chemicals or drugs to destroy cancer cells and cancer microenvironments are applied. Genomic studies such as those on *TP53, BCL2,* and *c-MYC* have accelerated the effective application of chemotherapy for developing anticancer drugs and reagents in cancer treatment [48–50]. Anticancer drugs, according to their mechanisms of action, are generally classified as either alkylating agents for damaging cancer cell DNA, antimetabolites for replacing the normal building blocks of RNA and DNA, or antibiotics for interfering with the enzymes involved in DNA replication [51–53].

Although observed therapeutic issues for NSCLC are still deemed to be unsatisfactory because of multidrug resistance and adverse effects [54,55], chemical drugs such as vinorelbine and cisplatin have been tested in NSCLC treatment [56,57]. To overcome these problems, the combined effects of two chemotherapy drugs including cisplatin or carboplatin plus one other drug have often been deployed to treat early-stage NSCLC. Despite many efforts, these chemotherapy-based regimens seem to have reached a therapeutic limit. Recently, many studies have reported the potential possibility of applying natural compounds in the treatment or control of various cancerous diseases. In previous studies, we demonstrated various anticancer effects of natural compounds [41,58,59]. Moreover, combination treatment using a chemotherapy drug and naturally derived drugs showed more effective anticancer effects, which imply that such might reduce the burden of adverse effects brought on by chemotherapy drugs alone [60]. However, a therapeutic strategy using natural compounds is difficult to apply without knowing the specific targets, which is one of the disadvantages of use. Thus, a targeted study focused on using natural compounds is essential to achieve more effective anticancer treatment. Many studies have investigated a phenolic natural compound, gallic acid, that acts as an anticancer agent against various cancers [16,17,19,20]. Nevertheless, these studies did not identify where the target position of GA is against various cancer cells or did they reveal detailed molecular mechanisms underlying the anticancer effects of GA in cancer cell death. In this study, we demonstrated that GA influences cancer cell viability and specifically binds to the tyrosine kinase receptor, EGFR in NSCLC cell lines.

EGFR is a cell-surface protein that binds with epidermal growth factor (EGF) [61]. EGFR often is mutated and/or overexpressed in several types of human cancers, including lung, ovary, breast, head, and neck cancer, and it serves to modulate the growth, differentiation, signaling, adhesion, migration, and survival of cancer cells. Usually, EGF-mediated EGFR phosphorylation induces three main signal transductions including JAK-STAT, KRAS-ERK, and PI3K-AKT-mTOR. These pathways are known to be involved in the growth, proliferation, inhibition of apoptosis, angiogenesis, and invasion of cancer cells [62,63]. For this reason, EGFR has been regarded as an attractive candidate for anticancer treatment because of its multifunctional role in tumorigenesis [38]. To date, two monoclonal antibodies, cetuximab and panitumumab, capable of inhibiting EGF or growth factor-mediated signaling pathways have been used for cancer therapy [64]. In addition, several TKIs such as erlotinib and gefitinib have been employed for the inhibition of EGFR phosphorylation. In this study, we demonstrated that GA inhibits EGFR phosphorylation by binding to EGFR in two NSCLC cells. Moreover, GA showed binding specificity and inhibited EGFR phosphorylation despite EGF-binding. These results may imply that GA is a selective and potent inhibitor against EGFR phosphorylation. Furthermore, the inhibition of EGFR phosphorylation by GA induced the downregulation of phosphorylated PI3K and AKT. Previous studies revealed that the inhibition of EGFR TKI-mediated EGFR phosphorylation induces the downregulation of phospho-PI3K and AKT [65,66]. Therefore, GA, which showed a similar effect to that of TKIs, may be a useful drug candidate for NSCLC treatment.

The tumor suppressor p53 is a transcription factor and plays a pivotal role in cell-cycle, DNA repair, senescence, and apoptosis [67–69]. Under various stresses such as DNA damage, p53 is phosphorylated and acetylated via posttranslational modification and then it is translocated to the nucleus for trans-activating numerous target genes that direct processes including cell-cycle arrest and/or apoptosis. Mutations of *TP53* have been discovered in more than 50% of human cancers and *p53* mutation leads to not only the loss of cancer suppressive functions but also the acquisition of additional oncogenic functions such as growth and survival [70]. Wild-type p53 proteins (WTp53) are frequently downregulated because of their function of tumor suppression in many cancer cells. Previous studies have identified that the downregulation of WTp53 is associated with EGFR signal-mediated PI3K/AKT pathway activation in cancer cells [65,66,71,72]. As mentioned above, we demonstrated that the downregulation of EGFR phosphorylation by GA leads to the inhibition of PI3K and AKT phosphorylation. The decrease in their phosphorylation by GA induced the upregulation of WTp53 protein and mRNA in A549 and H292 cells. Furthermore, the competitive activity of GA in an EGF-dependent condition suggested that binding of GA to EGFR, may associated with the upregulation of p53 through inhibiting EGFR/PI3K/AKT4 phosphorylation. These results also suggest that natural bioactive GA may have a potential role as a chemotherapeutic drug for NSCLC treatment. Although many studies have revealed that p53 is related to some immune responses including IFN signaling [73,74], the expression of inflammatory cytokines and Toll-like receptors [75–77], and the activation of T- and natural killer cells [78], the correlation of p53 and tumor immune evasion is poorly understood. Recently, some studies reported that p53 interacts with the apoptotic pathway by regulating miRNAs in cancer cells [79,80]. Furthermore, the effect on p53 was augmented in miR-34a expression, which leads to decreased expression levels of PD-L1 in NSCLC cells [33]. Interestingly, we found that bioactive GA decreased the protein and mRNA levels of PD-L1 as compared with the control experiment, and the expression levels of p53 and miR-34a were upregulated by GA in NSCLC cells. These results propose that GA controls the expression of PD-L1 by regulating the p53–miR-34a pathway.

Finally, studies have revealed that PD-L1 expression in cancer cells enhances cell proliferation and resistance toward pro-apoptotic stimuli [29,81]. Furthermore, PD-L1 expression in cancer also enhances PD-L1-mediated tumor immune resistance from cytotoxic cluster of differentiation (CD)8 T-cells through the PD-1/PD-L1 blockade [82]. Thus, inhibition of PD-L1 expression will activate cytotoxic CD8 T-cell responses to various cancers. This approach has been labeled as PD-1/PD-L1 based-immunotherapy. Recently, many clinical approaches and successes are emerging through PD-1/PD-L1 blockade therapy. As mentioned above, we found that GA decreases PD-L1 expression in A549 and H292 cells. In combination experiments with a human monoclonal anti-PD-1 mAb (nivolumab), GA exhibited a more effective effect regarding cancer cell viability. In accordance with the decreased expression levels of PD-L1 by GA, the experimental condition involving anti-PD-1 mAb decreased NSCLC cell viability and oppositely increased the level of IFN-γ in the NSCLC-cell and PBMC coculture system.

4. Materials and Methods

4.1. Cell Lines and Cell Culture

Roswell Park Memorial Institute (RPMI) 1640 media and a penicillin–streptomycin solution was purchased from Gibco (Gaithersburg, MD, USA). Fetal bovine serum (FBS) was purchased from Sigma-Aldrich (St. Louis, MO, USA). Trypsin ethylenediaminetetraacetic acid (0.05%) was obtained from Gibco (Gaithersburg, MD, USA). The human NSCLC cell lines H292 (no. 21848; Korean Cell Line Bank, Seoul, South Korea) and A549 (CCL-185; American Type Culture Collection, Manassas, VA, USA) were cultured in RPMI-1640 supplemented with 10% FBS and antibiotics (1% penicillin–streptomycin) at 37 °C with 5% CO_2. For each experiment, at 70% to 80% confluence, cells were gently washed twice with phosphate-buffered saline. Unless otherwise specified, cells were treated with 100 μM of GA (in H292 cells) or 400 μM of GA (in A549 cells) for 48 hours at 37°C under an atmosphere of 5% CO_2.

4.2. Immunoblotting

Whole-cell lysates were prepared by radioimmunoprecipitation assay buffer (EMD Millipore, Burlington, MA, USA) containing phosphatase and protease inhibitors. Antibodies specific for β-actin (sc-47778), p53 (sc-126) and secondary antibodies (antimouse (sc-516102), and antirabbit (sc-2357) antibody) were obtained from Santa Cruz Biotechnology, Inc. (Dallas, TX, USA). pEGFR (#2234), EGFR (#3776s), pAKT (#4060), AKT (#4691), pPI3K (#4228), and PI3K (#4257) antibodies were purchased from Cell Signaling Technology Inc. (Danvers, MA, USA). PD-L1 (R30949) antibody was purchased from NSJ Bioreagents (San Diego, CA, USA). Recombinant human EGF (AF-100-15) was purchased from PeproTech Inc. (Rocky Hill, NJ, USA).

4.3. Real Time Quantitative PCR (qPCR)

Total RNA was isolated with the RNeasy Mini Kit (Qiagen GmbH, Hilden, Germany) according to the manufacturer's protocol. The extracted RNA was quantified spectrophotometrically at 260 nm, and cDNA was synthesized at 42 °C for 1 h and 95 °C for 5 min with a first-strand cDNA synthesis kit (K-2041; Bioneer Corporation, Daejeon, Korea) and oligo d(T) primers. Real-time qPCR was conducted in a thermal cycler (C1000 Thermal Cycler, Bio-Rad, Hercules, CA) as follows: 2 μL diluted cDNA was added to diluted forward and reverse primers (1 μL each, 100 pM) and 10 μL TB Green Advantage Premix (Takara Bio, Japan) according to the manufacturer's instructions. We used the following primers for EGFR, sense 5′- TGGCAGTGTCTTAGCTGGTTGT -3′ and anti-sense 5′- TGCACTCAGAGAGCTCAGGA -3′, for PD-L1, sense 5′- TGCCAGGCATTGAATCTACA -3′ and anti-sense 5′- GGCCTATTTCCTCCTCTTGG -3′, for p53, sense 5′- AGGCCTTGGAACTCAAGGAT -3′ and anti-sense 5′- CAGTCTGAGTCAGGCCCTTC -3′, and for miR34a analysis: for miR34a, sense 5′- TGGCAGTGTCTTAGCTGGTTGT -3′. The measurement was carried out in triplicate. The relative expression of target genes was normalized to GAPDH or U6 snRNA.

4.4. Transfections of siRNA and miRNA

Lung cancer cells (1×10^5 cells) were seeded in six-well plates and grown to 60% confluence. The cells were then transfected with p53 siRNA (sc-29435; Santa Cruz Biotechnology, Dallas, TX, USA) or miR-34a inhibitor (AM 17000; Thermo Fisher Scientific, Inc., Waltham, MA, USA) using Lipofectamine transfection reagent (Thermo Fisher Scientific, Inc., Waltham, MA, USA). After 48 hours, transfected cells additionally were cultured with/without GA for an additional 48 hours under a cell culture condition.

4.5. NSCLC-Cell and PBMC Co-Culture Experiments

Lung cancer cells (5×10^4 cells) were seeded in 24-well plate until 70% to 80% confluence under a cell culture condition. Human PBMCs were isolated by Ficoll Paque density centrifugation from peripheral blood donated by healthy volunteers using Lymphoprep™ and SepMate™-50 (Stemcell Technologies, Vancouver, Canada). Then, the acquired PBMCs were added into each coculture system at a PBMCs/attached NSCLC cells ratio of 5:1. Some cocultured wells were treated with 5 μg/mL of anti-PD-1 mAb (nivolumab, #A1307; BioVision, Milpitas, CA, USA) and/or GA (A549: 200 μM and H292: 50 μM) and cultured for 48 hours. After 48 hours of co-culture, the culture supernatant was used to analyze the human IFN-γ level, while the viability of attached NSCLC cells was analyzed by MTT assay. The human IFN-γ level in cell-free supernatant was determined using an ELISA kit (#430104; BioLegend, San Diego, CA, USA) according to the manufacturer's protocol.

4.6. Statistical Analyses

All experiments were performed at least three times. Results are expressed as means ± standard errors of the mean. Statistical analyses were conducted using a one-way analysis of variance (ANOVA) or the Student's t-test. The one-way ANOVA was performed with Duncan's multiple-range test as a post-hoc test. Analyses were performed using the SAS 9.3 program (SAS Institute, Inc., Cary, NC, USA). A p-value of less than 0.05 was taken to indicate a statistically significant difference.

5. Conclusions

In summary, our results constitute the first study to disclose the detailed mechanism of PD-L1 downregulation, which could be mediated by bioactive natural GA in NSCLC cells. Moreover, we demonstrated that GA might not only directly inhibit cancer cell survival through the upregulation of tumor suppressor p53 but also indirectly enhance antitumor immunity through the downregulation of PD-L1. Thus, our findings additionally pave the way for further research on bioactive natural compounds to study its efficiency in combinations with immune checkpoint-based therapies and chemotherapeutic agents.

Supplementary Materials:
Figure S1: Effects of GA on A549 and H292 cell viability. (A) MTT-based evaluation of A549 and H292 cell viability in different time- and GA concentration-dependent manners. Data are representative of three independent experiments. *** $p < 0.001$ (t-test). (B) A549 and H292 cell lines were treated with increasing concentration of GA for 48 h and the viability was checked using the crystal violet method. Data are representative of three independent experiments. *** $p < 0.001$ (t-test). Figure S2: Effects of GA on Huvec cell viability. The cell survival rates of Huvec cells were examined after treatment with 400 μM GA, anti-PD-1 mAb (5 μg/mL), or both GA and anti-PD-1 mAb for 48 hours. Figure S3: Effect of GA in Jak2/STAT3 pathway. (A) The expression levels of pSTAT3 and pJAK2 protein in A549 and H292 cells were detected after GA treatment in concentrations indicated for 48 h. Data are representative of three independent experiments. * $p < 0.05$ (t-test). (B) Relative protein levels pJak2 and pSTAT3 were determined by densitometry analysis and normalized to β-actin. Data are representative of three independent experiments.

Author Contributions: K.-J.J. and Y.M.Y. designed the experiments. D.Y.K. and N.S. performed the most of experiments. E.S.J., A.R., and D.Y.H. helped on some of the experiments. K.-J.J., Y.M.Y., D.Y.K., N.S., H.G.L., J.-S.Y., and Q.L. analyzed the data, and K.-J.J. wrote the manuscript. All authors have read and agreed to the published version of the manuscript.

References

1. Reck, M.; Heigener, D.F.; Mok, T.; Soria, J.C.; Rabe, K.F. Management of non-small-cell lung cancer: Recent developments. *Lancet* **2013**, *382*, 709–719. [CrossRef]
2. Bender, E. Epidemiology: The dominant malignancy. *Nature* **2014**, *513*, S2–S3. [CrossRef] [PubMed]
3. Inamura, K. Lung Cancer: Understanding its molecular pathology and the 2015 WHO classification. *Front. Oncol.* **2017**, *7*, 193. [CrossRef] [PubMed]
4. Brambilla, E.; Travis, W.D.; Colby, T.V.; Corrin, B.; Shimosato, Y. The new World Health Organization classification of lung tumours. *Eur. Respir. J.* **2001**, *18*, 1059–1068. [CrossRef]
5. Ettinger, D.S.; Akerley, W.; Borghaei, H.; Chang, A.C.; Cheney, R.T.; Chirieac, L.R.; D'Amico, T.A.; Demmy, T.L.; Govindan, R.; Grannis, F.W.; et al. Non-Small Cell Lung Cancer, Version 2.2013 Featured Updates to the NCCN Guidelines. *J. Natl. Compr. Cancer Netw.* **2013**, *11*, 645–653. [CrossRef]
6. Di, S.Y.; Fan, C.X.; Yang, Y.; Jiang, S.; Liang, M.M.; Wu, G.L.; Wang, B.D.; Xin, Z.L.; Hu, W.; Zhu, Y.F.; et al. Activation of endoplasmic reticulum stress is involved in the activity of icariin against human lung adenocarcinoma cells. *Apoptosis* **2015**, *20*, 1229–1241. [CrossRef]
7. Ma, Z.Q.; Yang, Y.; Fan, C.X.; Han, J.; Wang, D.J.; Di, S.Y.; Hu, W.; Liu, D.; Li, X.F.; Reiter, R.J.; et al. Melatonin as a potential anticarcinogen for non-small-cell lung cancer. *Oncotarget* **2016**, *7*, 46768–46784. [CrossRef]
8. Aung, T.N.; Qu, Z.P.; Kortschak, R.D.; Adelson, D.L. Understanding the Effectiveness of Natural Compound Mixtures in Cancer through Their Molecular Mode of Action. *Int. J. Mol. Sci.* **2017**, *18*, 656. [CrossRef]
9. Shahrzad, S.; Aoyagi, K.; Winter, A.; Koyama, A.; Bitsch, I. Pharmacokinetics of gallic acid and its relative bioavailability from tea in healthy humans. *J. Nutr.* **2001**, *131*, 1207–1210. [CrossRef]
10. Abdelwahed, A.; Bouhlel, I.; Skandrani, I.; Valenti, K.; Kadri, M.; Guiraud, P.; Steiman, R.; Mariotte, A.M.; Ghedira, K.; Laporte, F.; et al. Study of antimutagenic and antioxidant activities of gallic acid and 1,2,3,4,6-pentagalloylglucose from Pistacia lentiscus. Confirmation by microarray expression profiling. *Chem. Biol. Interact.* **2007**, *165*, 1–13. [CrossRef]

11. Velderrain-Rodriguez, G.R.; Torres-Moreno, H.; Villegas-Ochoa, M.A.; Ayala-Zavala, J.F.; Robles-Zepeda, R.E.; Wall-Medrano, A.; Gonzalez-Aguilar, G.A. Gallic Acid Content and an Antioxidant Mechanism Are Responsible for the Antiproliferative Activity of 'Ataulfo' Mango Peel on LS180 Cells. *Molecules* **2018**, *23*, 695. [CrossRef] [PubMed]
12. Kim, S.W.; Han, Y.W.; Lee, S.T.; Jeong, H.J.; Kim, S.H.; Kim, I.H.; Lee, S.O.; Kim, D.G.; Kim, S.Z.; Park, W.H. A superoxide anion generator, pyrogallol, inhibits the growth of HeLa cells via cell cycle arrest and apoptosis. *Mol. Carcinog.* **2008**, *47*, 114–125. [CrossRef] [PubMed]
13. Sorrentino, E.; Succi, M.; Tipaldi, L.; Pannella, G.; Maiuro, L.; Sturchio, M.; Coppola, R.; Tremonte, P. Antimicrobial activity of gallic acid against food-related Pseudomonas strains and its use as biocontrol tool to improve the shelf life of fresh black truffles. *Int. J. Food Microbiol.* **2018**, *266*, 183–189. [CrossRef]
14. Lee, J.H.; Oh, M.; Seok, J.H.; Kim, S.; Lee, D.B.; Bae, G.; Bae, H.I.; Bae, S.Y.; Hong, Y.M.; Kwon, S.O.; et al. Antiviral Effects of Black Raspberry (Rubus coreanus) Seed and Its Gallic Acid against Influenza Virus Infection. *Viruses-Basel* **2016**, *8*, 157. [CrossRef] [PubMed]
15. Dludla, P.V.; Nkambule, B.B.; Jack, B.; Mkandla, Z.; Mutize, T.; Silvestri, S.; Orlando, P.; Tiano, L.; Louw, J.; Mazibuko-Mbeje, S.E. Inflammation and Oxidative Stress in an Obese State and the Protective Effects of Gallic Acid. *Nutrients* **2019**, *11*, 23. [CrossRef] [PubMed]
16. You, B.R.; Moon, H.J.; Han, Y.H.; Park, W.H. Gallic acid inhibits the growth of HeLa cervical cancer cells via apoptosis and/or necrosis. *Food Chem. Toxicol.* **2010**, *48*, 1334–1340. [CrossRef]
17. Subramanian, A.P.; Jaganathan, S.K.; Mandal, M.; Supriyanto, E.; Muhamad, I.I. Gallic acid induced apoptotic events in HCT-15 colon cancer cells. *World J. Gastroentero.* **2016**, *22*, 3952–3961. [CrossRef]
18. Tang, H.M.; Cheung, P.C.K. Gallic Acid Triggers Iron-Dependent Cell Death with Apoptotic, Ferroptotic, and Necroptotic Features. *Toxins* **2019**, *11*, 492. [CrossRef]
19. Phan, A.N.; Hua, T.N.; Kim, M.K.; Vo, V.T.; Choi, J.W.; Kim, H.W.; Rho, J.K.; Kim, K.W.; Jeong, Y. Gallic acid inhibition of Src-Stat3 signaling overcomes acquired resistance to EGF receptor tyrosine kinase inhibitors in advanced non-small cell lung cancer. *Oncotarget* **2016**, *7*, 54702–54713. [CrossRef]
20. Liao, C.C.; Chen, S.C.; Huang, H.P.; Wang, C.J. Gallic acid inhibits bladder cancer cell proliferation and migration via regulating fatty acid synthase (FAS). *J. Food Drug Anal.* **2018**, *26*, 620–627. [CrossRef]
21. Bhattacharya, S.; Muhammad, N.; Steele, R.; Peng, G.; Ray, R.B. Immunomodulatory role of bitter melon extract in inhibition of head and neck squamous cell carcinoma growth. *Oncotarget* **2016**, *7*, 33202–33209. [CrossRef] [PubMed]
22. Raina, K.; Rajamanickam, S.; Deep, G.; Singh, M.; Agarwal, R.; Agarwal, C. Chemopreventive effects of oral gallic acid feeding on tumor growth and progression in TRAMP mice. *Mol. Cancer Ther.* **2008**, *7*, 1258–1267. [CrossRef] [PubMed]
23. Baitsch, L.; Baumgaertner, P.; Devevre, E.; Raghav, S.K.; Legat, A.; Barba, L.; Wieckowski, S.; Bouzourene, H.; Deplancke, B.; Romero, P.; et al. Exhaustion of tumor-specific CD8(+) T cells in metastases from melanoma patients. *J. Clin. Investig.* **2011**, *121*, 2350–2360. [CrossRef] [PubMed]
24. Pauken, K.E.; Wherry, E.J. Overcoming T cell exhaustion in infection and cancer. *Trends Immunol.* **2015**, *36*, 265–276. [CrossRef]
25. Sharma, P.; Allison, J.P. The future of immune checkpoint therapy. *Science* **2015**, *348*, 56–61. [CrossRef]
26. Zou, W.; Wolchok, J.D.; Chen, L. PD-L1 (B7-H1) and PD-1 pathway blockade for cancer therapy: Mechanisms, response biomarkers, and combinations. *Sci. Transl Med.* **2016**, *8*, 328rv4–328rv4. [CrossRef]
27. Havel, J.J.; Chowell, D.; Chan, T.A. The evolving landscape of biomarkers for checkpoint inhibitor immunotherapy. *Nat. Rev. Cancer* **2019**, *19*, 133–150. [CrossRef]
28. Swaika, A.; Hammond, W.A.; Joseph, R.W. Current state of anti-PD-L1 and anti-PD-1 agents in cancer therapy. *Mol. Immunol.* **2015**, *67*, 4–17. [CrossRef]
29. Escors, D.; Gato-Canas, M.; Zuazo, M.; Arasanz, H.; Garcia-Granda, M.J.; Vera, R.; Kochan, G. The intracellular signalosome of PD-L1 in cancer cells. *Signal Transduct. Target. Ther.* **2018**, *3*, 26. [CrossRef]
30. Pascual, M.; Mena-Varas, M.; Robles, E.F.; Garcia-Barchino, M.J.; Panizo, C.; Hervas-Stubbs, S.; Alignani, D.; Sagardoy, A.; Martinez-Ferrandis, J.I.; Bunting, K.L.; et al. PD-1/PD-L1 immune checkpoint and p53 loss facilitate tumor progression in activated B-cell diffuse large B-cell lymphomas. *Blood* **2019**, *133*, 2401–2412. [CrossRef]

31. Cha, Y.J.; Kim, H.R.; Lee, C.Y.; Cho, B.C.; Shim, H.S. Clinicopathological and prognostic significance of programmed cell death ligand-1 expression in lung adenocarcinoma and its relationship with p53 status. *Lung Cancer* **2016**, *97*, 73–80. [CrossRef] [PubMed]
32. Thiem, A.; Hesbacher, S.; Kneitz, H.; di Primio, T.; Heppt, M.V.; Hermanns, H.M.; Goebeler, M.; Meierjohann, S.; Houben, R.; Schrama, D. IFN-gamma-induced PD-L1 expression in melanoma depends on p53 expression. *J. Exp. Clin. Cancer Res.* **2019**, *38*, 397. [CrossRef] [PubMed]
33. Cortez, M.A.; Ivan, C.; Valdecanas, D.; Wang, X.; Peltier, H.J.; Ye, Y.; Araujo, L.; Carbone, D.P.; Shilo, K.; Giri, D.K.; et al. PDL1 Regulation by p53 via miR-34. *J. Natl. Cancer Inst.* **2016**, *108*. [CrossRef] [PubMed]
34. Wang, X.; Cao, X.; Sun, R.; Tang, C.; Tzankov, A.; Zhang, J.; Manyam, G.C.; Xiao, M.; Miao, Y.; Jabbar, K.; et al. Clinical Significance of PTEN Deletion, Mutation, and Loss of PTEN Expression in De Novo Diffuse Large B-Cell Lymphoma. *Neoplasia* **2018**, *20*, 574–593. [CrossRef] [PubMed]
35. Xu, C.; Fillmore, C.M.; Koyama, S.; Wu, H.; Zhao, Y.; Chen, Z.; Herter-Sprie, G.S.; Akbay, E.A.; Tchaicha, J.H.; Altabef, A.; et al. Loss of Lkb1 and Pten leads to lung squamous cell carcinoma with elevated PD-L1 expression. *Cancer cell* **2014**, *25*, 590–604. [CrossRef]
36. Buchakjian, M.R.; Merritt, N.M.; Moose, D.L.; Dupuy, A.J.; Tanas, M.R.; Henry, M.D. A Trp53fl/flPtenfl/fl mouse model of undifferentiated pleomorphic sarcoma mediated by adeno-Cre injection and in vivo bioluminescence imaging. *PLoS ONE* **2017**, *12*, e0183469. [CrossRef]
37. Xu, L.; Zhang, Y.; Tian, K.; Chen, X.; Zhang, R.; Mu, X.; Wu, Y.; Wang, D.; Wang, S.; Liu, F.; et al. Apigenin suppresses PD-L1 expression in melanoma and host dendritic cells to elicit synergistic therapeutic effects. *J. Exp. Clin. Cancer Res.* **2018**, *37*, 261. [CrossRef]
38. Sigismund, S.; Avanzato, D.; Lanzetti, L. Emerging functions of the EGFR in cancer. *Mol. Oncol.* **2018**, *12*, 3–20. [CrossRef]
39. Bell, D.W.; Lynch, T.J.; Haserlat, S.M.; Harris, P.L.; Okimoto, R.A.; Brannigan, B.W.; Sgroi, D.C.; Muir, B.; Riemenschneider, M.J.; Iacona, R.B.; et al. Epidermal growth factor receptor mutations and gene amplification in non-small-cell lung cancer: Molecular analysis of the IDEAL/INTACT gefitinib trials. *J. Clin. Oncol.* **2005**, *23*, 8081–8092. [CrossRef]
40. Erlichman, C.; Hidalgo, M.; Boni, J.P.; Martins, P.; Quinn, S.E.; Zacharchuk, C.; Amorusi, P.; Adjei, A.A.; Rowinsky, E.K. Phase I study of EKB-569, an irreversible inhibitor of the epidermal growth factor receptor, in patients with advanced solid tumors. *J. Clin. Oncol.* **2006**, *24*, 2252–2260. [CrossRef]
41. Sp, N.; Kang, D.Y.; Joung, Y.H.; Park, J.H.; Kim, W.S.; Lee, H.K.; Song, K.D.; Park, Y.M.; Yang, Y.M. Nobiletin Inhibits Angiogenesis by Regulating Src/FAK/STAT3-Mediated Signaling through PXN in ER+ Breast Cancer Cells. *Int. J. Mol. Sci.* **2017**, *18*. [CrossRef] [PubMed]
42. Kang, D.Y.; Sp, N.; Kim, D.H.; Joung, Y.H.; Lee, H.G.; Park, Y.M.; Yang, Y.M. Salidroside inhibits migration, invasion and angiogenesis of MDAMB 231 TNBC cells by regulating EGFR/Jak2/STAT3 signaling via MMP2. *Int. J. Oncol.* **2018**, *53*, 877–885. [PubMed]
43. Chen, J.; Jiang, C.C.; Jin, L.; Zhang, X.D. Regulation of PD-L1: A novel role of pro-survival signalling in cancer. *Ann. Oncol.* **2016**, *27*, 409–416. [CrossRef] [PubMed]
44. Abdelhamed, S.; Ogura, K.; Yokoyama, S.; Saiki, I.; Hayakawa, Y. AKT-STAT3 Pathway as a Downstream Target of EGFR Signaling to Regulate PD-L1 Expression on NSCLC cells. *J. Cancer* **2016**, *7*, 1579–1586. [CrossRef] [PubMed]
45. Ogawara, Y.; Kishishita, S.; Obata, T.; Isazawa, Y.; Suzuki, T.; Tanaka, K.; Masuyama, N.; Gotoh, Y. Akt enhances Mdm2-mediated ubiquitination and degradation of p53. *J. Biol. Chem.* **2002**, *277*, 21843–21850. [CrossRef] [PubMed]
46. Gong, A.Y.; Zhou, R.; Hu, G.; Li, X.; Splinter, P.L.; O'Hara, S.P.; LaRusso, N.F.; Soukup, G.A.; Dong, H.; Chen, X.M. MicroRNA-513 regulates B7-H1 translation and is involved in IFN-gamma-induced B7-H1 expression in cholangiocytes. *J. Immunol.* **2009**, *182*, 1325–1333. [CrossRef]
47. Guo, W.; Tan, W.; Liu, S.; Huang, X.; Lin, J.; Liang, R.; Su, L.; Su, Q.; Wang, C. MiR-570 inhibited the cell proliferation and invasion through directly targeting B7-H1 in hepatocellular carcinoma. *Tumour Biol.* **2015**, *36*, 9049–9057. [CrossRef]
48. Lowe, S.W.; Bodis, S.; Mcclatchey, A.; Remington, L.; Ruley, H.E.; Fisher, D.E.; Housman, D.E.; Jacks, T. P53 Status and the Efficacy of Cancer-Therapy in-Vivo. *Science* **1994**, *266*, 807–810. [CrossRef]
49. Santoro, A.; Vlachou, T.; Luzi, L.; Melloni, G.; Mazzarella, L.; D'Elia, E.; Aobuli, X.; Pasi, C.E.; Reavie, L.; Bonetti, P.; et al. p53 Loss in Breast Cancer Leads to Myc Activation, Increased Cell Plasticity, and Expression of a Mitotic Signature with Prognostic Value. *Cell Rep.* **2019**, *26*, 624. [CrossRef]

50. Chiarugi, V.; Ruggiero, M. Role of three cancer "master genes" p53, bcl2 and c-myc on the apoptotic process. *Tumori* **1996**, *82*, 205–209.
51. Espinosa, E.; Zamora, P.; Feliu, J.; Baron, M.G. Classification of anticancer drugs - a new system based on therapeutic targets. *Cancer Treat. Rev.* **2003**, *29*, 515–523. [CrossRef]
52. Sun, J.C.; Wei, Q.; Zhou, Y.B.; Wang, J.Q.; Liu, Q.; Xu, H. A systematic analysis of FDA-approved anticancer drugs. *BMC Syst. Biol.* **2017**, *11*, 27–43. [CrossRef]
53. Xu, X.L.; Gu, H.; Wang, Y.; Wang, J.; Qin, P. Autoencoder Based Feature Selection Method for Classification of Anticancer Drug Response. *Front Genet.* **2019**, *10*, 233. [CrossRef] [PubMed]
54. Schiller, J.H.; Harrington, D.; Belani, C.P.; Langer, C.; Sandler, A.; Krook, J.; Zhu, J.M.; Johnson, D.H.; Grp, E.C.O. Comparison of four chemotherapy regimens for advanced non-small-cell lung cancer. *New Engl. J. Med.* **2002**, *346*, 92–98. [CrossRef]
55. Hanna, N.; Shepherd, F.A.; Fossella, F.V.; Pereira, J.R.; De Marinis, F.; von Pawel, J.; Gatzemeier, U.; Tsao, T.C.Y.; Pless, M.; Muller, T.; et al. Randomized phase III trial of pemetrexed versus docetaxel in patients with non-small-cell lung cancer previously treated with chemotherapy. *J. Clin. Oncol.* **2004**, *22*, 1589–1597. [CrossRef] [PubMed]
56. Winton, T.; Livingston, R.; Johnson, D.; Rigas, J.; Johnston, M.; Butts, C.; Cormier, Y.; Goss, G.; Inculet, R.; Vallieres, E.; et al. Vinorelbine plus cisplatin vs. observation in resected non-small-cell lung cancer. *New Engl. J. Med.* **2005**, *352*, 2589–2597. [CrossRef]
57. Le Chevalier, T.; Arriagada, R.; Le Pechoux, C.; Grunenwald, D.; Dunant, A.; Pignon, J.P.; Tarayre, M.; Abratt, R.; Arriagada, R.; Bergman, B.; et al. Cisplatin-based adjuvant chemotherapy in patients with completely resected non-small-cell lung cancer. *New Engl. J. Med.* **2004**, *350*, 351–360.
58. Sp, N.; Kang, D.Y.; Kim, D.H.; Park, J.H.; Lee, H.G.; Kim, H.J.; Darvin, P.; Park, Y.M.; Yang, Y.M. Nobiletin Inhibits CD36-Dependent Tumor Angiogenesis, Migration, Invasion, and Sphere Formation Through the Cd36/Stat3/Nf-Kb Signaling Axis. *Nutrients* **2018**, *10*, 772. [CrossRef]
59. Kang, D.Y.; Darvin, P.; Yoo, Y.B.; Joung, Y.H.; Sp, N.; Byun, H.J.; Yang, Y.M. Methylsulfonylmethane inhibits HER2 expression through STAT5b in breast cancer cells. *Int. J. Oncol.* **2016**, *48*, 836–842. [CrossRef]
60. Sp, N.; Darvin, P.; Yoo, Y.B.; Joung, Y.H.; Kang, D.Y.; Kim, D.N.; Hwang, T.S.; Kim, S.Y.; Kim, W.S.; Lee, H.K.; et al. The combination of methylsulfonylmethane and tamoxifen inhibits the Jak2/STAT5b pathway and synergistically inhibits tumor growth and metastasis in ER-positive breast cancer xenografts. *BMC Cancer* **2015**, *15*, 474. [CrossRef]
61. Schlessinger, J. Receptor Tyrosine Kinases: Legacy of the First Two Decades. *Cold Spring Harbor Perspect. Biol.* **2014**, *6*, a008912. [CrossRef] [PubMed]
62. Hynes, N.E.; Lane, H.A. ERBB receptors and cancer: The complexity of targeted inhibitors. *Nat. Rev. Cancer* **2005**, *5*, 341–354. [CrossRef] [PubMed]
63. Yarden, Y.; Sliwkowski, M.X. Untangling the ErbB signalling network. *Nat. Rev. Mol. Cell Biol.* **2001**, *2*, 127–137. [CrossRef] [PubMed]
64. Sforza, V.; Martinelli, E.; Ciardiello, F.; Gambardella, V.; Napolitano, S.; Martini, G.; Della Corte, C.; Cardone, C.; Ferrara, M.L.; Reginelli, A.; et al. Mechanisms of resistance to anti-epidermal growth factor receptor inhibitors in metastatic colorectal cancer. *World J. Gastroenterol.* **2016**, *22*, 6345–6361. [CrossRef] [PubMed]
65. Li, M.; Yang, J.Y.; Zhou, W.L.; Ren, Y.; Wang, X.X.; Chen, H.P.; Zhang, J.Y.; Chen, J.L.; Sun, Y.H.; Cui, L.J.; et al. Activation of an AKT/FOXM1/STMN1 pathway drives resistance to tyrosine kinase inhibitors in lung cancer. *Brit. J. Cancer* **2017**, *117*, 974–983. [CrossRef]
66. Jacobsen, K.; Bertran-Alamillo, J.; Molina, M.A.; Teixido, C.; Karachaliou, N.; Pedersen, M.H.; Castellvi, J.; Garzon, M.; Codony-Servat, C.; Codony-Servat, J.; et al. Convergent Akt activation drives acquired EGFR inhibitor resistance in lung cancer. *Nat. Commun.* **2017**, *8*, 1–14. [CrossRef]
67. Sionov, R.V.; Haupt, Y. The cellular response to p53: The decision between life and death. *Oncogene* **1999**, *18*, 6145–6157. [CrossRef]
68. Burns, T.F.; El-Deiry, W.S. The p53 pathway and apoptosis. *J. Cell Physiol.* **1999**, *181*, 231–239. [CrossRef]
69. Matsuda, K.; Tanikawa, C. The transcriptional landscape of p53 signaling pathway. *Cancer Res.* **2017**, *77*, 109–119.
70. Blandino, G.; Di Agostino, S. New therapeutic strategies to treat human cancers expressing mutant p53 proteins. *J. Exp. Clin. Cancer Res.* **2018**, *37*, 30. [CrossRef]

71. Zheng, L.; Ren, J.Q.; Ll, H.; Kong, Z.L.; Zhu, H.G. Downregulation of wild-type p53 protein by HER-2/neu mediated PI3K pathway activation in human breast cancer cells: Its effect on cell proliferation and implication for therapy. *Cell Res.* **2004**, *14*, 497–506. [CrossRef] [PubMed]
72. Zhang, Y.Z.; Han, C.Y.; Duan, F.G.; Fan, X.X.; Yao, X.J.; Parks, R.J.; Tang, Y.J.; Wang, M.F.; Liu, L.; Tsang, B.K.; et al. p53 sensitizes chemoresistant non-small cell lung cancer via elevation of reactive oxygen species and suppression of EGFR/PI3K/AKT signaling. *Cancer Cell Int.* **2019**, *19*, 188. [CrossRef] [PubMed]
73. Porta, C.; Hadj-Slimane, R.; Nejmeddine, M.; Pampin, M.; Tovey, M.G.; Espert, L.; Alvarez, S.; Chelbi-Alix, M.K. Interferons alpha and gamma induce p53-dependent and p53-independent apoptosis, respectively. *Oncogene* **2005**, *24*, 605–615. [CrossRef] [PubMed]
74. Takaoka, A.; Hayakawa, S.; Yanai, H.; Stoiber, D.; Negishi, H.; Kikuchi, H.; Sasaki, S.; Imai, K.; Shibue, T.; Honda, K.; et al. Integration of interferon-alpha/beta signalling to p53 responses in tumour suppression and antiviral defence. *Nature* **2003**, *424*, 516–523. [CrossRef] [PubMed]
75. Xue, W.; Zender, L.; Miething, C.; Dickins, R.A.; Hernando, E.; Krizhanovsky, V.; Cordon-Cardo, C.; Lowe, S.W. Senescence and tumour clearance is triggered by p53 restoration in murine liver carcinomas. *Nature* **2007**, *445*, 656–660. [CrossRef]
76. Menendez, D.; Shatz, M.; Azzam, K.; Garantziotis, S.; Fessler, M.B.; Resnick, M.A. The Toll-Like Receptor Gene Family Is Integrated into Human DNA Damage and p53 Networks. *PLos Genet.* **2011**, *7*, e1001360. [CrossRef]
77. Shatz, M.; Menendez, D.; Resnick, M.A. The Human TLR Innate Immune Gene Family Is Differentially Influenced by DNA Stress and p53 Status in Cancer Cells. *Cancer Res.* **2012**, *72*, 3948–3957. [CrossRef]
78. Textor, S.; Fiegler, N.; Arnold, A.; Porgador, A.; Hofmann, T.G.; Cerwenka, A. Human NK Cells Are Alerted to Induction of p53 in Cancer Cells by Upregulation of the NKG2D Ligands ULBP1 and ULBP2. *Cancer Res.* **2011**, *71*, 5998–6009. [CrossRef]
79. Quan, X.W.; Li, X.L.; Yin, Z.H.; Ren, Y.W.; Zhou, B.S. p53/miR-30a-5p/SOX4 feedback loop mediates cellular proliferation, apoptosis, and migration of non-small-cell lung cancer. *J. Cell Physiol.* **2019**, *234*, 22884–22895. [CrossRef]
80. Biamonte, F.; Battaglia, A.M.; Zolea, F.; Oliveira, D.M.; Aversa, I.; Santamaria, G.; Giovannone, E.D.; Rocco, G.; Viglietto, G.; Costanzo, F. Ferritin heavy subunit enhances apoptosis of non-small cell lung cancer cells through modulation of miR-125b/p53 axis. *Cell Death Dis.* **2018**, *9*. [CrossRef]
81. Wu, Y.L.; Chen, W.Y.; Xu, Z.P.; Gu, W.Y. PD-L1 Distribution and Perspective for Cancer Immunotherapy-Blockade, Knockdown, or Inhibition. *Front. Immunol.* **2019**, *10*, 2022. [CrossRef] [PubMed]
82. Pardoll, D.M. The blockade of immune checkpoints in cancer immunotherapy. *Nat. Rev. Cancer* **2012**, *12*, 252–264. [CrossRef] [PubMed]

10

Isorhamnetin Induces Cell Cycle Arrest and Apoptosis Via Reactive Oxygen Species-Mediated AMP-Activated Protein Kinase Signaling Pathway Activation in Human Bladder Cancer Cells

Cheol Park [1,†], Hee-Jae Cha [2,†], Eun Ok Choi [3,4], Hyesook Lee [3,4], Hyun Hwang-Bo [3,5], Seon Yeong Ji [3,5], Min Yeong Kim [3,4], So Young Kim [3,4], Su Hyun Hong [3,4], JaeHun Cheong [5], Gi-Young Kim [6], Seok Joong Yun [7], Hye Jin Hwang [8], Wun-Jae Kim [7,*] and Yung Hyun Choi [3,4,*]

1 Department of Molecular Biology, College of Natural Sciences, Dong-eui University, Busan 47340, Korea; parkch@deu.ac.kr

2 Department of Parasitology and Genetics, Kosin University College of Medicine, Busan 49267, Korea; hcha@kosin.ac.kr

3 Anti-Aging Research Center, Dong-eui University, Busan 47227, Korea; nakajo39@naver.com (E.O.C.); 14769@deu.ac.kr (H.L.); hbhyun2003@naver.com (H.H.-B.); 14602@deu.ac.kr (S.Y.J.); ilytoo365@deu.ac.kr (M.Y.K.); 14731@deu.ac.kr (S.Y.K.); hongsh@deu.ac.kr (S.H.H.)

4 Department of Biochemistry, Dong-eui University College of Korean Medicine, Busan 47227, Korea

5 Department of Molecular Biology, Pusan National University, Busan 46241, Korea; molecule85@pusan.ac.kr

6 Department of Marine Life Sciences, School of Marine Biomedical Sciences, Jeju National University, Jeju 63243, Korea; immunkim@jejunu.ac.kr

7 Department of Urology, College of Medicine, Chungbuk National University, Chungbuk 8644, Korea; sjyun@chungbuk.ac.kr

8 Department of Food and Nutrition, College of Nursing, Healthcare Sciences & Human Ecology, Dong-Eui University, Busan 47340, Korea; hhj2001@deu.ac.kr

* Correspondence: wjkim@chungbuk.ac.kr (W.-J.K.); choiyh@deu.ac.kr (Y.H.C.)

† Equally contributed.

Abstract: Isorhamnetin is an O-methylated flavonol that is predominantly found in the fruits and leaves of various plants, which have been used for traditional herbal remedies. Although several previous studies have reported that this flavonol has diverse health-promoting effects, evidence is still lacking for the underlying molecular mechanism of its anti-cancer efficacy. In this study, we examined the anti-proliferative effect of isorhamnetin on human bladder cancer cells and found that isorhamnetin triggered the gap 2/ mitosis (G2/M) phase cell arrest and apoptosis. Our data showed that isorhamnetin decreased the expression of Wee1 and cyclin B1, but increased the expression of cyclin-dependent kinase (Cdk) inhibitor p21$^{WAF1/CIP1}$, and increased p21 was bound to Cdk1. In addition, isorhamnetin-induced apoptosis was associated with the increased expression of the Fas/Fas ligand, reduced ratio of B-cell lymphoma 2 (Bcl-2)/Bcl-2 associated X protein (Bax) expression, cytosolic release of cytochrome *c*, and activation of caspases. Moreover, isorhamnetin inactivated the adenosine 5′-monophosphate-activated protein kinase (AMPK) signaling pathway by diminishing the adenosine triphosphate (ATP) production due to impaired mitochondrial function. Furthermore, isorhamnetin stimulated production of intracellular reactive oxygen species (ROS); however, the interruption of ROS generation using a ROS scavenger led to an escape from isorhamnetin-mediated G2/M arrest and apoptosis. Collectively, this is the first report to show that isorhamnetin inhibited the proliferation of human bladder cancer cells by ROS-dependent arrest of the cell cycle at the G2/M phase and induction of apoptosis. Therefore, our results provide an important basis for the interpretation of the anti-cancer mechanism of isorhamnetin in bladder cancer cells and support the rationale for the need to evaluate more precise molecular mechanisms and in vivo anti-cancer properties.

Keywords: isorhamnetin; G2/M arrest; apoptosis; ROS; AMPK

1. Introduction

Although new therapies for treating cancer patients are being developed, chemotherapy is still the main approach for the treatment of cancer. However, some limitations, such as adverse side effects, drug resistance, and limited efficacy, remain to be solved [1,2]. Therefore, urgent new therapeutic strategies that minimize these limitations and have high therapeutic efficacy are required. In this respect, there is an increasing interest in the importance of compounds derived from natural resources that have been traditionally used for the prevention and treatment of various diseases [3–5]. In particular, numerous naturally occurring agents have been reported to cause cell cycle arrest and induce apoptosis, which are important strategies for the control of proliferation in cancer cells, without inducing toxicity in normal cells [6,7]. These agents have also emerged as an alternative to chemopreventive and chemotherapeutic agents because they can specifically regulate various cellular signaling pathways in cancer cells [8,9].

Isorhamnetin (3′-methoxy-3,4′,5,7-tetrahydroxyflavone) is a flavonol aglycone found in some medicinal plants, such as *Hippophae rhamnoides* L., *Oenanthe javanica*, and *Ginkgo biloba* L., which are used as traditional medicines for the treatment of rheumatism, hemorrhage, cardiovascular disease, and cancer [10,11]. As one of the metabolites of quercetin, isorhamnetin is structurally similar to kaempferol, and is also called 3-O-methyl quercetin [12–14]. Isorhamnetin displays a number of biological properties due to its antioxidant, anti-inflammatory, and metabolic properties [15–19], and is also considered to have potential as an anti-cancer agent based on the results of various cancer cell models. For example, isorhamnetin has been reported to inhibit human leukemia, breast, colon, and cervical cancer cell proliferation through the gap 2/ mitosis (G2/M) phase arrest [20–23], and to induce mitotic block in non-small cell lung carcinoma cells, thus enhancing cisplatin- and carboplatin-induced G2/M arrest [24]. However, isorhamnetin induced S-phase arrest in some cancer cells [25,26], indicating that cell cycle arrest by isorhamnetin is dependent on the type of cancer cell line.

In addition, the anti-cancer effects of isorhamnetin in various cancer cell lines have been shown to involve the death receptor (DR)-dependent extrinsic and/or mitochondria-dependent intrinsic pathways [19,24,27–31], which are representative apoptosis inducing pathways. It was also found that the anti cancer effect of isorhamnetin was accompanied by the disturbance of various cellular signaling pathways [20,25,32]. Furthermore, isorhamnetin showed a strong cytotoxic effect through a reactive oxygen species (ROS)-dependent apoptosis pathway in breast cancer cells [26]. In particular, isorhamnetin was able to induce high cytotoxicity at low doses compared to quercetin in cancer cells, including hepatocellular carcinoma and leukemia cells [33,34]. Although the possibility of the growth inhibitory activity of isorhamnetin in bladder cancer cells has recently been proposed [35], no molecular mechanism has been reported to support its effect. Therefore, in this study, we investigated the anti-cancer efficacy of isorhamnetin in human bladder cancer cells, focusing on the mechanisms associated with the induction of cell cycle arrest and apoptosis.

2. Results

2.1. *Isorhamnetin Inhibited Cell Viability in Bladder Cancer Cells*

To examine the cytotoxic effect of isorhamnetin, four bladder cancer T24 cell lines (T24, 5637, and 2531J) were treated with various concentrations of isorhamnetin, and then the 3-(4,5-dimethyl-2-thiazolyl)-2,5-diphenyltetra-zolium bromide (MTT) assay was conducted. Although there are some differences depending on the cell line, the cell viability was significantly decreased in a concentration-dependent manner in isorhamnetin-treated cells (Figure 1A), without affecting normal cultured human keratinocyte HaCaT cells and Chang liver cells under the same conditions. In addition, the 50% inhibitory concentration (IC_{50}) values of isorhamnetin on T24 and

5637 cells were 127.86 μM and 145.75 μM, respectively. The microscopic examination demonstrated that the phenotypic characteristics of isorhamnetin-treated T24 and 5637 cells showed irregular cell outlines, a decrease of cell density, shrinkage, and an increase of detached cells (Figure 1B, upper panel). In addition, 2531J cells showed similar results from the isorhamnetin treatment.

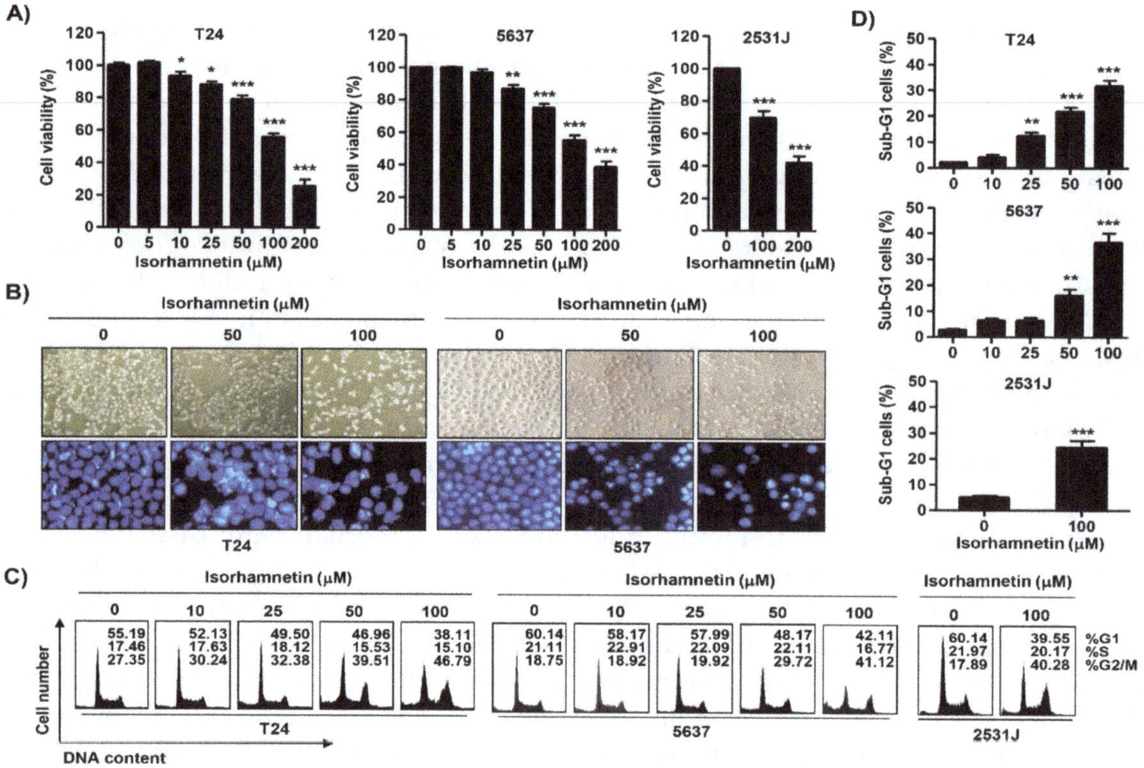

Figure 1. The inhibition of cell viability and induction of cell cycle arrest at gap 2/ mitosis (G2/M) phase using isorhamnetin in bladder cancer cells. T24, 5637, and 2531J cells were treated with the indicated concentrations of isorhamnetin for 48 h. (**A**) The cell viability was assessed using 3-(4,5-dimethyl-2-thiazolyl)-2,5-diphenyltetra-zolium bromide (MTT) assay. Each bar represents the mean ± standard deviation (SD) of three independent experiments (* $p < 0.05$ and *** $p < 0.0001$ compared to the control). (**B**, Upper panel) Morphological changes of T24 and 5637 cells were observed using phase-contrast microscopy. (B, Lower panel) The 4′,6-diamidino-2-phenylindole (DAPI)-stained nuclei were pictured under a fluorescence microscope. Representative photographs of the morphological changes are presented. (**C**,**D**) The cells were stained with propidium iodide (PI) solution for flow cytometry analysis. Quantification of the cell population (in percent) in different cell cycle phases of viable cells is shown. (D) Sub-G 1% was calculated as the percentage of the number of cells in the sub-G1 population relative to the number of total cells. Data were expressed as the mean ± SD of three independent experiments (* $p < 0.05$, ** $p < 0.001$, and *** $p < 0.0001$ compared to the control).

2.2. *Isorhamnetin Induced G2/M Phase Arrest and Apoptosis in Bladder Cancer Cells*

To examine the mechanism responsible for the isorhamnetin-induced anti-proliferative effect, the cell cycle distribution profile was examined. Flow cytometry data demonstrated that the percentage of cells arrested at G2/M phase was increased with increasing isorhamnetin treatment concentration, coupled with a decrease in the proportion of cells in the G1 and S phases (Figure 1C). Meanwhile, a significant increase of the cells in the sub-G1 phase, which was used as an index of apoptotic cells, was observed in isorhamnetin-treated cells (Figure 1D). Therefore, 4′,6-diamidino-2-phenylindole (DAPI) staining was performed to investigate whether apoptosis was involved in cell the growth inhibition induced by isorhamnetin. Figure 1B (lower panel) indicates that morphological changes of the nuclei, which were observed in apoptosis-inducing cells, such as nuclear fragmentation and chromatin condensation, were dominantly found in isorhamnetin-treated T24 and 5637 cells. Since 2531J cells also had the same results, the following experiments were performed on T24 and 5637 cells. To quantify the apoptosis triggered by isorhamnetin, an annexin V-fluorescein isothiocyanate (FITC)/propidium iodide (PI) double staining assay was conducted. As indicated in Figure 2A,B, after treatment with isorhamnetin, the populations of annexin V-staining positive cells were significantly increased, as compared to the control. On the other hand, T24 cells showed slightly increase in necrotic death upon 100 μM of isorhamnetin, but not 5637 cells (Figure 2B). Consistent with this, the results from agarose gel electrophoresis showed that as the isorhamnetin concentration increased and more fragmented DNA was observed (Figure 2C), indicating that an isorhamnetin-induced G2/M phase arrest was associated with the induction of apoptosis.

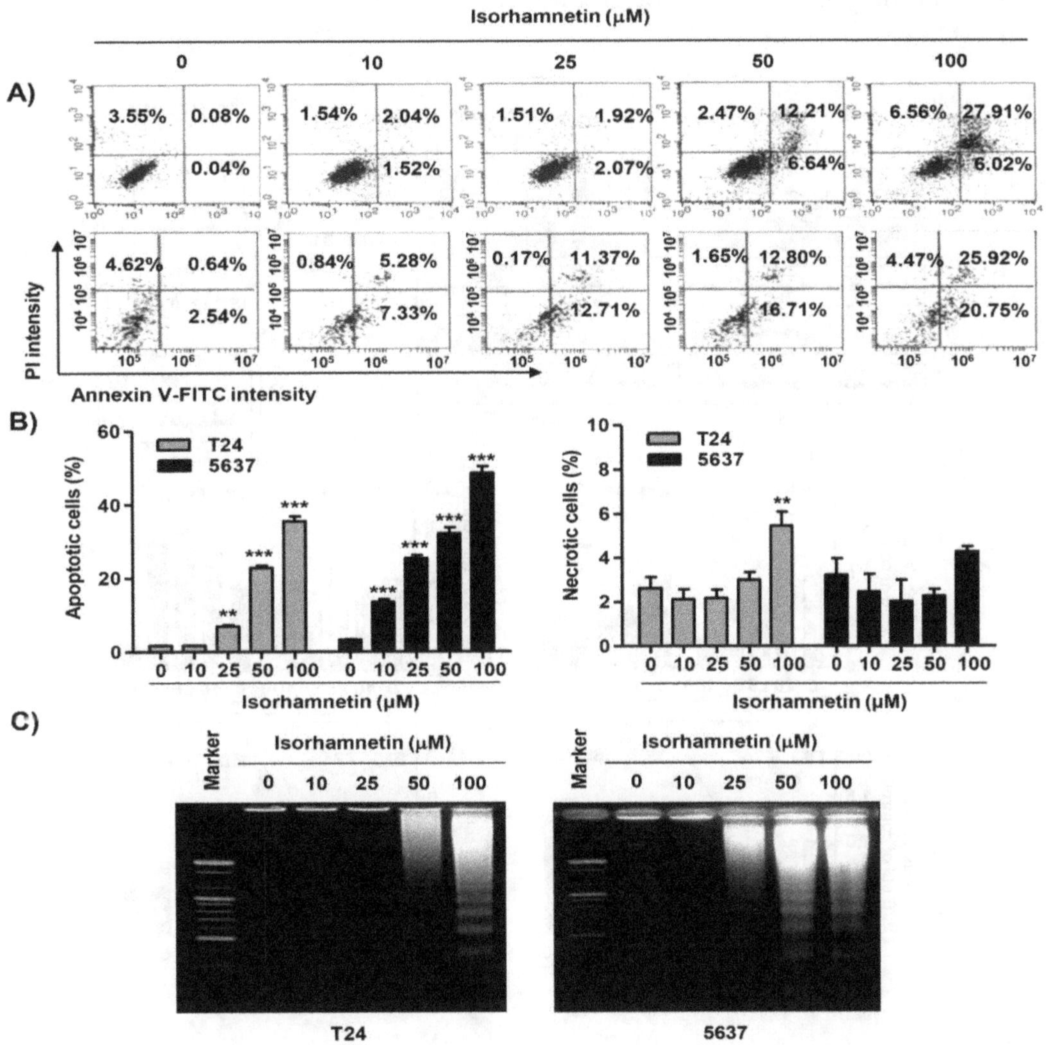

Figure 2. Induction of apoptosis using isorhamnetin in bladder cancer cells. (**A**,**B**) After treatment with different concentrations of isorhamnetin for 48 h, the cells were fixed and stained with annexin V-fluorescein isothiocyanate (FITC) and PI for flow cytometry analysis. (A) Representative profiles. The results show early apoptosis, defined as annexin V^+ and PI^- cells (lower right quadrant), and late apoptosis, defined as annexin V^+ and PI^+ (upper right quadrant) cells. (**B**) The percentages of apoptotic cells (left) and necrotic cells (right) were determined by expressing the numbers of Annexin V^+ cells as percentages of all the present cells. The results are presented as the mean ± SD of three independent experiments (** $p < 0.001$ and *** $p < 0.0001$ compared to the control). (**C**) DNA fragmentation in the cells cultured under the same conditions was analyzed via the extraction of genomic DNA, electrophoresis in agarose gel, and then visualization using ethidium bromide (EtBr) staining.

2.3. *Isorhamnetin Regulated the Expression of G2/M Phase-Associated Proteins in Bladder Cancer Cells*

To explore the biochemical event of the isorhamnetin-elicited cell cycle arrest, the levels of G2/M phase-associated proteins were analyzed. The immunoblotting results revealed that following isorhamnetin treatment, the levels of Wee1 and cyclin B1 were reduced, and the effect was concentration-dependent, while the expression of cyclin-dependent kinase (Cdk) 1 (also called cell division cycle 2, Cdc2) was maintained at the level of the control group (Figure 3A,B). However, the expression of Cdk inhibitor $p21^{WAF1/CIP1}$ was markedly increased in response to isorhamnetin exposure. Next, we performed co-immunoprecipitation to investigate the role of isorhamnetin-induced p21, and found that this increased p21 via treatment with isorhamnetin complexed with Cdk1 (Figure 3C). These results suggest that increased p21 protein in isorhamnetin-treated cells contributed to G2/M phase arrest by inhibiting its activity through binding to Cdk1.

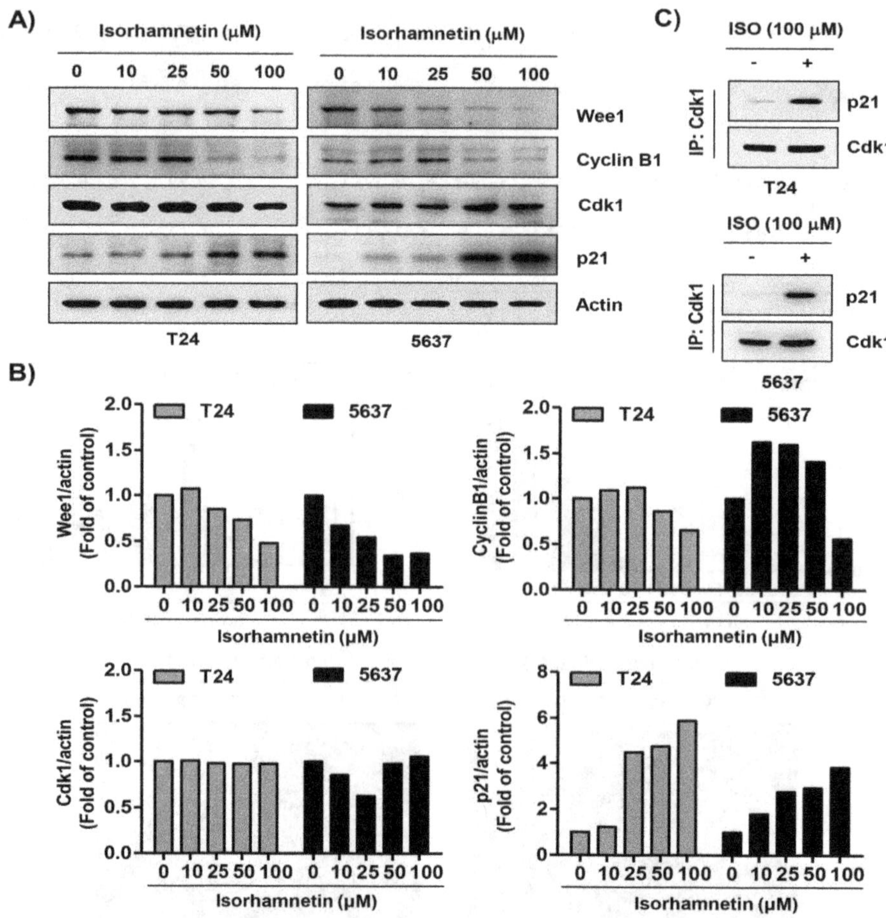

Figure 3. Effects of isorhamnetin on the levels of cell cycle regulatory proteins in bladder cancer cells. (**A**) T24 and 5637 cells were treated with the indicated concentrations of isorhamnetin for 48 h, and then total cell lysates were prepared. Western blotting was then performed using the indicated antibodies and an enhanced chemiluminescence (ECL) detection system. Actin was used as an internal control. (**B**) The expression of each protein was indicated as a fold change relative to the control. Quantitative analysis of mean pixel density was performed using the ImageJ® software. (**C**) Cells were incubated without or with 100 μM isorhamnetin for 48 h, and then equal amounts of proteins were immunoprecipitated with the anti-cyclin-dependent kinase (Cdk) 1 antibody. Western blotting using immunocomplexes was performed using anti-p21 or anti-Cdk1 antibodies and an ECL detection system (IP, immunoprecipitation).

2.4. *Isorhamnetin Modulated the Expression of Apoptosis-Regulatory Proteins in Bladder Cancer Cells*

To investigate the pathway of isorhamnetin-induced apoptosis, caspases activities were determined. Figure 4A,B shows that the protein levels of pro-caspase-8, -9, and -3 were concentration-dependently decreased, which was associated with the degradation of poly(ADP-ribose) polymerase (PARP). Therefore, we quantitatively assessed each caspase activity in the presence of isorhamnetin using fluorogenic substrates to determine whether these immunoblotting results were directly related to activation of the corresponding caspases and found that treatment with isorhamnetin significantly stimulated the activation of these caspases in a concentration-dependent manner in comparison with untreated control cells (Figure 4C). In addition, the effects of isorhamnetin on the expression of the Fas/Fas ligand (FasL) and B-cell lymphoma 2 (Bcl-2) family members were determined. Figure 4A,B shows that both Fas and FasL protein levels were up-regulated, and the level of Bcl-2-associated X protein (Bax), a pro-apoptotic protein, was also increased, while the level of Bcl-2, an anti-apoptotic protein, was reduced in isorhamnetin-treated cells. Furthermore, isorhamnetin promoted the release of cytochrome *c* from mitochondria into cytosol (Figure 4D).

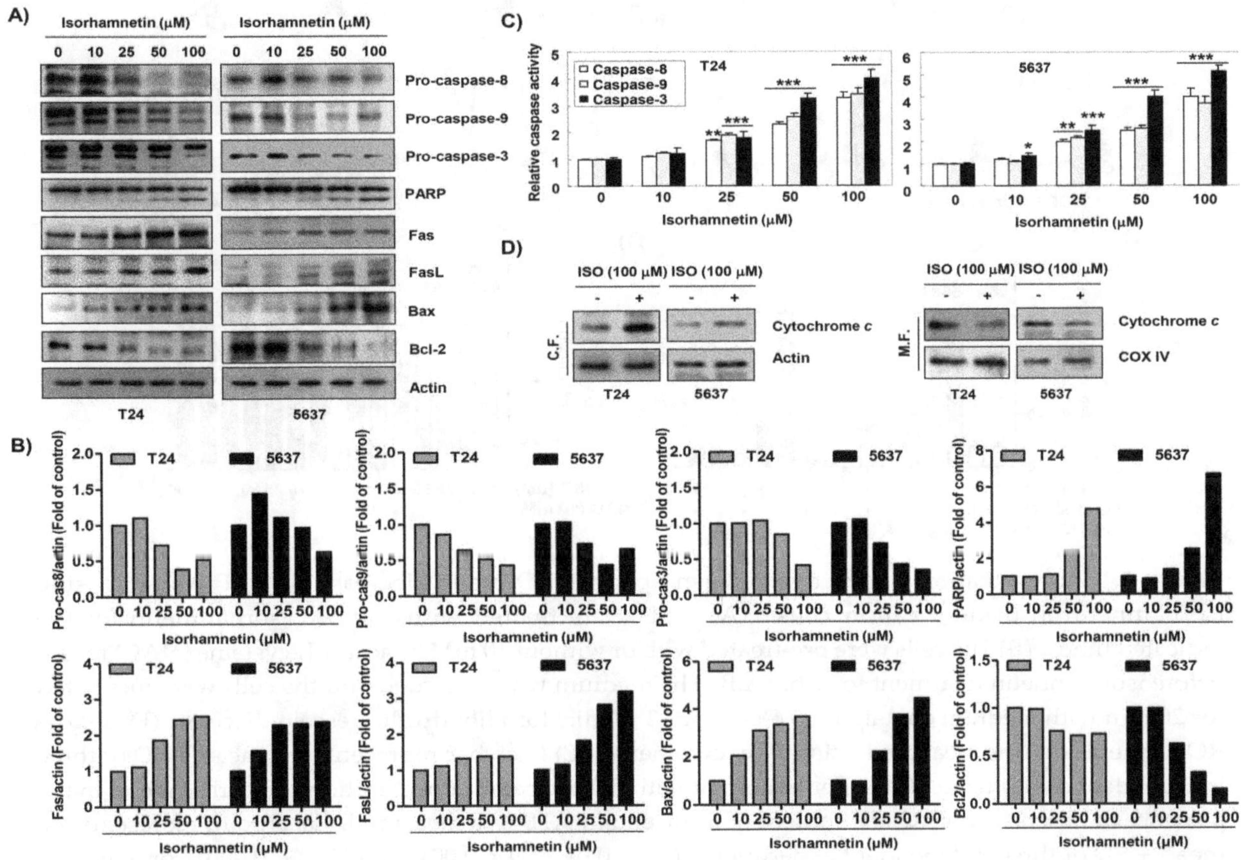

Figure 4. Modulation of apoptosis-regulatory factors using isorhamnetin in bladder cancer cells. (**A**) After treatment with isorhamnetin for 48 h, Western blotting was performed using the indicated antibodies and an ECL detection system. Actin was used as an internal control. (**B**) The expression of each protein was indicated as a fold change relative to the control. Quantitative analysis of mean pixel density was performed using the ImageJ® software. (**C**) The activities of caspases were evaluated using caspase colorimetric assay kits. The data were expressed as the mean ± SD of three independent experiments (* $p < 0.05$, ** $p < 0.001$, and *** $p < 0.0001$ compared to the control). (**D**) After treatment without or with 100 μM isorhamnetin for 48 h, cytosolic and mitochondrial proteins were prepared and analyzed for cytochrome *c* expression using Western blot analysis. Equal protein loading was confirmed via the analysis of actin and cytochrome oxidase subunit VI (COX VI) in each protein extract (C.F.—cytosolic fraction; M.F.—mitochondrial fraction).

2.5. Isorhamnetin Increased ROS Generation but Decreased ATP Content in Cancer Cells

To investigate the involvement of ROS on the cytotoxic effect of isorhamnetin, we performed flow cytometry analysis using a fluorescent probe, 5,6-carboxy-2′,7′-dichlorodihydrofluorescein diacetate (DCF-DA). Our data indicated that the production of ROS showed a significant increase within 1 h of the isorhamnetin treatment, and then gradually decreased, while the antioxidant N-acetyl-L-cysteine (NAC) suppressed it to the control level (Figure 5A–C). In addition, an ATP colorimetric assay kit was used to measure the content of mitochondrial ATP in the cells. Figure 5D shows that the concentration of ATP in the isorhamnetin-treated cells decreased in a concentration-dependent manner. However, under the condition that NAC existed, it was markedly weakened, indicating that the decrease in ATP levels was associated with ROS production.

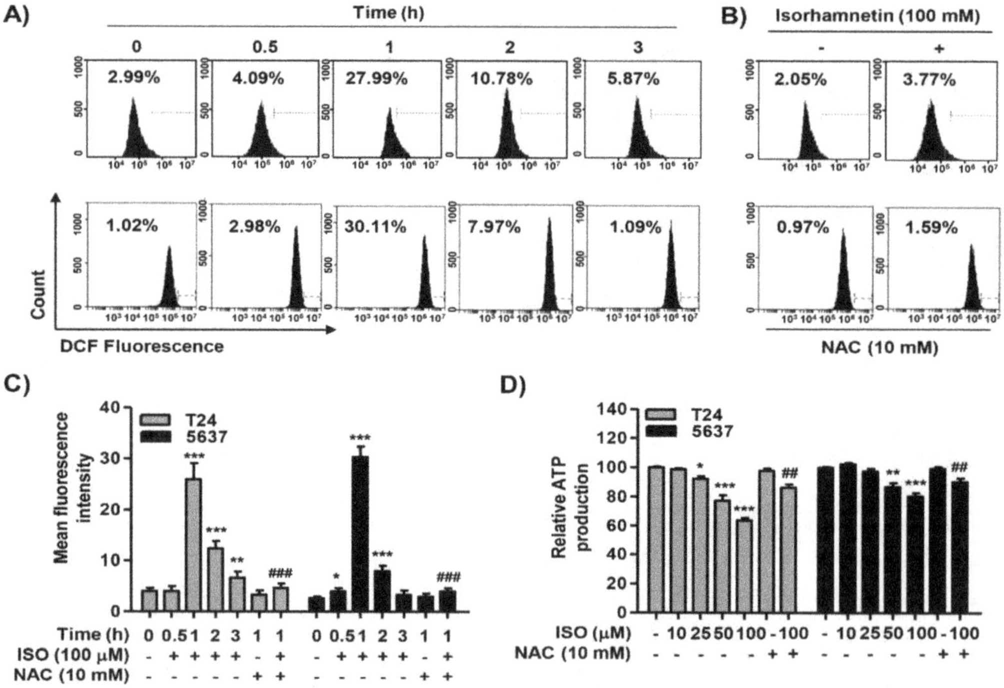

Figure 5. Accumulation of reactive oxygen species (ROS) and decrease of ATP content using isorhamnetin in bladder cancer cells. (**A**) Cells were treated with 100 μM isorhamnetin for the indicated times. (**B**) The cells were pre-treated with or without 10 mM N-acetyl-L-cysteine (NAC) for 1 h before isorhamnetin treatment for 1 h. (A,B) The medium was discarded and the cells were incubated for 20 min with medium containing 5,6-carboxy-2′,7′-dichlorodihydrofluorescein diacetate (DCF-DA). ROS generation was measured using flow cytometry. (**C**) Each bar represents the mean ± SD of three independent experiments. (**D**) After treatment with the indicated concentrations of isorhamnetin in the presence or absence of NAC, the content of intracellular ATP was measured. Each point represents the mean ± SD of three independent experiments (* $p < 0.05$, ** $p < 0.001$, and *** $p < 0.0001$ compared to control; ## $p < 0.001$ and ### $p < 0.0001$ compared to isorhamnetin-treated cells). ISO—isorhamnetin.

2.6. Isorhamnetin Reduced Mitochondrial Membrane Potential (MMP, ΔΨm) and Activated Adenosine 5′-Monophosphate-Activated Protein Kinase (AMPK) Signaling in Bladder Cancer Cells

We assessed the level of MMP to investigate whether the inhibition of ROS-dependent ATP production by isorhamnetin was associated with impaired mitochondrial function. According to the results of flow cytometry using 5,5′,6,6′-tetrachloro-1,1′,3,3′-tetraethylimidacarbocyanine iodide (JC-1) dyes, the formation of JC-1 aggregates in mitochondria was maintained at a relatively high rate in cells not treated with isorhamnetin, while the ratio of JC-1 monomers increased with increasing isorhamnetin treatment concentration, indicating a remarkable depletion of MMP after isorhamnetin treatment (Figure 6A,B). Furthermore, isorhamnetin increased the phosphorylated level of AMPK, as well as its downstream factor acetyl-CoA carboxylase (ACC) (Figure 6C,F), indicating that the AMPK signaling pathway was activated as a result of the loss of ATP. Additionally, we evaluated the effects of isorhamnetin on the phosphorylation of the mechanistic target of rapamycin (mTOR), p70S6K, and Unc-51-like kinase (ULK1), which are AMPK downstream molecules that regulate cell proliferation, apoptosis, and autophagy [36]. Exposure of T24 and 5637 cells with isorhamnetin led to down-regulation in the phosphorylation of mTOR and p76S6K in a dose-dependent manner (Figure 6F,G). Interestingly, we found the isorhamnetin inhibited autophagy via down-regulation of the expression and phosphorylation of ULK1. In addition, our supplementary result showed that the expression of autophagy-related markers was down-regulated using the isorhamnetin treatment, similar to ULK1 (Supplementary Figure S1). However, the presence of NAC or compound C, an antagonist of AMPK, significantly prevented the isorhamnetin-induced loss of MMP (Figure 6A,B), and NAC or compound C also markedly abolished enhanced activation of the AMPK signaling by isorhamnetin (Figure 6E). These data indicate that isorhamnetin-promoted mitochondrial dysfunction associated with the disturbance of ATP production was mediated through an ROS-dependent pathway.

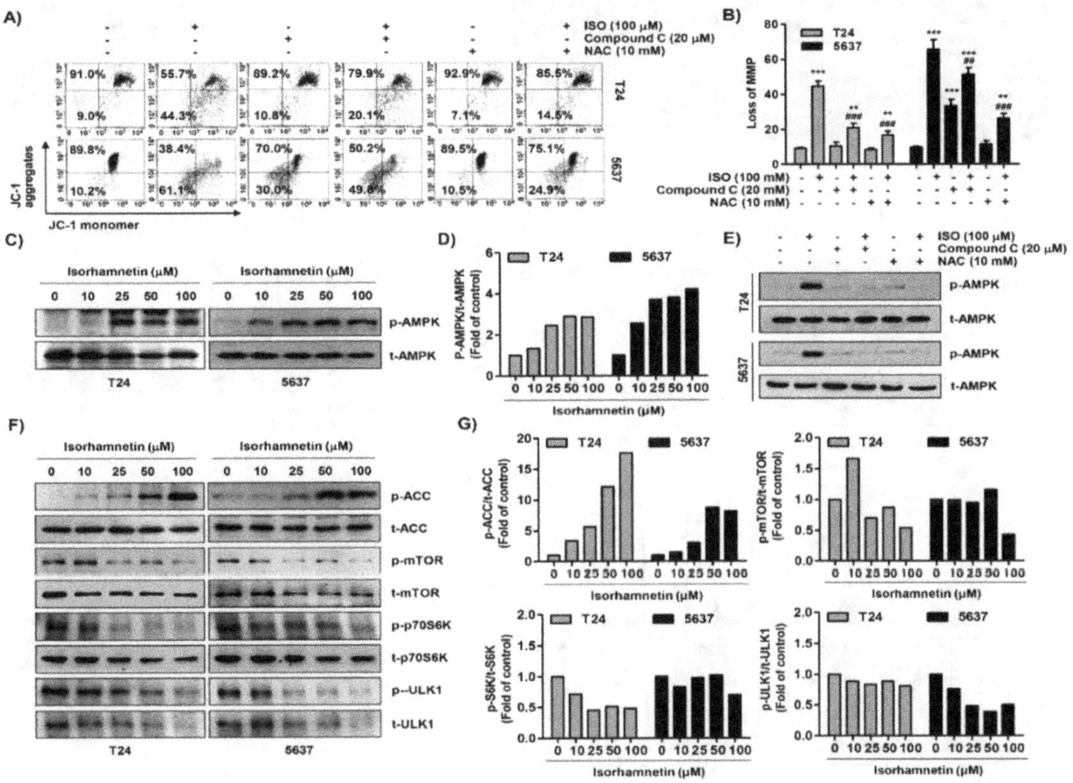

Figure 6. Mitochondrial dysfunction and activation of adenosine 5′-monophosphate-activated protein kinase (AMPK) signaling pathway using isorhamnetin in bladder cancer cells. (**A,B**) Cells were treated with 100 μM isorhamnetin for 48 h, or pre-treated with 20 μM compound C or 10 mM NAC for 1 h before isorhamnetin treatment for 48 h. (A) The cells were stained with 5,5′,6,6′-tetrachloro-1,1′,3,3′-tetraethylimidacarbocyanine iodide (JC-1) dye, and were then analyzed using flow cytometry in order to evaluate the changes in mitochondrial membrane potential (MMP). (**B**) Each bar represents the percentage of cells with JC-1 monomers (mean ± SD of triplicate determinations, ** $p < 0.001$ and *** $p < 0.0001$ compared to the control; ## $p < 0.001$ and ### $p < 0.0001$ compared to the isorhamnetin-treated cells). (**C,F**) After treatment with the indicated concentrations of isorhamnetin for 48 h, total cell lysates were prepared and Western blotting was then performed using the indicated antibodies and an ECL detection system. (**D,G**) The expression of each protein was indicated as a fold change relative to the control. Quantitative analysis of mean pixel density was performed using the ImageJ® software. (**E**) The cells cultured under the same conditions as A and B were collected, and Western blotting was then performed.

2.7. ROS Acted as an Upstream Regulator of Isorhamnetin-Mediated Apoptosis and Cell Cycle Blockade in Bladder Cancer Cells

The effect of ROS on isorhamnetin-mediated apoptosis and G2/M phase arrest was further investigated to determine the role of ROS in the anti-cancer activity of isorhamnetin. As depicted in the results of the DAPI staining and flow cytometry analysis, artificially blocking the production of ROS using NAC drastically attenuated isorhamnetin-induced apoptosis (Figure 7A–C). In parallel, pretreatment with NAC protected isorhamnetin-mediated G2/M arrest, which was related to a decrease in the number of sub-G1 phase cells (Figure 7E). Consistent with these results, inhibiting ROS production greatly restored reduced cell viability using isorhamnetin (Figure 7F), demonstrating that ROS generation was shown to be necessary for the contribution of apoptosis and G2/M arrest using isorhamnetin.

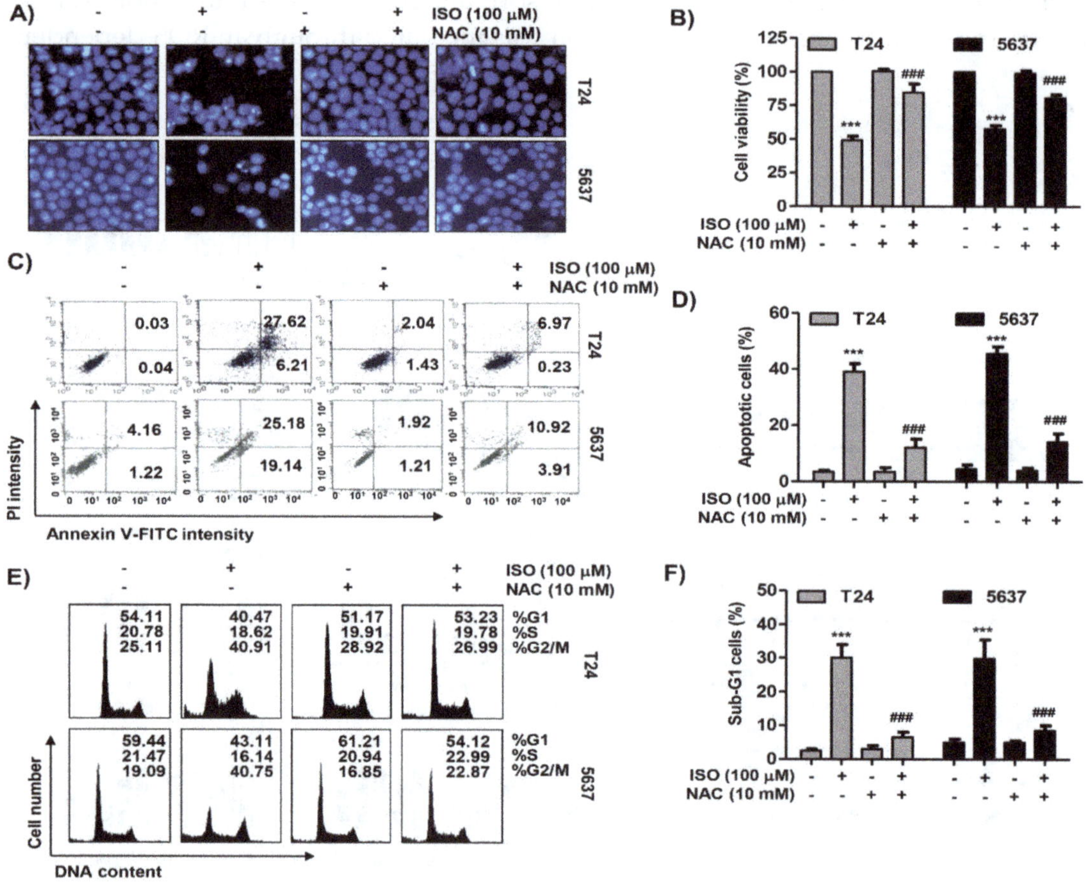

Figure 7. Roles of ROS in isorhamnetin-induced apoptosis and cell cycle arrest in bladder cancer cells. Cells were either treated with 100 µg/mL isorhamnetin for 48 h or pre-treated with 10 mM NAC for 1 h before isorhamnetin treatment, and were then collected. (**A**) The DAPI-stained nuclei were pictured under a fluorescence microscope. (**B,C**) The cells were stained with annexin V-FITC and PI for flow cytometry analysis. (B) Representative profiles. The results show early apoptosis, defined as annexin V^+ and PI^- cells (lower right quadrant), and late apoptosis, defined as annexin V^+ and PI^+ (upper right quadrant) cells. (C) The percentages of apoptotic cells were determined by expressing the numbers of Annexin V^+ cells as percentages of all the present cells. (**D**) The cells were stained with PI solution for flow cytometry analysis. Quantification of the cell population (in percent) in different cell cycle phases of viable cells is shown. (**E**) The percentages of apoptotic sub-G1 were calculated as the percentage of the number of cells in the sub-G1 population relative to the number of total cells. (**F**) The cell viability was assessed using an MTT assay. Each bar represents the mean ± SD of three independent experiments (*** $p < 0.0001$ compared to the control; $^{\#\#\#}$ $p < 0.0001$ compared to the isorhamnetin-treated cells).

3. Discussion

In many previous studies, it is clear that the induction of apoptosis by many anti-cancer agents is associated with cell cycle arrest at specific checkpoints [6,37]. In particular, the deregulation of cell cycle control is clearly implicated in the development and progression of most tumors, and the interruption of this progression is considered to be an important strategy to inhibit the proliferation of cancer cells [6,37]. Therefore, we first investigated whether the suppression of bladder cancer cell proliferation by isorhamnetin was associated with cell cycle arrest. The results of flow cytometry analysis showed that isorhamnetin caused G2/M phase arrest, similar to the results of previous studies in several human cancer cell lines [20–23], suggesting that G2/M phase arrest is one of the mechanisms of the growth inhibitory effects of isorhamnetin in human bladder cancer cells. The progression of the cell cycle in eukaryotic cells is tightly controlled by the interaction of cyclins and Cdks with their inhibitory factors [38,39]. In this process, the transition from G2 to M phase is achieved through the increased activity of Cdk1 by cyclin B1 complexing with Cdk1. In addition, Wee1 is a tyrosine kinase that induces phosphorylation of Cdk1, resulting in inhibition of cyclin B-Cdk1 activity and preventing cell mitotic entry [40,41]. In the current study, exposure of bladder cancer cells to isorhamnetin markedly reduced the expression of cyclin B1 and Wee1, without significant changes in the expression of Cdk1.

p21, a typical Cdk inhibitor belonging to the kinase inhibitory protein/ CDK interacting protein (KIP/CIP) family, has a broad-spectrum of specificity in the cell cycle proteins [38,39]. p21 was first reported to be a major inducer of tumor suppressor p53-dependent cell cycle arrest induced by DNA damage, but it could act as a mediator of p53-independent cell arrest in various types of cancer cells [42,43]. As a Cdk inhibitor, when p21 expression increases, it forms complexes with Cdks, reducing their kinase activity and inhibiting cell cycle progression [42,44]. According to our data, isorhamnetin dramatically increased p21 levels with increasing treatment concentration, and increased p21 complexed with Cdk1, which might have contributed to the inhibition of Cdk1 kinase activity. In addition, since T24 and 5637 cells are mutant p53 gene-bearing cell lines [45], increased p21 expression using isorhamnetin was thought to contribute to G2/M arrest, regardless of p53 gene status. Collectively, our data suggest that isorhamnetin-triggered G2/M arrest was due to the decreased expression of Wee1 and cyclin B1, and inactivation of p53-independent p21-mediated Cdk1 kinase.

Because the induction of apoptosis in cancer cells along with cell cycle arrest is a promising approach to cancer therapy, we assessed whether G2/M arrest using isorhamnetin was associated with apoptosis induction. Based on the results of morphological changes, DNA fragmentation, and flow cytometry analysis, we found that the cytotoxic effect of isorhamnetin was achieved through the induction of apoptosis associated with G2/M arrest. As is well known, apoptosis can be largely categorized into extrinsic and intrinsic pathways in mammalian cells [37,46]. The extrinsic pathway is characterized by the activation of caspase-8 by the formation of the death-inducing signal complex through the binding of death ligands to the cell surface DRs. For example, when FasL, one of the typical death ligands, binds to the corresponding DR, Fas, caspase-8 is sequentially activated [46,47]. On the other hand, the intrinsic pathway begins via the activation of caspase-9 through the release of mitochondrial pro-apoptotic proteins, such as cytochrome *c*, from mitochondria to cytoplasm due to increased mitochondrial permeability. This pathway is tightly regulated by the Bcl-2 protein family that includes pro- and anti-apoptotic proteins, which guard mitochondrial integrity and control the release of cytochrome *c* through the mitochondrial transition pore [48,49]. Caspases-8 and -9, which correspond to the initiator caspases of each pathway, ultimately activate apoptosis through the cleavage of various cellular substrates, such as PARP, by activating downstream executioner caspases, including caspase-3 and -7 [37,50]. In addition, these pathways are strictly controlled by a variety of cellular signaling pathways and regulatory molecules [50,51]. Our results show that isorhamnetin increased the expression of Fas and FasL; activated caspase-8, -9, and -3; and induced the cleavage of PARP. In addition, consistent with previous studies in non-small cell lung cancer cells and Lewis lung cancer cells [31,52], mitochondrial dysfunction was induced, as confirmed by the loss of MMP in isorhamnetin-treated cells. Moreover, the loss of MMP was accompanied by a down-regulation in the Bcl-2/Bax ratio and the promotion of cytosolic release of cytochrome *c*. Therefore, based on those observations, we speculated that the pro-apoptotic effect of isorhamnetin in bladder cancer cells could occur by simultaneously activating extrinsic and intrinsic pathways.

Growing evidence demonstrates that many anti-cancer agents induce apoptosis through pro-oxidant properties, such as increasing ROS accumulation or destroying cellular antioxidant systems [8,53]. In particular, mitochondria are the major subcellular organelles responsible for the production of ROS in the cells and are also a major target of ROS [54,55]. Therefore, elevating intracellular levels of ROS production is considered to be one of the ideal mechanisms for killing cancer cells through the activation of intrinsic pathways. Intriguingly, in various cell types, ROS are involved in activating the signaling system of AMPK, a key sensor that regulates energy balance and cell fate [56–58]. Mitochondrial dysfunction, due to excessive production of ROS, leads to a loss of function of the respiratory chain in the mitochondrial inner membrane, which can lower intracellular ATP levels and activate AMPK [56,57]. Choi et al. first reported that ROS induces concentration-dependent activation of AMPK [59]. More recently, it has been described that AMPK can be activated by ROS, thereby leading to an increase of glycolysis [60,61]. Furthermore, Corton et al. reported that hypoxic activation of AMPK was dependent on the levels of the mitochondrial ROS [62], and Tavazzi et al. demonstrated that AMPK activation was caused by ROS-mediated intracellular ATP depletion [63]. On the contrary, it has been reported that treatment of the potent ROS scavengers, including NAC and dimethyl sulfoxide (DMSO), significantly abolished oxidative stress-induced AMPK activation and ATP depletion [60,61,64]. Consistent with a previous study in breast cancer cells [22], our results show that isorhamnetin treatment markedly increased the levels of ROS production; however, the ROS scavenger, NAC, greatly weakened the accumulation of ROS by isorhamnetin. The quenching of ROS generation also significantly diminished the isorhamnetin-induced disruption of MMP to the control level, followed by significant ATP restoration, indicating that ROS act as upstream signaling molecules to enhance isorhamnetin-mediated mitochondrial dysfunction. Our results also demonstrate that the activation of the AMPK signaling pathway was increased in cells exposed to isorhamnetin, probably due to decreased ATP content. Furthermore, the presence of NAC markedly attenuated isorhamnetin-induced phosphorylation of AMPK, while their total protein levels were kept at an equivalent level, suggesting that the isorhamnetin-induced activation of AMPK signaling pathway is dependent on ROS production. Subsequently, NAC pretreatment also significantly reversed the enhanced apoptosis, G2/M phase arrest, and viability reduction induced by isorhamnetin, confirming that increasing ROS may serve as a key contributor to the anti-cancer effects of isorhamnetin. The AMPK acts as a metabolic mater switch that controls cell fate, such as cell survival, apoptosis, and autophagy [65]. Indeed, fatty acid synthesis is a critical energy-consuming process for the differentiation of tumor cells, and it has been demonstrated that AMPK inhibits lipid synthesis by the phosphorylation and inactivation of acetyl-CoA carboxylase 1 (ACC1) [65]. Furthermore, AMPK directly inhibits mTOR complex I, which regulates p70S6K, an enhancer of protein synthesis. In this sense, AMPK plays a critical role as a cell growth suppressor by inhibiting protein, rRNA, and lipid synthesis [65,66]. In the present study, we conjecture that the AMPK-mediated interruption of the mTOR/p70S6K/ACC1 signaling pathway may contribute to isorhamnetin-induced cell cycle arrest and apoptosis. On the other hand, there are conflicting opinions on the relationship between AMPK and autophagy. Although increasing evidence described that AMPK activation can induce the autophagy through the inhibition of mTOR and phosphorylation of ULK1 [67,68], a few studies reported that ROS attenuated autophagy by the down-regulation of ULK-1 [69,70]. Interestingly, based on our results, we found the isorhamnetin inhibited autophagy by down-regulation of the expression and phosphorylation of ULK1. Therefore, our data suggested that isorhamnetin-induced ROS activates AMPK, and subsequently down-regulates the mTOR/ACC1/ULK1 signaling pathway, which results in promoting cell apoptosis and inhibits autophagy at the same time.

The current results lead us to suggest that the production of ROS by isorhamnetin plays a critical role in the induction of G2/M arrest and apoptosis through simultaneous initiation of both extrinsic and intrinsic pathways in human bladder cancer cells. In addition, ROS act as an upstream signal related to the effect of isorhamnetin on the activation of the AMPK signaling pathway. However, further studies are warranted to identify the molecular mechanisms of isorhamnetin-mediated activation of AMPK signaling on autophagy and mitochondrial energy metabolism in bladder cancer cells. In addition, further studies are required to identify and understand the role of intracellular organelles involved in ROS generation by isorhamnetin, including in vivo animal experiments.

4. Materials and Methods

4.1. Cell Culture and Isorhamnetin Treatment

The human bladder cancer cell lines (T24, 5637, 2531J, and EJ) were purchased from the American Type Culture Collection (Manassas, MD, USA). The cells were cultured in Dulbecco's modified Eagle's medium supplemented with 10% fetal bovine serum and 1% penicillin-streptomycin (100 U/mL penicillin and 100 μg/mL streptomycin, all from WelGENE Inc., Daegu, Republic of Korea) at 37 °C under a humidified 5% CO_2. The cells were sub-cultured every 3–4 days to maintain logarithmic growth, and were allowed to grow for 24 h before treatments were applied. Isorhamnetin was obtained from Sigma-Aldrich Chemical Co. (St. Louis, MO, USA), and was dissolved in dimethyl sulfoxide (DMSO, Sigma-Aldrich Chemical Co.) to a final concentration of 100 M. Prior to use, the stock solution was diluted with culture medium to the desired concentration.

4.2. Cell Viability Assay

Cell viability was determined using an MTT assay, as previously described [71]. Briefly, cells (1×10^4 cells/well) were seeded onto 96-well plates in 100 μL medium. After overnight incubation, the cells were exposed to a series of concentrations of isorhamnetin for 48 h. Thereafter, the MTT reagent (Sigma-Aldrich Chemical Co.) at 50 μg/mL final concentration was added to each well and cells were incubated continuously at 37 °C for 2 h. The medium was then removed and 100 μL DMSO was added to each well to dissolve the formed blue formazan crystals, followed by measurement at 540 nm in a microplate reader (Molecular Device Co., Sunnyvale, CA, USA). All results were performed in three independent experiments and the cell survival rate was expressed as a percentage of the control. The morphological changes of cells were directly observed and photographed using phase-contrast microscopy (Carl Zeiss, Oberkochen, Germany).

4.3. Determination of Cell Cycle Distribution Using Flow Cytometric Analysis

PI staining was applied to analyze the DNA content and cell cycle distribution. In brief, cells were exposed to different concentrations of isorhamnetin for 48 h, and then the cells were harvested and fixed gently in 70% ice-cold ethanol (in phosphate-buffered saline, PBS, WelGENE Inc., Daegu, Korea) at 4 °C for 30 min. The cells were re-suspended in PBS containing 40 μg/mL PI, 100 μg/mL RNase A, and 0.1% triton X-100 (all from Sigma-Aldrich Chemical Co.) in a dark room at 37 °C for 30 min, and subjected to flow cytometry (BD Biosciences, San Jose, CA, USA), to determine the cell cycle distribution and apoptotic cells (sub-G1 phase).

4.4. Determination of Apoptotic Cell Death by Flow Cytometric Analysis

The Annexin V-FITC staining kit from BD Biosciences (San Jose, CA, USA) was used to determine and quantify the apoptotic cells using flow cytometry, according to the manufacturer's instruction. In brief, the collected cells were suspended in the supplied binding buffer, and then stained with FITC-conjugated annexin V and PI at room temperature (RT) for 20 min in the dark. The fluorescent intensities of the cells were detected using flow cytometry, and the annexin V^+/PI^- and annexin V^+/PI^+ cell populations were considered indicators of apoptotic cells.

4.5. Nuclear Staining and Deoxyribonucleic Acid (DAN) Fragmentation Assay

The changes of nuclear morphology for assessing apoptosis were assessed using DAPI staining. Briefly, cells were cultured with or without different concentrations of isorhamnetin for 48 h, and were then fixed with 4% paraformaldehyde (Sigma-Aldrich Chemical Co.) for 10 min at RT. The cells were rinsed with PBS, and incubated with 1 μg/mL DAPI solution (Sigma-Aldrich Chemical Co.) at 37 °C for 10 min. Stained cells were visualized and photographed using fluorescence microscopy (Carl Zeiss, Oberkochen, Germany). For DNA fragmentation assay, the collected cells were lysed in a buffer containing 10 mM Tris-HCl (pH 7.4), 150 mM NaCl, 5 mM ethylenediaminetetraacetic acid, and 0.5% Triton X-100 for 30 min. The fragmented DNA in the supernatant was extracted using an equal volume of neutral phenol:chloroform:isoamyl alcohol (25:24:1, Sigma-Aldrich Chemical Co.), analyzed electrophoretically on 1% agarose gel containing EtBr (Sigma-Aldrich Chemical Co.), and photographed under a Fusion FX Image system (Vilber Lourmat, Torcy, France).

4.6. Protein Extraction, Co-Immunoprecipitation, and Western Blot Analysis

After treatment, both adherent and floating cells were harvested, and the whole cellular proteins were prepared using the Bradford protein assay kit (Bio-Rad Laboratories, Hercules, CA, USA), according to the manufacturer's protocol. For the preparation of mitochondrial and cytosolic proteins from the cells, NE-PER nuclear and cytoplasmic extraction reagents (Thermo Fisher Scientific Inc., Waltham, UT, USA) were applied. Protein concentration was measured using the Bio-Rad protein assay kit (Bio-Rad Laboratories, Hercules, CA, USA), according to the manufacturer's instructions. For the co-immunoprecipitation assay, the 500 μg of cell lysates from each sample was precleaned with normal rabbit immunoglobulin G (IgG) and a protein-A-sepharose bead slurry (Amersham, Arlington Heights, IL, USA), and immunoprecipitation was conducted using 1 μg of anti-Cdk1 antibody (Santa Cruz Biotechnology, Inc., Santa Cruz, CA, USA) and protein-A-sepharose (Sigma-Aldrich Chemical Co.). The protein complex was then prepared according to the previously described method [62]. For Western blot analysis, equal amounts of protein samples or immunoprecipitated proteins were separated using sodium dodecyl sulphate-polyacrylamide gel electrophoresis and transferred to polyvinylidene difluoride membranes (Millipore, Bedford, MA, USA) (whole blot figures can be found at the Supplementary). The membranes were blocked with Tris-buffered saline (10 mM Tris-Cl, pH 7.4) containing 0.5% Tween-20 and 5% nonfat dry milk for 1 h at RT, and then probed with the indicated primary antibodies (Santa Cruz Biotechnology, Inc., and Cell Signaling Technology, Danvers, MA, USA), to react with the blotted membranes at 4 °C overnight. Afterwards, the membranes were incubated with the corresponding horseradish peroxidase-conjugated secondary antibodies (Santa Cruz Biotechnology, Inc.), developed using an ECL detection kit (GE Healthcare Life Sciences, Little Chalfont, U.K.), and then visualized using a Fusion FX Image system. Densitometric analysis of the data was performed using the ImageJ® software (v1.48, NIH, Bethesda, MD, USA).

4.7. Caspase Activity Assay

The activity of caspases was measured according to the manufacturer's instructions for the Caspase colorimetric assay kits (R&D Systems, Minneapolis, MN, USA). Briefly, cells were harvested and lysed in the lysis buffer provided in the kit on ice for 10 min, and then centrifuged at 10,000× *g* for 1 min. The supernatants containing equal proteins were incubated with the supplied reaction mixtures, including the fluorogenic peptide substrate (Asp-Glu-Val-Asp specific for caspase-3, Ile-Glu-Thr-Asp for caspase-8, and Leu-Glu-His-Asp specific for caspase-9) labeled with p-nitroaniline (pNA) for 1 h at 37 °C in the dark. The amounts of released pNA was measured using a microplate reader using excitement at 405 nm and emitting at 510 nm.

4.8. Measurement of ROS Production and MMP

The production of ROS was measured using DCF-DA, as described previously [72]. At the end of the treatment with isorhamnetin for defined periods in the presence or absence of NAC (Sigma-Aldrich Chemical Co.), cells were washed with PBS and incubated with 10 μM DCF-DA (Invitrogen, Carlsbad, CA, USA) in the dark at 37 °C for 20 min. Subsequently, cells were analyzed for DCF fluorescence using flow cytometry at 480 nm/520 nm. To measure MMP, JC-1 staining was performed according to the manufacturer's instructions. After treatment with isorhamnetin for 48 h in the presence or absence of NAC or compound C, cells were exposed to 10 μM JC-1 (Invitrogen) for 30 min at 37 °C, and then analyzed using flow cytometry at 488 nm/575 nm, as previously described [73].

4.9. Detection of ATP Levels

The firefly luciferase-based ATP Bioluminescence assay kit (Roche Applied Science, Indianapolis, IN, USA) was used for the detection of intracellular ATP levels, according to the manufacturer's instructions. Briefly, cells treated with isorhamnetin for 48 h with or without NAC were lysed with the lysis buffer provided in the kit, and the supernatants were collected via centrifugation at 12,000× *g* for 10 min at 4 °C. Subsequently, an equal amount of supernatants and ATP detection reagent, which catalyzed the light production from ATP and luciferin, were mixed. Firefly luciferase activity was immediately measured using a luminometer and the ATP level was calculated according to the ATP standard curve. Intracellular ATP levels were calculated as a percentage of the untreated control.

4.10. Statistical Analysis

All experiments were performed at least three times. Data were analyzed using GraphPad Prism software (version 5.03; GraphPad Software, Inc., La Jolla, CA, USA), and expressed as the mean ± standard deviation (SD). Differences between groups were assessed using analysis of variance, followed by ANOVA-Tukey's post hoc test, and $p < 0.05$ was considered to indicate a statistically significant difference.

5. Conclusions

Our findings demonstrate that isorhamnetin exerted an anti-proliferative effect on human bladder cancer cells through the induction of cell cycle arrest during the G2/M phase and apoptosis. Isorhamnetin-induced G2/M arrest was attributed to the decrease in Wee1 and cyclin B1 expression and the upregulation of p21. Isorhamnetin also induced apoptosis by activating caspase-8 and -9, which belong to the initiator caspases of the extrinsic and intrinsic pathways, respectively, followed by the activation of effector caspase-3, leading to the degradation of PARP. In addition, isorhamnetin enhanced the mitochondrial dysfunction, which was associated with an increase in Bax/Bcl-2 expression ratio and cytochrome *c* release into the cytoplasm. Moreover, the induction of G2/M arrest and apoptosis by isorhamnetin was accompanied by activation of the AMPK signaling pathway, and excessive production of ROS. However, artificial interception of the AMPK signaling pathway attenuated isorhamnetin-induced apoptosis, and the interruption of ROS generation led cells to escape from G2/M arrest and apoptosis. Based on these finding, we suggest that isorhamnetin has chemopreventive potential by inducing G2/M arrest and apoptosis through ROS-dependent activation of the AMPK signaling pathway in bladder cancer cells.

Author Contributions: Y.H.C., C.P., and W.-J.K. conceived and designed the experiments; H.-J.C., E.O.C., H.L., H.H.-B., S.Y.J., M.Y.K., S.Y.K., and S.H.H. performed the experiments; G.-Y.K., S.J.Y., J.H.C., and H.J.H. analyzed the data; C.P. wrote the paper; and Y.H.C. edited the paper.

References

1. Kumar, A.; Jaitak, V. Natural products as multidrug resistance modulators in cancer. *Eur. J. Med. Chem.* **2019**, *176*, 268–291. [CrossRef] [PubMed]
2. Fu, B.; Wang, N.; Tan, H.Y.; Li, S.; Cheung, F.; Feng, Y. Multi-component herbal products in the prevention and treatment of chemotherapy-associated toxicity and side effects: A review on experimental and clinical evidences. *Front. Pharmacol.* **2018**, *9*, 1394. [CrossRef] [PubMed]
3. Butler, M.S.; Robertson, A.A.; Cooper, M.A. Natural product and natural product derived drugs in clinical trials. *Nat. Prod. Rep.* **2014**, *31*, 1612–1661. [CrossRef] [PubMed]
4. Nobili, S.; Lippi, D.; Witort, E.; Donnini, M.; Bausi, L.; Mini, E.; Capaccioli, S. Natural compounds for cancer treatment and prevention. *Pharmacol. Res.* **2009**, *59*, 365–378. [CrossRef]
5. Efferth, T.; Fu, Y.J.; Zu, Y.G.; Schwarz, G.; Konkimalla, V.S.; Wink, M. Molecular target-guided tumor therapy with natural products derived from traditional Chinese medicine. *Curr. Med. Chem.* **2007**, *14*, 2024–2032. [CrossRef]
6. Medema, R.H.; Macůrek, L. Checkpoint control and cancer. *Oncogene* **2012**, *31*, 2601–2613. [CrossRef]
7. Hanahan, D.; Weinberg, R.A. Hallmarks of cancer: The next generation. *Cell* **2011**, *144*, 646–674. [CrossRef]
8. Bolhassani, A. Cancer chemoprevention by natural carotenoids as an efficient strategy. *Anticancer Agents Med. Chem.* **2015**, *15*, 1026–1231. [CrossRef]
9. Schnekenburger, M.; Dicato, M.; Diederich, M. Plant-derived epigenetic modulators for cancer treatment and prevention. *Biotechnol. Adv.* **2014**, *32*, 1123–1132. [CrossRef]
10. Gu, Q.; Duan, G.; Yu, X. Bioconversion of flavonoid glycosides from *Hippophae rhamnoides* leaves into flavonoid aglycones by *Eurotium amstelodami*. *Microorganisms* **2019**, *7*, 122. [CrossRef]
11. Zhang, Q.; Cui, H. Simultaneous determination of quercetin, kaempferol, and isorhamnetin in phytopharmaceuticals of *Hippophae rhamnoides* L. by high-performance liquid chromatography with chemiluminescence detection. *J. Sep. Sci.* **2005**, *28*, 1171–1178. [CrossRef] [PubMed]
12. Chen, C.; Xu, X.M.; Chen, Y.; Yu, M.Y.; Wen, F.Y.; Zhang, H. Identification, quantification and antioxidant activity of acylated flavonol glycosides from sea buckthorn (*Hippophae rhamnoides* ssp. sinensis). *Food Chem.* **2013**, *141*, 1573–1579. [CrossRef] [PubMed]
13. Castrillo, J.L.; Vanden Berghe, D.; Carrasco, L. 3-Methylquercetin is a potent and selective inhibitor of poliovirus RNA synthesis. *Virology* **1986**, *152*, 219–227. [CrossRef]
14. Rösch, D.; Krumbein, A.; Mügge, C.; Kroh, L.W. Structural investigations of flavonol glycosides from sea buckthorn (*Hippophaë rhamnoides*) pomace by NMR spectroscopy and HPLC-ESI-MS(n). *J. Agric. Food Chem.* **2004**, *52*, 4039–4046. [CrossRef] [PubMed]
15. Qi, F.; Sun, J.H.; Yan, J.Q.; Li, C.M.; Lv, X.C. Anti-inflammatory effects of isorhamnetin on LPS-stimulated human gingival fibroblasts by activating Nrf2 signaling pathway. *Microb. Pathog.* **2018**, *120*, 37–41. [CrossRef] [PubMed]
16. Abdallah, H.M.; Esmat, A. Antioxidant and anti-inflammatory activities of the major phenolics from *Zygophyllum simplex* L. *J. Ethnopharmacol.* **2017**, *205*, 51–56. [CrossRef]
17. Seo, S.; Seo, K.; Ki, S.H.; Shin, S.M. Isorhamnetin inhibits reactive oxygen species-dependent hypoxia inducible factor (HIF)-1α accumulation. *Biol. Pharm. Bull.* **2016**, *39*, 1830–1838. [CrossRef]
18. Yang, J.H.; Kim, S.C.; Kim, K.M.; Jang, C.H.; Cho, S.S.; Kim, S.J.; Ku, S.K.; Cho, I.J.; Ki, S.H. Isorhamnetin attenuates liver fibrosis by inhibiting TGF-β/Smad signaling and relieving oxidative stress. *Eur. J. Pharmacol.* **2016**, *783*, 92–102. [CrossRef]
19. Luo, Y.; Sun, G.; Dong, X.; Wang, M.; Qin, M.; Yu, Y.; Sun, X. Isorhamnetin attenuates atherosclerosis by inhibiting macrophage apoptosis via PI3K/AKT activation and HO-1 induction. *PLoS ONE* **2015**, *10*, e0120259. [CrossRef]
20. Zhang, H.W.; Hu, J.J.; Fu, R.Q.; Liu, X.; Zhang, Y.H.; Li, J.; Liu, L.; Li, Y.N.; Deng, Q.; Luo, Q.S.; et al. Flavonoids inhibit cell proliferation and induce apoptosis and autophagy through downregulation of III9K$_{\gamma}$ mediated PI3K/AKT/mTOR/p70S6K/ULK signaling pathway in human breast cancer cells. *Sci. Rep.* **2018**, *8*, 11255. [CrossRef]
21. Wei, J.; Su, H.; Bi, Y.; Li, J.; Feng, L.; Sheng, W. Anti-proliferative effect of isorhamnetin on HeLa cells through inducing G2/M cell cycle arrest. *Exp. Ther. Med.* **2018**, *15*, 3917–3923. [CrossRef] [PubMed]

22. Wu, X.; Chen, X.; Dan, J.; Cao, Y.; Gao, S.; Guo, Z.; Zerbe, P.; Chai, Y.; Diao, Y.; Zhang, L. Characterization of anti-leukemia components from *Indigo naturalis* using comprehensive two-dimensional K562/cell membrane chromatography and in silico target identification. *Sci. Rep.* **2016**, *6*, 25491. [CrossRef] [PubMed]
23. Li, C.; Yang, X.; Chen, C.; Cai, S.; Hu, J. Isorhamnetin suppresses colon cancer cell growth through the PI3K-Akt-mTOR pathway. *Mol. Med. Rep.* **2014**, *9*, 935–940. [CrossRef] [PubMed]
24. Zhang, B.Y.; Wang, Y.M.; Gong, H.; Zhao, H.; Lv, X.Y.; Yuan, G.H.; Han, S.R. Isorhamnetin flavonoid synergistically enhances the anticancer activity and apoptosis induction by cisplatin and carboplatin in non-small cell lung carcinoma (NSCLC). *Int. J. Clin. Exp. Pathol.* **2015**, *8*, 25–37. [PubMed]
25. Wang, J.L.; Quan, Q.; Ji, R.; Guo, X.Y.; Zhang, J.M.; Li, X.; Liu, Y.G. Isorhamnetin suppresses PANC-1 pancreatic cancer cell proliferation through S phase arrest. *Biomed. Pharmacother.* **2018**, *108*, 925–933. [CrossRef] [PubMed]
26. Wu, Q.; Kroon, P.A.; Shao, H.; Needs, P.W.; Yang, X. Differential effects of quercetin and two of its derivatives, isorhamnetin and isorhamnetin-3-glucuronide, in inhibiting the proliferation of human breast-cancer MCF-7 cells. *J. Agric. Food Chem.* **2018**, *66*, 7181–7189. [CrossRef]
27. Sak, K.; Lust, H.; Kase, M.; Jaal, J. Cytotoxic action of methylquercetins in human lung adenocarcinoma cells. *Oncol. Lett.* **2018**, *15*, 1973–1978. [CrossRef]
28. Huang, S.P.; Ho, T.M.; Yang, C.W.; Chang, Y.J.; Chen, J.F.; Shaw, N.S.; Horng, J.C.; Hsu, S.L.; Liao, M.Y.; Wu, L.C.; et al. Chemopreventive potential of ethanolic extracts of luobuma leaves (*Apocynum venetum* L.) in androgen insensitive prostate cancer. *Nutrients* **2017**, *9*, 948. [CrossRef]
29. Li, Q.; Ren, F.Q.; Yang, C.L.; Zhou, L.M.; Liu, Y.Y.; Xiao, J.; Zhu, L.; Wang, Z.G. Anti-proliferation effects of isorhamnetin on lung cancer cells in vitro and in vivo. *Asian Pac. J. Cancer. Prev.* **2015**, *16*, 3035–3042. [CrossRef]
30. Antunes-Ricardo, M.; Moreno-García, B.E.; Gutiérrez-Uribe, J.A.; Aráiz-Hernández, D.; Alvarez, M.M.; Serna-Saldivar, S.O. Induction of apoptosis in colon cancer cells treated with isorhamnetin glycosides from *Opuntia ficusindica* pads. *Plant Foods Hum. Nutr.* **2014**, *69*, 331–336. [CrossRef]
31. Lee, H.J.; Lee, H.J.; Lee, E.O.; Ko, S.G.; Bae, H.S.; Kim, C.H.; Ahn, K.S.; Lu, J.; Kim, S.H. Mitochondria-cytochrome *c*-caspase-9 cascade mediates isorhamnetin-induced apoptosis. *Cancer Lett.* **2008**, *270*, 342–353. [CrossRef]
32. Hu, S.; Huang, L.; Meng, L.; Sun, H.; Zhang, W.; Xu, Y. Isorhamnetin inhibits cell proliferation and induces apoptosis in breast cancer via Akt and mitogen-activated protein kinase kinase signaling pathways. *Mol. Med. Rep.* **2015**, *12*, 6745–6751. [CrossRef] [PubMed]
33. Choi, K.C.; Chung, W.T.; Kwon, J.K.; Yu, J.Y.; Jang, Y.S.; Park, S.M.; Lee, S.Y.; Lee, J.C. Inhibitory effects of quercetin on aflatoxin B1-induced hepatic damage in mice. *Food Chem. Toxicol.* **2010**, *48*, 2747–2753. [CrossRef] [PubMed]
34. Hibasami, H.; Mitani, A.; Katsuzaki, H.; Imai, K.; Yoshioka, K.; Komiya, T. Isolation of five types of flavonol from seabuckthorn (*Hippophae rhamnoides*) and induction of apoptosis by some of the flavonols in human promyelotic leukemia HL-60 cells. *Int. J. Mol. Med.* **2005**, *15*, 805–809. [CrossRef] [PubMed]
35. Prasain, J.K.; Rajbhandari, R.; Keeton, A.B.; Piazza, G.A.; Barnes, S. Metabolism and growth inhibitory activity of cranberry derived flavonoids in bladder cancer cells. *Food Funct.* **2016**, *7*, 4012–4019. [CrossRef]
36. Ebrahimi, S.; Hosseini, M.; Shahidsales, S.; Maftouh, M.; Ferns, G.A.; Ghayour-Mobarhan, M.; Hassanian, S.M.; Avan, A. Targeting the Akt/PI3K Signaling Pathway as a Potential Therapeutic Strategy for the Treatment of Pancreatic Cancer. *Curr. Med. Chem.* **2017**, *24*, 1321–1331. [CrossRef] [PubMed]
37. Hassan, M.; Watari, H.; AbuAlmaaty, A.; Ohba, Y.; Sakuragi, N. Apoptosis and molecular targeting therapy in cancer. *Biomed. Res. Int.* **2014**, *2014*, 150845. [CrossRef]
38. Bai, J.; Li, Y.; Zhang, G. Cell cycle regulation and anticancer drug discovery. *Cancer Biol. Med.* **2017**, *14*, 348–362.
39. Sánchez-Martínez, C.; Gelbert, L.M.; Lallena, M.J.; De Dios, A. Cyclin dependent kinase (CDK) inhibitors as anticancer drugs. *Bioorg. Med. Chem. Lett.* **2015**, *25*, 3420–3435. [CrossRef]
40. Matheson, C.J.; Backos, D.S.; Reigan, P. Targeting WEE1 kinase in cancer. *Trends Pharmacol. Sci.* **2016**, *37*, 872–881. [CrossRef]
41. Bulavin, D.V.; Demidenko, Z.N.; Phillips, C.; Moody, S.A.; Fornace, A.J., Jr. Phosphorylation of Xenopus Cdc25C at Ser285 interferes with ability to activate a DNA damage replication checkpoint in pre-midblastula embryos. *Cell Cycle* **2003** 2, 263–266. [CrossRef]

42. Karimian, A.; Ahmadi, Y.; Yousefi, B. Multiple functions of p21 in cell cycle, apoptosis and transcriptional regulation after DNA damage. *DNA Repair* **2016**, *42*, 63–71. [CrossRef] [PubMed]
43. Reinhardt, H.C.; Schumacher, B. The p53 network: Cellular and systemic DNA damage responses in aging and cancer. *Trends Genet.* **2012**, *28*, 128–136. [CrossRef] [PubMed]
44. Hydbring, P.; Malumbres, M.; Sicinski, P. Non-canonical functions of cell cycle cyclins and cyclin-dependent kinases. *Nat. Rev. Mol. Cell Biol.* **2016**, *17*, 280–292. [CrossRef] [PubMed]
45. Cooper, M.J.; Haluschak, J.J.; Johnson, D.; Schwartz, S.; Morrison, L.J.; Lippa, M.; Hatzivassiliou, G.; Tan, J. p53 mutations in bladder carcinoma cell lines. *Oncol. Res.* **1994**, *6*, 569–579. [PubMed]
46. Pfeffer, C.M.; Singh, A.T.K. Apoptosis: A target for anticancer therapy. *Int. J. Mol. Sci.* **2018**, *19*, 448. [CrossRef]
47. Kantari, C.; Walczak, H. Caspase-8 and bid: Caught in the act between death receptors and mitochondria. *Biochim. Biophys. Acta* **2011**, *1813*, 558–563. [CrossRef] [PubMed]
48. Edlich, F. BCL-2 proteins and apoptosis: Recent insights and unknowns. *Biochem. Biophys. Res. Commun.* **2018**, *500*, 26–34. [CrossRef]
49. Birkinshaw, R.W.; Czabotar, P.E. The BCL-2 family of proteins and mitochondrial outer membrane permeabilisation. *Semin. Cell Dev. Biol.* **2017**, *72*, 152–162. [CrossRef]
50. Kiraz, Y.; Adan, A.; Kartal Yandim, M.; Baran, Y. Major apoptotic mechanisms and genes involved in apoptosis. *Tumour Biol.* **2016**, *37*, 8471–8486. [CrossRef]
51. Schultz, D.R.; Harrington, W.J., Jr. Apoptosis: Programmed cell death at a molecular level. *Semin. Arthritis Rheum.* **2003**, *32*, 345–369. [CrossRef] [PubMed]
52. Ruan, Y.; Hu, K.; Chen, H. Autophagy inhibition enhances isorhamnetin-induced mitochondria-dependent apoptosis in non-small cell lung cancer cells. *Mol. Med. Rep.* **2015**, *12*, 5796–5806. [CrossRef] [PubMed]
53. Badrinath, N.; Yoo, S.Y. Mitochondria in cancer: In the aspects of tumorigenesis and targeted therapy. *Carcinogenesis* **2018**, *39*, 1419–1430. [CrossRef] [PubMed]
54. Moloney, J.N.; Cotter, T.G. ROS signalling in the biology of cancer. *Semin. Cell Dev. Biol.* **2018**, *80*, 50–64. [CrossRef] [PubMed]
55. Galadari, S.; Rahman, A.; Pallichankandy, S.; Thayyullathil, F. Reactive oxygen species and cancer paradox: To promote or to suppress? *Free Radic. Biol. Med.* **2017**, *104*, 144–164. [CrossRef] [PubMed]
56. Thirupathi, A.; De Souza, C.T. Multi-regulatory network of ROS: The interconnection of ROS, PGC-1 alpha, and AMPK-SIRT1 during exercise. *J. Physiol. Biochem.* **2017**, *73*, 487–494. [CrossRef]
57. Wu, S.B.; Wu, Y.T.; Wu, T.P.; Wei, Y.H. Role of AMPK-mediated adaptive responses in human cells with mitochondrial dysfunction to oxidative stress. *Biochim. Biophys. Acta* **2014**, *1840*, 1331–1344. [CrossRef] [PubMed]
58. Zou, M.H.; Kirkpatrick, S.S.; Davis, B.J.; Nelson, J.S.; Wiles, W.G., 4th; Schlattner, U.; Neumann, D.; Brownlee, M.; Freeman, M.B.; Goldman, M.H. Activation of the AMP-activated protein kinase by the anti-diabetic drug metformin in vivo. Role of mitochondrial reactive nitrogen species. *J. Biol. Chem.* **2004**, *279*, 43940–43951. [CrossRef]
59. Choi, S.L.; Kim, S.J.; Lee, K.T.; Kim, J.; Mu, J.; Birnbaum, M.J.; Soo Kim, S.; Ha, J. The regulation of AMP activated protein kinase by H_2O_2. *Biochem. Biophys. Res. Commun.* **2001**, *287*, 92–97. [CrossRef]
60. Wu, S.B.; Wei, Y.H. AMPK-mediated Increase of glycolysis as an adaptive response to oxidative stress in human cells: Implication of the cell survival in mitochondrial diseases. *Biochim. Biophys. Acta* **2012**, *1822*, 233–247. [CrossRef]
61. Cao, C.; Lu, S.; Jiang, Q.; Wang, W.J.; Song, X.; Kivlin, R.; Wallin, B.; Bagdasarian, A.; Tamakloe, T.; Chu, W.M.; et al. EGFR activation confers protections against UV-induced apoptosis in cultured mouse skin dendritic cells. *Cell Signal* **2018**, *20*, 1830–1838. [CrossRef]
62. Corton, J.M.; Gillespie, J.G.; Hardi, D.G. Role of the AMP-activated protein kinase in the cellular stress response. *Curr. Biol.* **1994**, *4*, 315–324. [CrossRef]
63. Tavazzi, B.; Di Pierro, D.; Amorini, A.M.; Fazzina, G.; Tuttobene, M.; Giardina, B.; Lazzarino, G. Energy metabolism and lipid peroxidation of human erythrocytes as a function of increased oxidative stress. *Eur. J. Biochem.* **2000**, *267*, 684–689. [CrossRef] [PubMed]
64. Chen, L.; Xu, B.; Liu, L.; Luo, Y.; Yin, J.; Zhou, H.; Chen, W.; Shen, T.; Han, X.; Huang, S. Hydrogen peroxide inhibits mTOR signaling by activation of AMPK alpha leading to apoptosis of neuronal cells. *Lab. Investig.* **2010** *90*, 762–773. [CrossRef] [PubMed]

65. Vara-Ciruelos, D.; Russell, F.M.; Hardie, D.G. The strange case of AMPK and cancer: Dr Jekyll or Mr Hyde? *Open Biol.* **2019**, *9*, 190099. [CrossRef]
66. Vander Heiden, M.G.; Cantley, L.C.; Thompson, C.B. Understanding the Warburg effect: The metabolic requirements of cell proliferation. *Science* **2009**, *324*, 1029–1033. [CrossRef] [PubMed]
67. Kim, J.; Kundu, M.; Viollet, B.; Guan, K.L. AMPK and mTOR regulate autophagy through direct phosphorylation of Ulk1. *Nat. Cell Biol.* **2011**, *13*, 132–141. [CrossRef] [PubMed]
68. Egan, D.F.; Shackelford, D.B.; Mihaylova, M.M.; Gelino, S.; Kohnz, R.A.; Mair, W.; Vasquez, D.S.; Joshi, A.; Gwinn, D.M.; Taylor, R.; et al. Phosphorylation of ULK1 (hATG1) by AMP-activated protein kinase connects energy sensing to mitophagy. *Science* **2011**, *331*, 456–461. [CrossRef]
69. Wong, C.H.; Iskandar, K.B.; Yadav, S.K.; Hirpara, J.L.; Loh, T.; Pervaiz, S. Simultaneous induction of non-canonical autophagy and apoptosis in cancer cells by ROS-dependent ERK and JNK activation. *PLoS ONE* **2010**, *5*, e9996. [CrossRef] [PubMed]
70. Ci, Y.; Shi, K.; An, J.; Yang, Y.; Hui, K.; Wu, P.; Shi, L.; Xu, C. ROS inhibit autophagy by downregulating ULK1 mediated by the phosphorylation of p53 in selenite-treated NB4 cells. *Cell Death Dis.* **2014**, *5*, e1542. [CrossRef]
71. Park, C.; Jeong, N.Y.; Kim, G.Y.; Han, M.H.; Chung, I.M.; Kim, W.J.; Yoo, Y.H.; Choi, Y.H. Momilactone B induces apoptosis and G1 arrest of the cell cycle in human monocytic leukemia U937 cells through downregulation of pRB phosphorylation and induction of the cyclin-dependent kinase inhibitor p21Waf1/Cip1. *Oncol. Rep.* **2014**, *31*, 1653–1660. [CrossRef] [PubMed]
72. Koh, E.M.; Lee, E.K.; Song, C.H.; Song, J.; Chung, H.Y.; Chae, C.H.; Jung, K.J. Ferulate, an active component of wheat germ, ameliorates oxidative stress-induced PTK/PTP imbalance and PP2A inactivation. *Toxicol. Res.* **2018**, *34*, 333–341. [CrossRef] [PubMed]
73. Kim, D.Y.; Kim, J.H.; Lee, J.C.; Won, M.H.; Yang, S.R.; Kim, H.C.; Wie, M.B. Zinc oxide nanoparticles exhibit both cyclooxygenase- and lipoxygenase-mediated apoptosis in human bone marrow-derived mesenchymal stem cells. *Toxicol. Res.* **2019**, *35*, 83–91. [CrossRef] [PubMed]

11

Cancer Glycolytic Dependence as a New Target of Olive Leaf Extract

Jessica Ruzzolini [1], Silvia Peppicelli [1], Francesca Bianchini [1], Elena Andreucci [1], Silvia Urciuoli [2], Annalisa Romani [2], Katia Tortora [3], Giovanna Caderni [3], Chiara Nediani [1,*] and Lido Calorini [1,4,*]

1 Department of Experimental and Clinical Biomedical Sciences "Mario Serio", University of Florence, 50134 Florence, Italy; jessica.ruzzolini@unifi.it (J.R.); silvia.peppicelli@unifi.it (S.P.); francesca.bianchini@unifi.it (F.B.); e.andreucci@unifi.it (E.A.)
2 PHYTOLAB (Pharmaceutical, Cosmetic, Food Supplement Technology and Analysis)-DiSIA, Scientific and Technological Pole, University of Florence, 50019 Sesto Fiorentino (Florence), Italy; silvia.urciuoli@gmail.com (S.U.); annalisa.romani@unifi.it (A.R.)
3 NEUROFARBA Department, Pharmacology and Toxicology Section, University of Florence, 50139 Florence, Italy; katia.tortora@unifi.it (K.T.); giovanna.caderni@unifi.it (G.C.)
4 Center of Excellence for Research, Transfer and High Education DenoTHE University of Florence, 50134 Florence, Italy
* Correspondence: chiara.nediani@unifi.it (C.N.); lido.calorini@unifi.it (L.C.)

Abstract: Oleuropein (Ole), the main bioactive phenolic component of *Olea europaea* L. has recently attracted the scientific attention for its several beneficial properties, including its anticancer effects. This study is intended to investigate whether an olive leaf extract enriched in Ole (OLEO) may counteract the aerobic glycolysis exploited by tumor cells. We found that OLEO decreased melanoma cell proliferation and motility. OLEO was also able to reduce the rate of glycolysis of human melanoma cells without affecting oxidative phosphorylation. This reduction was associated with a significant decrease of glucose transporter-1, protein kinase isoform M2 and monocarboxylate transporter-4 expression, possible drivers of such glycolysis inhibition. Extending the study to other tumor histotypes, we observed that the metabolic effects of OLEO are not confined to melanoma, but also confirmed in colon carcinoma, breast cancer and chronic myeloid leukemia. In conclusion, OLEO represents a natural product effective in reducing the glycolytic metabolism of different tumor types, revealing an extended metabolic inhibitory activity that may be well suited in a complementary anti-cancer therapy.

Keywords: olive leaf extract; oleuropein; Seahorse analysis; cancer metabolism; glycolytic markers

1. Introduction

The Pasteur effect describes the inhibition of glycolysis by oxygen, through the inhibition of phosphofructokinase-1, the most important controlling enzyme of glycolysis, by ATP and citrate [1]. Otto Warburg, for the first time, showed that cancer cells do not follow this principle, since even under normoxic condition they prefer to exploit the glycolytic pathway, producing lactic acid from glucose. Indeed, while normal cells in the presence of oxygen use the oxidative phosphorylation, most cancer cells prefer the glycolysis, a phenomenon termed "Warburg effect" or aerobic glycolysis [2]. This is of a special importance for proliferating cancer cells which may regenerate NAD^+, increase the availability of glycolytic biosynthetic intermediates and lactate production. Lactate may contribute to sustain proliferation either by stimulating the production of vascular endothelial growth factor or by promoting cellular motility, two favorable aspects for proliferating cancer cells, e.g., generation of new blood vessels and expansion in neighboring tissues [3]. Lactic acid production and its release into the tumor microenvironment helps reduce the local extracellular pH, which might be instrumental for tumor progression, by promoting the invasive abilities of cancer cells [4], their resistance to apoptotic stimuli as well as chemo- and target therapies [5], by inducing anoikis resistance thus favouring tumor cell survival into the circulatory system [6], and importantly, by inhibiting the immune response supporting tumor cell escape [7]. The Warburg phenotype is regulated by numerous oncogenes, e.g., MYC transcription factor has been found to activate lactate dehydrogenase (LDH)A [8], and promote the switch from pyruvate kinase muscle isozyme 1 (PKM1) to 2 (PKM2), a limiting glycolytic enzyme of the final step of glycolysis, involved in the pyruvate and ATP production from phosphoenolpyruvate [9]. PKM2, in its less active dimeric form, reduces ATP generation leading to the production of lactate and several glycolytic intermediates, used as building blocks for the biosynthesis of cellular macromolecules, such as amino acids, lipids and nucleotides. In addition, mammalian target of rapamycin (mTOR) was demonstrated to be a key activator of the Warburg effect, as it induces under normoxic conditions several glycolytic enzymes, including PKM2 [10].

Recently, plant-derived compounds have drawn the attention of the scientific community for their several beneficial properties. In particular, polyphenols have been subjected to numerous studies and they showed anti-oxidant, anti-inflammatory, cardio- and neuro-protective functions as well as anti-cancer activity [11–15]. Moreover, their anti-cancer activity has been proved in a broad range of cancer models, so that some of these natural compounds have been included in clinical trials [16,17], as they showed promising effects in terms of promoting the anti-cancer response and decreasing at the same time the toxicity of conventional therapies [18–22].

Oleuropein (Ole) is the main bioactive phenolic compound of *Olea europaea* L. that has attracted great interest in the prevention and therapy of several non–communicable diseases, including cancer [23]. As to its anti-cancer properties, Ole affects and modulates multiple different biochemical processes and pathways involved in carcinogenesis. Indeed, Ole exerts an inhibitory effect on cancer cell proliferation, tumor growth and angiogenesis; it reduces inflammation and induces apoptosis [23–25]. In our previous study we found that Ole affects both the proliferation and the viability of A375 BRAF melanoma cells and potentiates their therapy response through pAKT/mTOR pathway [26]. In addition, we observed that an olive leaf extract enriched in Ole (OLEO), used at equimolar Ole concentration, was more effective to potentiate the cytotoxic effect, co-administered with conventional chemotherapeutic agents, compared to Ole alone [26]. Following this line of research, we decided to investigate if OLEO could be able to inhibit the metabolism of BRAF melanoma cells, that are usually glycolysis-addicted. The existence of a strong link between tumor-specific signalling pathways and metabolic adaptations is well known. Therefore, interfering with metabolic processes and metabolic enzymes may be a key strategy for cancer therapy. In this context, significant efforts have been recently done to elucidate how plant-derived natural compounds may act as modulators of tumor cell metabolism and, in this way, exert their anti-cancer activity [27].

Gerhauser, revising the knowledge on tumor metabolism and epigenetic variation of glycolytic genes, discovered that several of these processes are influenced by natural compounds [28]. Then, Gao and Chen underlined how several natural compounds may regulate HIF-1α-dependent anaerobic glycolysis of tumor cells: this actually represents a great contribution underlining the ability of natural products to inhibit one of the most critical transcription factors, i.e., HIF-1α, in cancer progression [29]. In this study, we proved that OLEO is able to reduce the glycolytic rate of both primary and metastatic melanoma cells, reducing the expression levels of critical glucose and lactate transporters (glucose transporter-1 (GLUT1) and monocarboxylate transporter-4 (MCT4), respectively) and enzymes, such as PKM2. Extending the study to other tumor types, we observed that OLEO is able to inhibit the glycolytic metabolism also in colorectal, breast and chronic myeloid leukemia cancer cells.

2. Results

In a previous work, with the aim to verify whether Ole might potentiate drug efficiency on BRAF mutant melanoma cells, we decided to use a non-toxic 250 μM dose able to reduce cell proliferation rate without affecting cancer cell viability and apoptosis. We found that Ole potentiates the cytotoxic effect of everolimus against BRAF melanoma cells inhibiting pAKT/mTOR pathway, as measured by the decrease of pAKT/S6. This effect was also demonstrated using an olive leaf extract enriched in an equimolar concentration of Ole [26]. Here, we confirmed that a similar OLEO, at a 200 μM dose, reduces the viability of A375 melanoma cells in a very limited amount (see the 48 and 72 h of treatment), as cell proliferation without modifying cell cycle phase distribution (Figure 1A–C). The same concentration of the extract does not modify viability of human mesenchymal stem cells at each time point of the experiments (see Figure S1). Further, the OLEO, at a 200 μM dose, significantly reduced the closure of a wound (Figure 1D), which was used as an assay of cell motility. The reduced closure of wounds of OLEO-treated melanoma cells discloses the ability of this natural product to inhibit cell motility. These findings prompted to investigate effects of OLEO on melanoma metabolism. We know that V600E mutant BRAF melanoma cells are strictly addicted to glycolysis, the so-called Warburg effect, thus it was possible that a reduction of the glycolytic pathway may have a role in the decreased proliferation and motility of OLEO-treated melanoma cells.

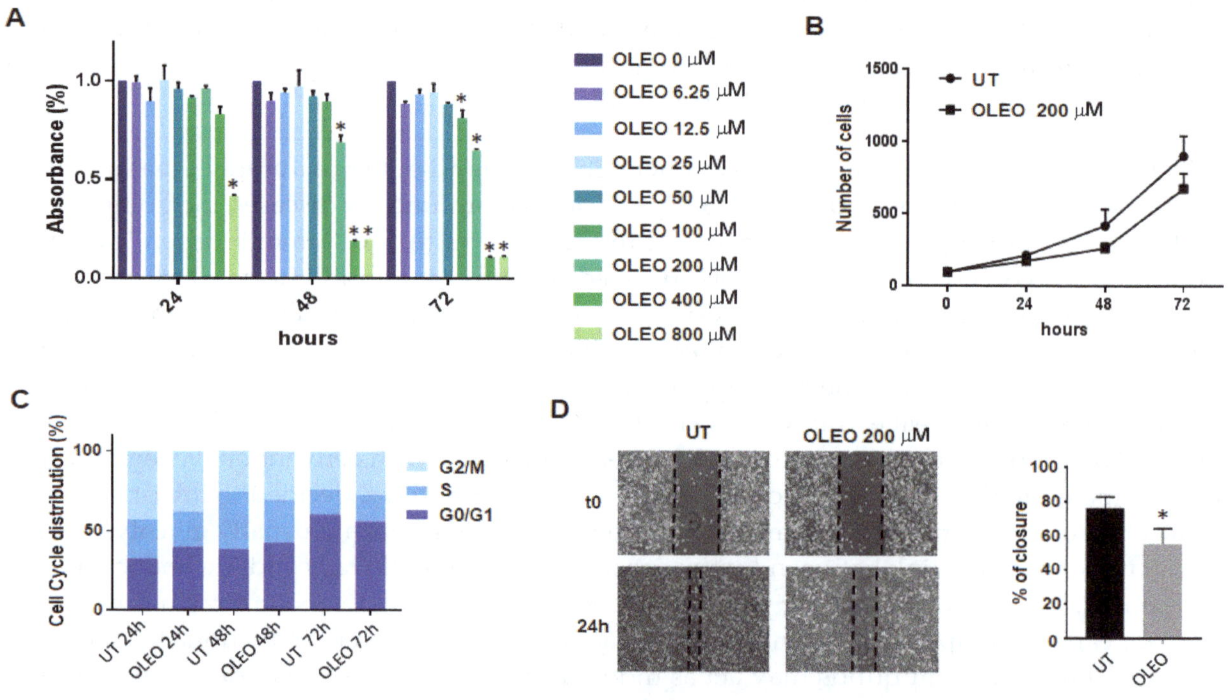

Figure 1. Effects of Ole-enriched leaf extract (OLEO) on A375 melanoma cells. (**A**) Dose-time response evaluated by MTT assay. Significance is indicated with *; (**B**) Cell growth of A375 human melanoma cells treated with OLEO 200 μM; (**C**) Cell cycle distribution analyzed using FACS; (**D**) Effect of OLEO 200 μM on the motility of A375 cells evaluated by scratch wound healing assay. Significance is indicated with *.

We evaluated the metabolic profile of melanoma cells after 200 μM OLEO administration through Seahorse Bioanalyzer XF96 analysis, thereafter studying the metabolic markers through real time PCR and Western Blot analysis.

We first tested the effect of OLEO extract on the glycolytic activity of A375 melanoma cells using a glycostress standard assay. Overall, OLEO impairs glycolysis rate without modifying glycolytic capacity and reserve of melanoma cells (Figure 2A). On the other hand, Mito stress analysis indicates that OLEO does not modify the respiration of melanoma cells.

To add information on OLEO-driven glycolysis inhibition, we exploited the Seahorse Bioanalyzer XF96 to check the metabolism of A375 melanoma cells exposed for 24 h to an equimolar concentration of pure Oleuropein, and we found an equivalent reducing effect on the glycolysis rate (Figure 2B), without any modification of respiration of these cells.

Further, to sustain the inhibitory role on the glycolytic metabolism of melanoma cells by OLEO, we tested its glycolysis inhibitory effect on a metastatic clone of A375 melanoma cells, called A375-M6, isolated from the lung of immunodeficient animals. In line with the previous results, we observed that OLEO exerts the same inhibitory effect on glycolysis of these metastatic cells, as showed in the glycostress analysis (Figure 2C). Overall, OLEO is able to repress the aerobic glycolysis of primary and metastatic melanoma cells.

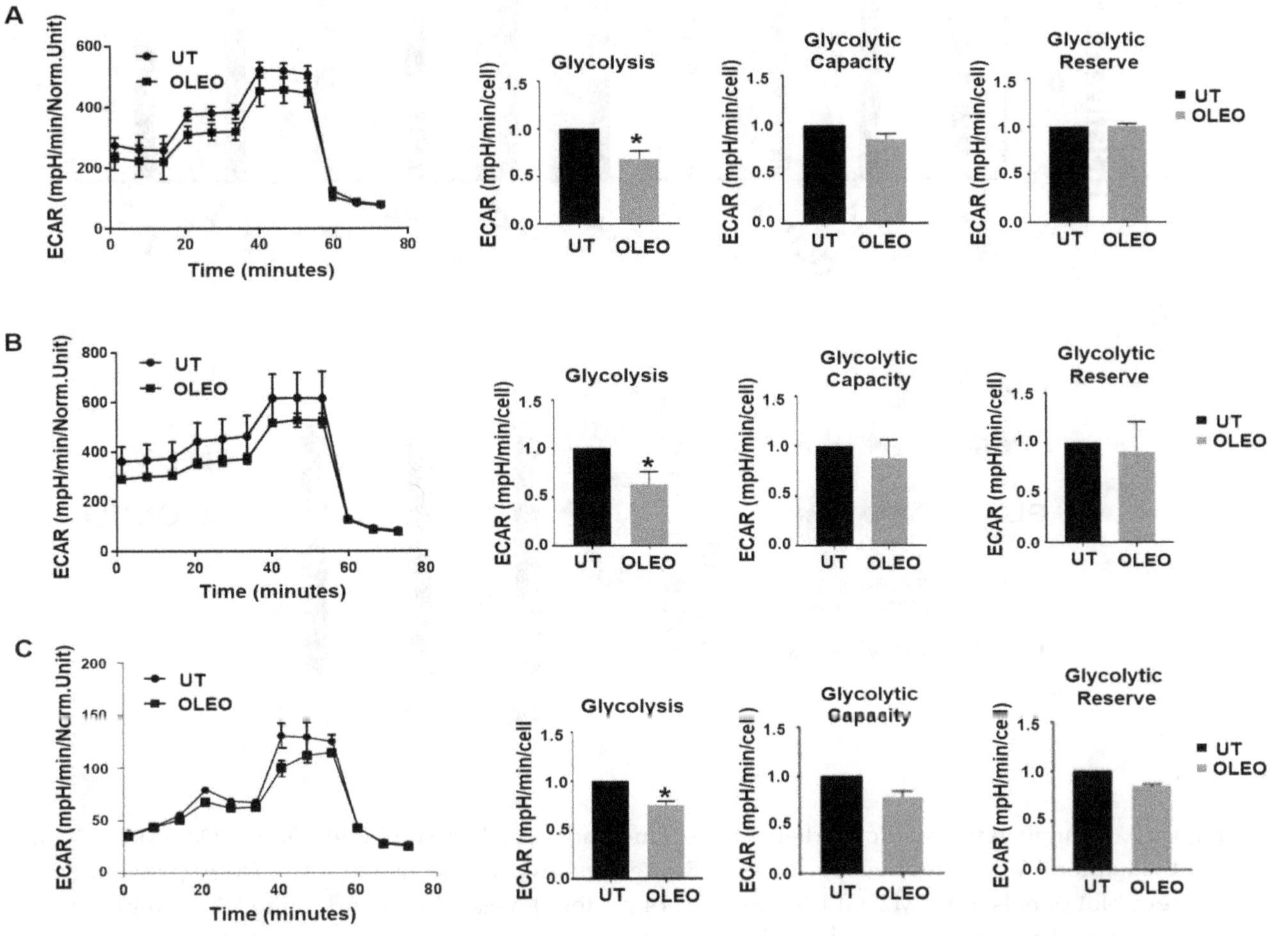

Figure 2. Representative results of a glucose stress test of A375 melanoma cells treated with 200 μM OLEO (**A**) or 200 μM Ole (**B**) for 24 h, and of A375-M6 melanoma cells treated with 200 μM OLEO for 24 h (**C**). Plots on the right represent glycolysis, glycolytic reserve and glycolytic capacity extracted from glycolysis stress assay results obtained using the Seahorse Analyzer. Significance is indicated with *.

Along with the dynamic investigation of metabolism expressed by A375 and A375-M6 melanoma cells following OLEO treatment, we identified a series of glycolytic biomarkers down regulated by our nutraceutical product. Testing both mRNA and protein levels, we observed that glucose transporter isoform 1 (GLUT1), pyruvate kinase isozymes M2 (PKM2) and monocarboxylate transporter 4 (MCT4) of OLEO-treated A375 melanoma cells are reduced by a 50% compared to control (i.e., untreated melanoma cells) (Figure 3). To underline the importance of these three key glycolytic biomarkers inhibited by OLEO: (1) GLUT1 is the major glucose transporter in cancer cells; (2) PKM2 is a modulator of glucose metabolism sustaining building block generation needed for cell proliferation; (3) MCT4 exports lactate and protons produced by glycolysis, preventing the inhibition of glycolytic enzymes such as phosphofructokinase activity, that is reduced by intracellular acidification.

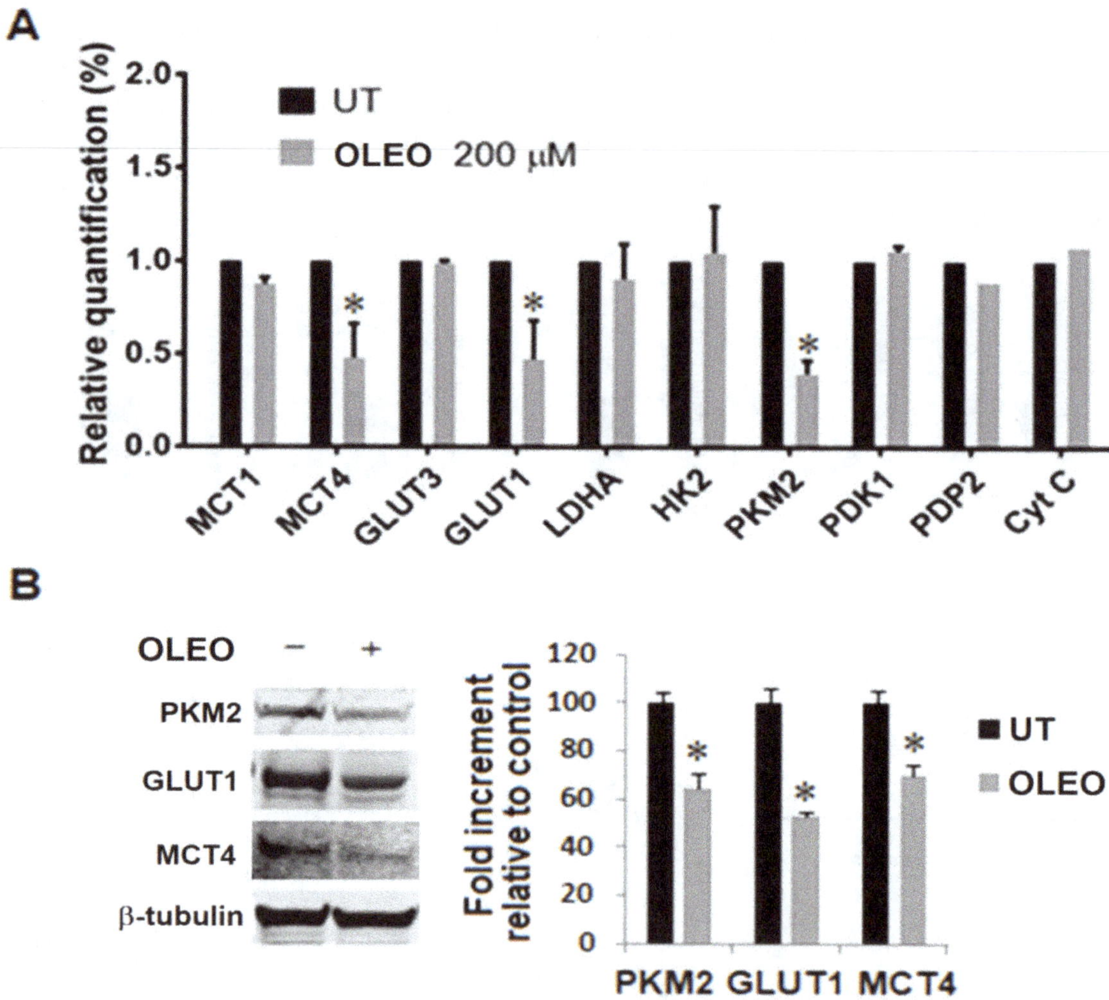

Figure 3. Change in metabolic markers of A375 melanoma cells treated with OLEO 200 μM for 24 h. (**A**) Evaluation by quantitative real-time PCR of genes involved in metabolism; (**B**) Representative Western blot panels of PKM2, GLUT1 and MCT4 protein levels. Each band in the Western blot was quantified by densitometric analysis and the corresponding histogram was constructed by normalizing the density of each band to that of β-tubulin. Values presented are means ± SEM of three independent experiments. Significance is indicated with *.

To extend our investigation on OLEO metabolic inhibition in cancer cells, we also tested HCT116 (a human colorectal carcinoma cell line), MDA-MB-231 (an undifferentiated triple-negative breast cancer cell line) and K562 cells (a chronic myeloid leukemia cell line) through the Seahorse Bioanalyzer XF96. OLEO does not modify substantially number and viability of colorectal, breast and leukemia cancer cells (Figure 4A,C,E), but was effective in reducing glycolysis rate of all these type of cancer cells; a higher dose of OLEO was needed to inhibit glycolysis of K562 cells. Overall, these results demonstrate a metabolic inhibitory activity of OLEO on a wide array of cancer histotypes, including that of malignant cells of a clonal disorder of hematopoietic stem cells (Figure 4B,D,F).

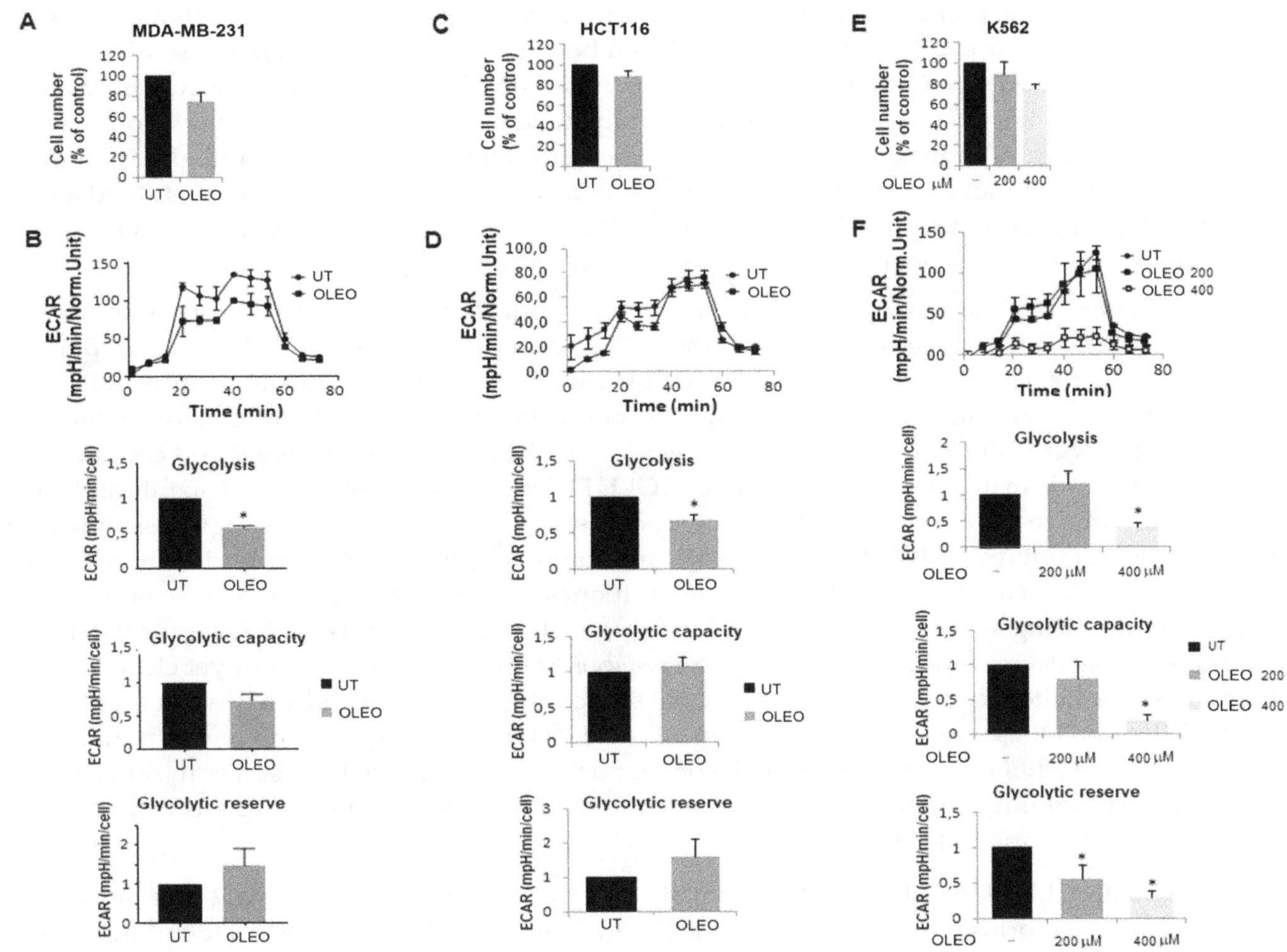

Figure 4. Effect of OLEO on glycolytic metabolism of breast cancer, colon carcinoma and myeloid leukemia cells. Cell number (**A**,**C**,**E**) and representative results of a glucose stress test of MDA-MB-231 (**B**), HCT116 (**D**), and K562 (**F**) cells, treated with 200 or 400 μM OLEO for 48 h. Plots on the right represent glycolysis, glycolytic reserve and glycolytic capacity extracted from glycolysis stress assay results obtained using the Seahorse Analyzer. Significance is indicated with *.

3. Discussion

It is well known that cancer cells, compared to normal tissues, are characterized by a high rate of glycolytic metabolism. They indeed prefer to use glycolysis even in the presence of enough oxygen to sustain the oxidative phosphorylation (the so-called "Warburg effect" or aerobic glycolysis, to be distinguished from the anaerobic glycolysis exploited under hypoxic conditions). The higher glycolytic rate of cancer cells ensures them an adequate amount of energy and an ample availability of intermediate macromolecules useful to sustain a rapid cell proliferation and tumor mass expansion [3]. Nowadays, the deregulated metabolism is considered a hallmark of cancer and the identification of new compounds able to modulate tumor metabolism is under intense investigation. For this reason, natural agents can be a great importance, in particular because they demonstrated to interfere with most of the activities of cancer cells, at the same time showing, very low toxic effects on normal cells [11,18,30]. To sum up, several authors have underlined how plant-derived natural products interfere with tumor metabolism [22].

Here we show that OLEO is able to exert a significant inhibitory effect on cancer cell glycolysis. In particular, by a dynamic evaluation of cancer cell metabolism through the Seahorse Bioanalyzer XF96 platform, we observed that OLEO reduces the glycolytic rate of primary and metastatic melanoma cells, but also of colorectal, breast and chronic myeloid leukemia cancer cells. In line with our results, Sharma and colleagues showed that morin and/or esculetin impaired glycolysis and glutaminolysis preventing colon carcinogenesis [31]. Moreover, Gomez de Cedron and colleagues identified a new series of polyphenols characterized by a galloyl based "head" and a hydrophobic N-acyl "tail", able to inhibit glycolysis and mitochondrial respiration in colon cancer cells [32].

We observed that the glycolytic reduction exerted by our OLEO in melanoma cells is associated with a decreased GLUT1 expression, at both the mRNA and protein levels. GLUT1 is an important target in cancer treatment, being over-expressed by a wide range of tumor cells. Cancer cells may indeed take great advantages of the GLUT1 rapid response and its high affinity for glucose, in order to overcome the several stress conditions encountered in the host microenvironment and continue the progression towards malignancy. The K_M value of GLUT1 for glucose is near 1 mM, a significantly less amount compared to the normal glucose level found in serum, allowing a relentless glucose transport into the cells. Of interest, GLUT1 represents the predominant glucose transporter isoform of fetus tissues, which exhibit a higher growth rate than adult ones, at comparable levels to those observed in tumor cells, requiring an increased supply of energy-producing substrates [32]. After birth, GLUT1 expression levels decrease and, even though the reasons behind its decline are not yet clear, it could occur a possible switch form a carbohydrate to a fat source of fuel that may induce this change in some organs [33]. For all these reasons, the development of new clinical strategies involving natural GLUT1 inhibitors such as OLEO, in combination with conventional anticancer agents, deserves the attention of the scientific community, sounding as promising combined therapeutic strategy, as recently reported for other natural compounds [34,35].

Along with GLUT1, we showed that OLEO is also able to down regulate PKM2, one of the four pyruvate kinase isoforms which is highly expressed in rapidly proliferating tissues including cancer. This metabolic enzyme is regulated by oncogenic tyrosine kinases which usually lead to an increase glycolytic rate in tumor cells. Despite, tyrosine phosphorylation of glycolytic enzymes usually increases the activities of a majority of glycolytic enzymes, the tyrosine phosphorylation of PKM2 paradoxically results in a decreased PKM2 activity that in turn promotes the Warburg effect [36]. It is possible that the OLEO-driven PKM2 reduction may reduce its glycolytic promotion [37]. PKM2 overexpression was observed in melanoma human samples compared to naevi, showing a gradient of increased expression from radial growth phase to metastatic melanoma. Furthermore, recent studies have shown that PKM2 is also able to act as a protein kinase using phosphoenolpyruvate as a substrate to promote tumorigenesis [36]. Then, Zhang and colleagues found that miR-625-5p regulates PKM2 expression at both mRNA and protein levels in melanoma cells, disclosing a miR/PKM2 role in glucose metabolism of melanoma cells [38]. PKM2 expression has been shown to be also reduced by other natural products such as resveratrol and curcumin. In particular, resveratrol inhibits aerobic glycolysis and PKM2 enzyme in HeLa (human cervical cancer), HepG2 (human liver cancer) and MCF-7 (human breast cancer) cancer cells through the inhibition of mTOR signaling [39]. Resveratrol was also demonstrated to impair hexokinase-2 enzyme in human non-small cell lung cancer cells inhibiting Akt signaling pathway [40], and pyruvate dehydrogenase complex in colon cancer cells [41]. Curcumin, a further well-known phytopolyphenolic compound, has been shown to decrease glucose uptake and lactate production in several cancer cells (lung, breast, cervical, prostate and embryonic kidney cancer cell lines) down-regulating PKM2 expression, interfering with the mTOR-HIF-1α axis [42].

MCT4 is the other glycolytic marker that we found to be inhibited by OLEO in melanoma cells. This monocarboxylate transporter acquires a key role in the metabolic activity of glycolytic cells through the proton-coupled transport of monocarboxylates, such as L-lactate, ketone bodies and pyruvate. An immunohistochemical study of the expression of MCT4 in 356 melanoma-bearing patients revealed that this glycolytic marker is significantly increased in metastatic lesions and associated with a poor prognosis [43].

To conclude, in this study we demonstrated that OLEO is able to reduce the high glycolytic activity of various solid tumors, like melanoma, colorectal and breast cancer, but also of chronic myeloid leukemia cells, suggesting a possible usage of this natural product in combination with conventional therapy for a wide range of malignancy.

4. Materials and Methods

4.1. Olive Leaf Extract's Preparation and Toxicity

The OLEO used to treat normal and cancer cells was prepared and characterized as previously described ([26], see Figures S3 and S4). *Olea europaea* L. (cultivar Leccino), organic green leaves, were collected in April 2018 in Tuscany (Vinci, Florence, Italy) and immediately processed. The extraction using 15% of *Olea* leaves (45 g leaves/300 g double-distilled and purified water), was performed in water at a temperature of 50 °C for 60 min and at room temperature over the night (12 h) [44]. The final powder is obtained by lyophilization with a LYOVAC GT 2 system (Leybold GmbH, Cologne, Germany), freeze-drying yield 1.85%. The identity of the phenolic compounds of *Olea* dry extract powder and the composition of the solution used for the test in vitro, enriched in oleuropein, was ascertained using data from the HPLC/DAD and HPLC/mass spectrometry analyses, in accordance with a previous paper [45].

All the solvents (HPLC grade) and formic acid (ACS reagent) were purchased from Aldrich Chemical Company Inc. (Milwaukee, WI, USA). Tyrosol, luteolin 7-O-glucoside, chlorogenic and Ole were obtained from Extrasynthese S.A. (Genay, France). The HPLC-grade water was obtained via double-distillation and purification with a Labconco Water Pro PS polishing station (Labconco Corporation, Kansas City, MO, USA).

The OLEO used in our study has been tested in a sub-acute test of toxicity (7 days) on female F344 rats fed a diet containing 2.7 g of extract/kg of diet (corresponding to a dosage of 100 mg of extract/kg of b.w.) without inducing any change of body weight.

This lack of toxicity is in agreement with a recent study of Guex et al., which showed that an olive leaf extract, in vivo tested up to 2000 mg/kg, had no toxic or unwanted effects on rats [46]. Moreover, Sepporta et al. [47]'s paper demonstrated absence of toxicity in mice administered 125 mg of Ole/kg (b.w.). The standard dose of Ole used in vivo animal model, from 10 to 125 mg/kg, did not induce toxic effects, evaluated in terms of viability of the animals [48] or liver biomarkers, such as alanine and aspartate aminotransferase activities [49].

4.2. Cell Lines and Culture Conditions

In this study we used A375 human melanoma cell lines, obtained from American Type Culture Collection (ATCC, Rockville, MD, USA), A375M6, isolated in our laboratory from lung metastasis of SCID bg/bg mice i.v. injected with A375 [5]; human colorectal carcinoma cell line HT116, a kind gift of Dr. Matteo Lulli (Department of Clinical and Experimental Biomedical Sciences, University of Florence, Italy); human breast carcinoma cells MDA-MB-231, obtained from American Type Culture Collection (ATCC); human leukemia cells K562, a kind gift of Prof. Persio Dello Sbarba (Department of Clinical and Experimental Biomedical Sciences, University of Florence) and human mesenchymal stem cells (MSC) obtained from bone marrow aspirates of donors which signed informed consent [50]. A375, A375M6, HCT116 and MDA-MB-231 were cultured in Dulbecco's Modified Eagle Medium high glucose (DMEM 4500, EuroClone, Milan, Italy) supplemented with 10% fetal bovine serum (FBS, EuroClone); K562 were cultured in Roswell Park Memorial Institute 1640 medium (RPMI, EuroClone) supplemented with 10% FBS; MSC were expanded in Dulbecco's modified Eagle's medium with low glucose (DMEM 1000; Gibco, Life Technologies, Monza, Italy) supplemented with 20% FBS. Cells were maintained at 37 °C in humidified atmosphere containing 90% air and 10% CO_2 and they were harvested from subconfluent cultures by incubation with a trypsin-EDTA solution (EuroClone), and propagated every three days. Viability of the cells was determined by trypan blue exclusion test. Cultures were periodically monitored for mycoplasma contamination using Chen's fluorochrome test. Cells were treated with OLEO for 24–72 h.

4.3. MTT Assay

Cell viability was assessed using MTT (3-(4,5-dimethylthiazol-2-yl)-2,5-diphenyltetrazolium bromide) tetrazolium reduction assay (Sigma Aldrich, Milan, Italy) as described in [26]. Cells were plated into 96-multiwell plates in complete medium without red phenol. The treatment was added to the medium colture at different dose and times, according to the experiment. Then the MTT reagent was added to the medium and plates were incubated at 37 °C. After 2 h, MTT was removed and the blue MTT–formazan product was solubilized with dimethyl sulfoxide (DMSO, Sigma Aldrich). The absorbance of the formazan solution was read at 595 nm using the microplate reader (Bio-Rad, Milan, Italy).

4.4. Cell Cycle Analysis

Cell cycle distribution was analyzed by the DNA content using propidium iodide (PI) staining method. Cells were centrifugated and stained with a mixture of 50 µg/mL PI (Sigma-Aldrich, St. Louis, MO, USA), 0.1% trisodium citrate and 0.1% NP40 (or triton x-100) in the dark at 4°C for 30 min. The stained cells were analyzed by flow cytometry (BD-FACS Canto, BD-Biosciences, San Jose, CA, USA) using red propidium-DNA fluorescence as previously described [5].

4.5. Wound Healing Assay

Cell migration was evaluated by an in vitro wound healing assay as previously described [6]. Cells were treated for 24 h with the extract, then cells have been detached and sown in 35 mm dishes at high confluence; cell monolayer was wounded with a sterile 200 mL pipette tip, washed with PBS and incubated in 1% FBS culture medium. Wound was analyzed following a 24-h incubation and photographed using phase contrast microscopy.

4.6. Seahorse Analysis

Seahorse analysis has been performed as previously described [51]. The extracellular acidification rate (ECAR) and the Oxygen Consumption Rate (OCR) were determined using the Seahorse XF96 Extracellular Flux Analyzer (Seahorse Bioscience, Billerica, MA, USA) through Seahorse XF Glycolysis Stress Test Kit (Agilent Technologies, Santa Clara, CA, USA), measuring preferentially the glycolytic function in cells, or Seahorse XF Mito Stress Test Kit (Agilent Technologies), measuring the dependence of cells on the oxidative metabolism. Cells were counted and seeded in XF96 Seahorse® microplates precoated with poly-D-lysine (ThermoFisher Scientific, Waltham, MA, USA). Cells were suspended in XF Assay Medium supplemented with 1 mM glutamine (from EuroClone, Paington, UK) in order to assess ECAR, in XF Assay Medium supplemented with 2 mM glutamine in order to assess OCR. Cells were left to adhere for a minimum of 30 min at 37 °C. The plate was left to equilibrate in a CO_2-free incubator before being transferred to the Seahorse XF96 analyzer. The pre-hydrated cartridge was filled with the indicated compounds and calibrated for 30 min in the Seahorse Analyzer. All the experiments were performed at 37 °C. Normalization to protein content was performed after each experiment. The Seahorse XF Report Generator automatically calculated the parameters from Wave data that have been exported to Excel or Graphpad.

4.7. RNA Isolation and Quantitative PCR (qPCR)

Total RNA was isolated from cells by using TRI Reagent (Sigma, Milan, Italy). The amount and purity of RNA were determined spectrophotometrically. cDNAwas obtained by incubating 2 µg of total

RNA with 4 U/μL of M-MLV reverse transcriptase (Promega, San Luis Obispo, CA, USA) according to the manufacturer's instructions. Quantitative real time PCR (qPCR) was performed as reported in [51] using the GoTaq® Probe Systems (Promega). The qPCR analysis was carried out in triplicate using an Applied Biosystems 7500 Sequence Detector with the default PCR setting: 40 cycles at 95 °C for 15 s, 60 °C for 60 s. mRNA was quantified with the DDCt method as described [52]. mRNA levels were normalized to β2 microglobulin as an endogenous control. The primer sequences used are listed in Table 1.

Table 1. Primer sequences for PCR.

Gene	FW	RV
MCT1	5′-GTGGCTCAGCTCCGTATTGT-3′	5′-GAGCCGACCTAAAAGTGGTG-3′
MCT4	5′-CAGTTCGAGGTGCTCATGG-3′	5′-ATGTAGAGGTGGGTCGCATC-3′
GLUT1	5′-CGGGCCAAGAGTGTGCTAAA-3′	5′-TGACGATACCGGAGCCAATG-3′
GLUT3	5′-CGAACTTCCTAGTCGGATTG-3′	5′-AGGAGGCACGACTTAGACAT-3′
LDHA	5′-AGCCCGATTCCGTTACCT-3′	5′-CACCAGCAACATTCATTCCA-3′
PKM2	5′-CAGAGGCTGCCATCTACCAC-3′	5′-CCAGACTTGGTGAGGACGAT-3′
PDK1	5′-CCAAGACCTCGTGTTGAGACC-3′	5′-AATACAGCTTCAGGTCTCCTTGG-3′
HK2	5′- CAAAGTGACAGTGGGTGTGG-3′	5′- GCCAGGTCCTTCACTGTCTC-3′
18s	5′-CGCCGCTAGAGGTGAAATTCT-3′	5′-CGAACCTCCGA CTTTCGTTCT-3′
PDP2	5′-ACCACCTCCGTGTCTATTGG-3′	5′-CCAGCGAGATGTCAGAATCC-3′
CytC	5′-TTGCACTTACACCGGTACTTAAGC-3′	5′-ACGTCCCCACTCTCTAAGTCCAA-3
GLS1	5′-TGCTACCTGTCTCCATGGCTT-3′	5′-CTTAGATGGCACCTCCTTTGG-3′

4.8. Western Blotting Analysis

Cells were lysed and separated using electrophoresis as previously described [5]. Cells were washed with ice cold PBS containing 1 mM Na4VO3, and lysed in 100 mL of cell RIPA lysis buffer (Merck Millipore, Vimodrone, Milan, Italy) containing PMSF (Sigma-Aldrich), sodium orthovanadate (Sigma-Aldrich) and protease inhibitor cocktail (Calbiochem). Aliquots of supernatants containing equal amounts of protein (40 mg) in Laemmli buffer were separated on Bolt® Bis-Tris Plus gels 4e12% precast polyacrylamide gels (Life Technologies, Monza, Italy). Fractionated proteins were transferred from the gel to a PVDF (polyvinylidene difluoride) membrane using iBlot 2 system (Life Technologies, Monza, Italy). Blots were stained with Ponceau red to ensure equal loading and complete transfer of proteins, and then they were blocked for 1 h, at room temperature, with Odyssey blocking buffer (Dasit Science, Cornaredo, Milan, Italy). Subsequently, the membrane was probed at 4 °C overnight with primary antibodies diluted in a solution of 1:1 Odyssey blocking buffer/T-PBS buffer. The primary antibodies were: rabbit anti-PKM2 (1:1000, Cell Signaling Technology, Danvers, MA, USA), rabbit anti-MCT-4 (1:1000, Santa Cruz Biotechnology, Santa Cruz, CA, USA), rabbit anti-GLUT1 (1:1000, Cell Signaling Technology). The membrane was washed in T-PBS buffer, incubated for 1 h at room temperature with goat anti-rabbit IgG Alexa Flour 750 antibody or with goat antimouse IgG Alexa Fluor 680 antibody (Invitrogen, Monza, Italy), and then visualized by an Odyssey Infrared Imaging System (LI-COR® Bioscience, Lincoln, NE, USA). Mouse anti-β tubulin monoclonal antibody (1:1000, Cell Signaling Technology) was used to assess equal amount of protein loaded in each lane.

4.9. Statistical Analysis

Densitometric data are expressed as means ± standard errors of the mean (SEM) depicted by vertical bars from representative experiment of at least three independent experiments. Statistical analysis of the data was performed by ANOVA and Tukey's multiple comparisons test, and $p \leq 0.05$ was considered statistically significant.

5. Conclusions

The rapid growth of cancer cells mainly depends on their high glycolytic metabolism. Indeed, tumor cells, compared to normal tissues, prefer to exploit the glycolytic pathway even in the presence of sufficient oxygen to sustain the oxidative phosphorylation. This is likely due to the fact that glycolysis guarantees a rapid availability of metabolic intermediates, assuring not only sufficient energy for their survival, but also an efficient production of nucleotides, amino acids and lipids needed to duplicate cell content before mitosis. In this study we show that the natural product OLEO is able to reduce the glycolytic rate of a wide range of solid and liquid tumor cells, without affecting their basal respiration but rather down-regulating the expression of three key effectors of the glycolytic pathway, i.e., GLUT-1, PKM2 and MCT4, likely resulting in a decreased glucose entrance and biomass production. Thus, the inhibition of glycolysis by OLEO acquires a great significance for the targeting of cancer cell growth and expansion. Our findings, together with previous evidence showing the anti-cancer effects exerted by OLEO, pure Ole and analogs [23,53,54], reinforce the hypothesis to propose the use of these natural compounds in combination with conventional therapy used in the treatment of cancer.

Author Contributions: Conceptualization, J.R., C.N. and L.C.; validation, S.P., E.A., F.B.; formal analysis, J.R., S.P., E.A.; investigation, J.R., S.P., F.B., G.C., K.T.; resources, S.U., A.R., C.N., L.C.; writing—original draft preparation, J.R., S.P., L.C.; writing—review and editing, F.B., E.A., C.N., A.R., S.U., G.C.; visualization, J.R., S.P.; supervision, L.C., J.R.; project administration, L.C., C.N.; funding acquisition, L.C., C.N., A.R. All authors have read and agreed to the published version of the manuscript.

References

1. Barker, J.; Khan, M.A.; Solomos, T. Mechanism of the Pasteur effect. *Nature* **1964**, *201*, 1126–1127. [CrossRef]
2. Warburg, O. On respiratory impairment in cancer cells. *Science* **1956**, *124*, 269–270. [PubMed]
3. Vander Heiden, M.G.; Cantley, L.C.; Thompson, C.B. Understanding the Warburg effect: The metabolic requirements of cell proliferation. *Science* **2009**, *324*, 1029–1033. [CrossRef] [PubMed]
4. Peppicelli, S.; Bianchini, F.; Torre, E.; Calorini, L. Contribution of acidic melanoma cells undergoing epithelial-to-mesenchymal transition to aggressiveness of non-acidic melanoma cells. *Clin. Exp. Metastasis* **2014**, *31*, 423–433. [CrossRef] [PubMed]
5. Ruzzolini, J.; Peppicelli, S.; Andreucci, E.; Bianchini, F.; Margheri, F.; Laurenzana, A.; Fibbi, G.; Pimpinelli, N.; Calorini, L. Everolimus selectively targets vemurafenib resistant BRAFV600E melanoma cells adapted to low pH. *Cancer Lett.* **2017**, *408*, 43–54. [CrossRef] [PubMed]
6. Peppicelli, S.; Ruzzolini, J.; Bianchini, F.; Andreucci, E.; Nediani, C.; Laurenzana, A.; Margheri, F.; Fibbi, G.; Calorini, L. Anoikis Resistance as a Further Trait of Acidic-Adapted Melanoma Cells. *J. Oncol.* **2019**, *2019*, 1–13. [CrossRef] [PubMed]
7. Peppicelli, S.; Bianchini, F.; Calorini, L. Extracellular acidity, a "reappreciated" trait of tumor environment driving malignancy: Perspectives in diagnosis and therapy. *Cancer Metastasis Rev.* **2014**, *33*, 823–832. [CrossRef] [PubMed]
8. Shim, H.; Dolde, C.; Lewis, B.C.; Wu, C.S.; Dang, G.; Jungmann, R.A.; Dalla-Favera, R.; Dang, C.V. c-Myc transactivation of LDH-A: Implications for tumor metabolism and growth. *Proc. Natl. Acad. Sci. USA* **1997**, *94*, 6658–6663. [CrossRef]
9. Dong, G.; Mao, Q.; Xia, W.; Xu, Y.; Wang, J.; Xu, L.; Jiang, F. PKM2 and cancer: The function of PKM2 beyond glycolysis. *Oncol. Lett.* **2016**, *11*, 1980–1986. [CrossRef]
10. Sun, Q.; Chen, X.; Ma, J.; Peng, H.; Wang, F.; Zha, X.; Wang, Y.; Jing, Y.; Yang, H.; Chen, R.; et al. Mammalian target of rapamycin up-regulation of pyruvate kinase isoenzyme type M2 is critical for aerobic glycolysis and tumor growth. *Proc. Natl. Acad. Sci. USA* **2011**, *108*, 4129–4134. [CrossRef]

11. Del Rio, D.; Rodriguez-Mateos, A.; Spencer, J.P.; Tognolini, M.; Borges, G.; Crozier, A. Dietary (poly)phenolics in human health: Structures, bioavailability, and evidence of protective effects against chronic diseases. *Antioxid. Redox Signal.* **2013**, *18*, 1818–1892. [CrossRef] [PubMed]
12. Romani, A.; Ieri, F.; Urciuoli, S.; Noce, A.; Marrone, G.; Nediani, C.; Bernini, R. Health Effects of Phenolic Compounds Found in Extra-Virgin Olive Oil, By-Products, and Leaf of Olea europaea L. *Nutrients* **2019**, *11*, 1776. [CrossRef] [PubMed]
13. Castelli, V.; Grassi, D.; Bocale, R.; d'Angelo, M.; Antonosante, A.; Cimini, A.; Ferri, C.; Desideri, G. Diet and Brain Health: Which Role for Polyphenols? *Curr. Pharm. Des.* **2018**, *24*, 227–238. [CrossRef] [PubMed]
14. Boss, A.; Bishop, K.S.; Marlow, G.; Barnett, M.P.; Ferguson, LR. Evidence to Support the Anti-Cancer Effect of Olive Leaf Extract and Future Directions. *Nutrients* **2016**, *8*, 513. [CrossRef]
15. Milanizadeh, S.; Reza Bigdeli, M. Pro-Apoptotic and Anti-Angiogenesis Effects of Olive Leaf Extract on Spontaneous Mouse Mammary Tumor Model by Balancing Vascular Endothelial Growth Factor and Endostatin Levels. *Nutr. Cancer* **2019**, *71*, 1374–1381. [CrossRef] [PubMed]
16. Butler, M.S.; Robertson, A.A.B.; Cooper, M.A. Natural product and natural product derived drugs in clinical trials. *Nat. Prod. Rep.* **2014**, *31*, 1612–1661. [CrossRef]
17. Seca, A.; Pinto, D. Plant Secondary Metabolites as Anticancer Agents: Successes in Clinical Trials and Therapeutic Application. *Int. J. Mol. Sci.* **2018**, *19*, 263. [CrossRef]
18. Goldsmith, C.D.; Bond, D.R.; Jankowski, H.; Weidenhofer, J.; Stathopoulos, C.E.; Roach, P.D.; Scarlett, C.J. The Olive Biophenols Oleuropein and Hydroxytyrosol Selectively Reduce Proliferation, Influence the Cell Cycle, and Induce Apoptosis in Pancreatic Cancer Cells. *Int. J. Mol. Sci.* **2018**, *19*, 1937. [CrossRef]
19. Siddique, A.B.; Ayoub, N.M.; Tajmim, A.; Meyer, S.A.; Hill, R.A.; El Sayed, K.A. (−)-Oleocanthal Prevents Breast Cancer Locoregional Recurrence After Primary Tumor Surgical Excision and Neoadjuvant Targeted Therapy in Orthotopic Nude Mouse Models. *Cancers* **2019**, *11*, 637. [CrossRef]
20. Zhou, Q.; Pan, H.; Li, J. Molecular Insights into Potential Contributions of Natural Polyphenols to Lung Cancer Treatment. *Cancers* **2019**, *11*, 1565. [CrossRef]
21. Juli, G.; Oliverio, M.; Bellizzi, D.; Gallo Cantafio, M.E.; Grillone, K.; Passarino, G.; Colica, C.; Nardi, M.; Rossi, M.; Procopio, A.; et al. Anti-tumor Activity and Epigenetic Impact of the Polyphenol Oleacein in Multiple Myeloma. *Cancers* **2019**, *11*, 990. [CrossRef] [PubMed]
22. De Stefanis, D.; Scimè, S.; Accomazzo, S.; Catti, A.; Occhipinti, A.; Bertea, C.M.; Costelli, P. Anti-Proliferative Effects of an Extra-Virgin Olive Oil Extract Enriched in Ligstroside Aglycone and Oleocanthal on Human Liver Cancer Cell Lines. *Cancers* **2019**, *11*, 1640. [CrossRef] [PubMed]
23. Nediani, C.; Ruzzolini, J.; Romani, A.; Calorini, L. Oleuropein, a Bioactive Compound from Olea europaea L., as a Potential Preventive and Therapeutic Agent in Non-Communicable Diseases. *Antioxidants* **2019**, *8*, 578. [CrossRef] [PubMed]
24. Shamshoum, H.; Vlavcheski, F.; Tsiani, E. Anticancer effects of oleuropein. *BioFactors* **2017**, *43*, 517–528. [CrossRef]
25. Margheri, F.; Menicacci, B.; Laurenzana, A.; Del Rosso, M.; Fibbi, G.; Cipolleschi, M.G.; Ruzzolini, J.; Nediani, C.; Mocali, A.; Giovannelli, L. Oleuropein aglycone attenuates the pro-angiogenic phenotype of senescent fibroblasts: A functional study in endothelial cells. *J. Funct. Foods* **2019**, *53*, 219–226. [CrossRef]
26. Ruzzolini, J.; Peppicelli, S.; Andreucci, E.; Bianchini, F.; Scardigli, A.; Romani, A.; la Marca, G.; Nediani, C.; Calorini, L. Oleuropein, the Main Polyphenol of Olea europaea Leaf Extract, Has an Anti-Cancer Effect on Human BRAF Melanoma Cells and Potentiates the Cytotoxicity of Current Chemotherapies. *Nutrients* **2018**, *10*, 1950. [CrossRef] [PubMed]
27. Guerra, A.R.; Duarte, M.F.; Duarte, I.F. Targeting Tumor Metabolism with Plant-Derived Natural Products: Emerging Trends in Cancer Therapy. *J. Agric. Food Chem.* **2018**, *66*, 10663–10685. [CrossRef]
28. Gerhäuser, C. Cancer cell metabolism, epigenetics and the potential influence of dietary components-A perspective. *Biomed. Res.* **2012**, *23*, 69–89.
29. Gao, J.L.; Chen, Y.G. Natural compounds regulate glycolysis in hypoxic tumor microenvironment. *Biomed. Res. Int.* **2015**, *2015*, 354143. [CrossRef]
30. Salehi, B.; Zucca, P.; Sharifi-Rad, M.; Pezzani, R.; Rajabi, S.; Setzer, W.N.; Varoni, E.M.; Iriti, M.; Kobarfard, F.; Sharifi-Rad, J. Phytotherapeutics in cancer invasion and metastasis. *Phytother. Res.* **2018**, *32*, 1425–1449. [CrossRef]

31. Sharma, S.H.; Thulasingam, S.; Chellappan, D.R.; Chinnaswamy, P.; Nagarajan, S. Morin and Esculetin supplementation modulates c-myc induced energy metabolism and attenuates neoplastic changes in rats challenged with the procarcinogen 1,2-dimethylhydrazine. *Eur. J. Pharmacol.* **2017**, *796*, 20–31. [CrossRef] [PubMed]
32. Gómez de Cedrón, M.; Vargas, T.; Madrona, A.; Jiménez, A.; Pérez-Pérez, M.J.; Quintela, J.C.; Reglero, G.; San-Félix, A.; Ramírez de Molina, A. Novel Polyphenols That Inhibit Colon Cancer Cell Growth Affecting Cancer Cell Metabolism. *J. Pharmacol. Exp. Ther.* **2018**, *366*, 377–389. [CrossRef] [PubMed]
33. Simmons, R.A. Cell Glucose Transport and Glucose Handling During Fetal and Neonatal Development. In *Fetal and Neonatal Physiology*, 5th ed.; Elsevier: Amsterdam, The Netherlands, 2017; pp. 428–435.
34. Barbosa, A.M.; Martel, F. Targeting Glucose Transporters for Breast Cancer Therapy: The Effect of Natural and Synthetic Compounds. *Cancers* **2020**, *12*, 154. [CrossRef] [PubMed]
35. Zambrano, A.; Molt, M.; Uribe, E.; Salas, M. Glut 1 in Cancer Cells and the Inhibitory Action of Resveratrol as A Potential Therapeutic Strategy. *Int. J. Mol. Sci.* **2019**. [CrossRef]
36. Wiese, E.K.; Hitosugi, T. Tyrosine Kinase Signaling in Cancer Metabolism: PKM2 Paradox in the Warburg Effect. *Front. Cell Dev. Biol.* **2018**, *6*, 79. [CrossRef]
37. Nájera, L.; Alonso-Juarranz, M.; Garrido, M.; Ballestín, C.; Moya, L.; Martínez-Díaz, M.; Carrillo, R.; Juarranz, A.; Rojo, F.; Cuezva, J.M.; et al. Prognostic implications of markers of the metabolic phenotype in human cutaneous melanoma. *Br. J. Dermatol.* **2019**, *181*, 114–127. [CrossRef]
38. Zhang, H.; Feng, C.; Zhang, M.; Zeng, A.; Si, L.; Yu, N.; Bai, M. miR-625-5p/PKM2 negatively regulates melanoma glycolysis state. *J. Cell Biochem.* **2019**, *120*, 2964–2972. [CrossRef]
39. Iqbal, M.A.; Bamezai, R.N. Resveratrol inhibits cancer cell metabolism by down regulating pyruvate kinase M2 via inhibition of mammalian target of rapamycin. *PLoS ONE* **2012**, *7*, e36764. [CrossRef]
40. Li, W.; Ma, X.; Li, N.; Liu, H.; Dong, Q.; Zhang, J.; Yang, C.; Liu, Y.; Liang, Q.; Zhang, S.; et al. Resveratrol inhibits Hexokinases II mediated glycolysis in non-small cell lung cancer via targeting Akt signaling pathway. *Exp. Cell Res.* **2016**, *349*, 320–327. [CrossRef]
41. Saunier, E.; Antonio, S.; Regazzetti, A.; Auzeil, N.; Laprévote, O.; Shay, J.W.; Coumoul, X.; Barouki, R.; Benelli, C.; Huc, L.; et al. Resveratrol reverses the Warburg effect by targeting the pyruvate dehydrogenase complex in colon cancer cells. *Sci. Rep.* **2017**, *7*, 6945. [CrossRef]
42. Siddiqui, F.A.; Prakasam, G.; Chattopadhyay, S.; Rehman, A.U.; Padder, R.A.; Ansari, M.A.; Irshad, R.; Mangalhara, K.; Bamezai, R.N.K.; Husain, M.; et al. Curcumin decreases Warburg effect in cancer cells by down-regulating pyruvate kinase M2 via mTOR-HIF1α inhibition. *Sci. Rep.* **2018**, *8*, 8323. [CrossRef]
43. Pinheiro, C.; Miranda-Gonçalves, V.; Longatto-Filho, A.; Vicente, A.L.; Berardinelli, G.N.; Scapulatempo-Neto, C.; Costa, R.F.; Viana, C.R.; Reis, R.M.; Baltazar, F.; et al. The metabolic microenvironment of melanomas: Prognostic value of MCT1 and MCT4. *Cell Cycle* **2016**, *15*, 1462–1470. [CrossRef]
44. Romani, A.; Mulas, S.; Heimler, D. Polyphenols and secoiridoids in raw material (Olea europaea L. leaves) and commercial food supplements. *Eur. Food Res. Technol.* **2017**, *243*, 429–435. [CrossRef]
45. Romani, A.; Scardigli, A.; Pinelli, P. An environmentally friendly process for the production of extracts rich in phenolic antioxidants from *Olea europaea* L. and *Cynara scolymus* L. matrices. *Eur. Food Res. Technol.* **2017**, *243*, 1229–1238. [CrossRef]
46. Guex, C.G.; Reginato, F.Z.; Figueredo, K.C.; da Silva, A.R.H.D.; Pires, F.B.; Jesus, R.D.S.; Lhamas, C.L.; Lopes, G.H.H.; Bauermann, L.F. Safety assessment of ethanolic extract of Olea europaea L. leaves after acute and subacute administration to Wistar rats. *Regul. Toxicol. Pharmacol.* **2018**, *95*, 395–399. [CrossRef]
47. Sepporta, M.V.; Fuccelli, R.; Rosignoli, P.; Ricci, G.; Servili, M.; Fabiani, R. Oleuropein Prevents Azoxymethane-Induced Colon Crypt Dysplasia and Leukocytes DNA Damage in A/J Mice. *J. Med. Food* **2016**, *19*, 983–989. [CrossRef]
48. Giner, E.; Recio, M.C.; Ríos, J.L.; Cerdá-Nicolás, J.M.; Giner, R.M. Chemopreventive effect of oleuropein in colitis-associated colorectal cancer in c57bl/6 mice. *Mol. Nutr. Food Res.* **2016**, *60*, 242–255. [CrossRef]
49. Park, S.; Choi, Y.; Um, S.J.; Yoon, S.K.; Park, T. Oleuropein attenuates hepatic steatosis induced by high-fat diet in mice. *J. Hepatol.* **2011**, *54*, 984–993. [CrossRef]
50. Peppicelli, S.; Bianchini, F.; Toti, A.; Laurenzana, A.; Fibbi, G.; Calorini, L. Extracellular acidity strengthens mesenchymal stem cells to promote melanoma progression. *Cell Cycle* **2015**, *14*, 3088–3100. [CrossRef]

51. Peppicelli, S.; Ruzzolini, J.; Andreucci, E.; Bianchini, F.; Kontos, F.; Yamada, T.; Ferrone, S.; Calorini, L. Potential Role of HLA Class I Antigens in the Glycolytic Metabolism and Motility of Melanoma Cells. *Cancers* **2019**, *11*, 1249. [CrossRef]
52. Livak, K.J.; Schmittgen, T.D. Analysis of Relative Gene Expression Data Using Real-Time Quantitative PCR and the $2-\Delta\Delta CT$ Method. *Methods* **2001**, *25*, 402–408. [CrossRef]
53. Acquaviva, R.; Di Giacomo, C.; Sorrenti, V.; Galvano, F.; Santangelo, R.; Cardile, V.; Gangia, S.; D'Orazio, N.; Abraham, N.G.; Vanella, L. Antiproliferative effect of oleuropein in prostate cell lines. *Int. J. Oncol.* **2012**, *41*, 31–38. [CrossRef]
54. Samara, P.; Christoforidou, N.; Lemus, C.; Argyropoulou, A.; Ioannou, K.; Vougogiannopoulou, K.; Aligiannis, N.; Paronis, E.; Gaboriaud-Kolar, N.; Tsitsilonis, O.; et al. New semi-synthetic analogs of oleuropein show improved anticancer activity in vitro and in vivo. *Eur. J. Med. Chem.* **2017**, *137*, 11–29. [CrossRef]

Permissions

All chapters in this book were first published by MDPI; hereby published with permission under the Creative Commons Attribution License or equivalent. Every chapter published in this book has been scrutinized by our experts. Their significance has been extensively debated. The topics covered herein carry significant findings which will fuel the growth of the discipline. They may even be implemented as practical applications or may be referred to as a beginning point for another development.

The contributors of this book come from diverse backgrounds, making this book a truly international effort. This book will bring forth new frontiers with its revolutionizing research information and detailed analysis of the nascent developments around the world.

We would like to thank all the contributing authors for lending their expertise to make the book truly unique. They have played a crucial role in the development of this book. Without their invaluable contributions this book wouldn't have been possible. They have made vital efforts to compile up to date information on the varied aspects of this subject to make this book a valuable addition to the collection of many professionals and students.

This book was conceptualized with the vision of imparting up-to-date information and advanced data in this field. To ensure the same, a matchless editorial board was set up. Every individual on the board went through rigorous rounds of assessment to prove their worth. After which they invested a large part of their time researching and compiling the most relevant data for our readers.

The editorial board has been involved in producing this book since its inception. They have spent rigorous hours researching and exploring the diverse topics which have resulted in the successful publishing of this book. They have passed on their knowledge of decades through this book. To expedite this challenging task, the publisher supported the team at every step. A small team of assistant editors was also appointed to further simplify the editing procedure and attain best results for the readers.

Apart from the editorial board, the designing team has also invested a significant amount of their time in understanding the subject and creating the most relevant covers. They scrutinized every image to scout for the most suitable representation of the subject and create an appropriate cover for the book.

The publishing team has been an ardent support to the editorial, designing and production team. Their endless efforts to recruit the best for this project, has resulted in the accomplishment of this book. They are a veteran in the field of academics and their pool of knowledge is as vast as their experience in printing. Their expertise and guidance has proved useful at every step. Their uncompromising quality standards have made this book an exceptional effort. Their encouragement from time to time has been an inspiration for everyone.

The publisher and the editorial board hope that this book will prove to be a valuable piece of knowledge for researchers, students, practitioners and scholars across the globe.

List of Contributors

Yathsoeung Ho, Krai Daowtak, Pachuen Potup, Yordhathai Thongsri and Kanchana Usuwanthim
Cellular and Molecular Immunology Research Unit, Faculty of Allied Health Sciences, Naresuan University, Phitsanulok 65000, Thailand

Nungruthai Suphrom
Department of Chemistry, Faculty of Science and Center of Excellence for Innovation in Chemistry, Naresuan University, Phitsanulok 65000, Thailand

Rafael Vicentini Popin, Jouni Jokela, Matti Wahlsten, David P. Fewer and Kaarina Sivonen
Department of Microbiology, University of Helsinki, Viikinkaari 9, FI-00014 Helsinki, Finland

Tania Keiko Shishido
Department of Microbiology, University of Helsinki, Viikinkaari 9, FI-00014 Helsinki, Finland
Institute of Biotechnology, University of Helsinki, Viikinkaari 5D, FI-00014 Helsinki, Finland

Marli Fatima Fiore
Center for Nuclear Energy in Agriculture, University of São Paulo, Avenida Centenário 303, 13400-970 Piracicaba, São Paulo, Brazil

Lars Herfindal
Centre for Pharmacy, Department of Clinical Science, University of Bergen, 5020 Bergen, Norway

Yuefei Wang
Tea Science Institute, Zhejiang University, Hangzhou 310058, China

Robert M. Hackman
Department of Nutrition, University of California, Davis, CA 95616, USA

Ran Wei
Tea Science Institute, Zhejiang University, Hangzhou 310058, China
Department of Nutrition, University of California, Davis, CA 95616, USA

Gerardo G. Mackenzie
Department of Nutrition, University of California, Davis, CA 95616, USA
Davis Comprehensive Cancer Center, University of California, Sacramento, CA 95817, USA

Chon Phin Ong, Wai Leong Lee, Yin Quan Tang and Wei Hsum Yap
School of Biosciences, Faculty of Health and Medical Sciences, Taylor's University Lakeside Campus, No. 1, Jalan Taylor's, Subang Jaya 47500, Malaysia

Jyh-Horng Wu
Department of Forestry, National Chung Hsing University, Taichung 402, Taiwan

Shang-Tse Ho
Department of Forestry, National Chung Hsing University, Taichung 402, Taiwan
Agricultural Biotechnology Research Center, Academia Sinica, Taipei 115, Taiwan

Chi-Chen Lin
Institute of Biomedical Science, National Chung Hsing University, Taichung 402, Taiwan

Yu-Tang Tung
Graduate Institute of Metabolism and Obesity Sciences, Taipei Medical University, Taipei 110, Taiwan
Nutrition Research Center, Taipei Medical University Hospital, Taipei 110, Taiwan
Cell Physiology and Molecular Image Research Center, Wan Fang Hospital, Taipei Medical University, Taipei 116, Taiwan

Giada Juli, Maria Eugenia Gallo Cantafio, Katia Grillone, Marco Rossi, Pierosandro Tagliaferri, Pierfrancesco Tassone and Nicola Amodio
Department of Experimental and Clinical Medicine, Magna Graecia University of Catanzaro, 88100 Catanzaro, Italy

Manuela Oliverio, Monica Nardi and Antonio Procopio
Department of Health Science, Magna Graecia University of Catanzaro, 88100 Catanzaro, Italy

Dina Bellizzi and Giuseppe Passarino
Department of Biology, Ecology and Earth Sciences (DiBEST), University of Calabria, 87036 Arcavacata di Rende, Italy

Carmela Colica
CNR, IBFM UOS of Germaneto, Magna Graecia University of Catanzaro, 88100, Catanzaro, Italy

Qingyu Zhou
Department of Pharmaceutical Sciences, Taneja College of Pharmacy, University of South Florida, Tampa, FL 33612, USA

Hua Pan
Department of Cardiovascular Sciences, Mossani College of Medicine, University of South Florida, Tampa, FL 33612, USA

Jing Li
Karmanos Cancer Institute, Wayne State University School of Medicine, Detroit, MI 48201, USA

Danilo Predes, Luiz F. S. Oliveira, Laís S. S. Ferreira, Lorena A. Maia, João M. A. Delou, Anderson Faletti, Igor Oliveira, Nathalia G. Amado, Alice H. Reis, Carlos A. M. Fraga, Fabio A. Mendes, Helena L. Borges and Jose G. Abreu
Program of Cell and Developmental Biology, Institute of Biomedical Sciences, Federal University of Rio de Janeiro, Rio de Janeiro 21941-902, Brazil

Ricardo Kuster
Department of Chemistry, Federal University of Espírito Santo, Espírito Santo 29075-910, Brazil

Dong Young Kang, Nipin Sp, Eun Seong Jo, Alexis Rugamba, Kyoung-Jin Jang and Young Mok Yang
Department of Pathology, School of Medicine, Institute of Biomedical Science and Technology, Konkuk University, Seoul 05029, Korea

Dae Young Hong
Department of Emergency Medicine, School of Medicine, Konkuk University, Seoul 05029, Korea

Hong Ghi Lee
Division of Hematology-Oncology, Department of Internal Medicine, Konkuk University Medical Center, Seoul 05029, Korea

Ji-Seung Yoo
Department of Immunology, Hokkaido University Graduate School of Medicine, Sapporo 060-0808, Japan

Qing Liu
Jilin Green Food Engineering Research Institute, Changchun 130000, Jilin, China

Cheol Park
Department of Molecular Biology, College of Natural Sciences, Dong-eui University, Busan 47340, Korea

Hee-Jae Cha
Department of Parasitology and Genetics, Kosin University College of Medicine, Busan 49267, Korea

Eun Ok Choi, Hyesook Lee, Min Yeong Kim, So Young Kim, Su Hyun Hong and Yung Hyun Choi
Anti-Aging Research Center, Dong-eui University, Busan 47227, Korea
Department of Biochemistry, Dong-eui University College of Korean Medicine, Busan 47227, Korea

Hyun Hwang-Bo and Seon Yeong Ji
Anti-Aging Research Center, Dong-eui University, Busan 47227, Korea
Department of Molecular Biology, Pusan National University, Busan 46241, Korea

JaeHun Cheong
Department of Molecular Biology, Pusan National University, Busan 46241, Korea

Gi-Young Kim
Department of Marine Life Sciences, School of Marine Biomedical Sciences, Jeju National University, Jeju 63243, Korea

Seok Joong Yun and Wun-Jae Kim
Department of Urology, College of Medicine, Chungbuk National University, Chungbuk 8644, Korea

Hye Jin Hwang
Department of Food and Nutrition, College of Nursing, Healthcare Sciences & Human Ecology, Dong-Eui University, Busan 47340, Korea

Jessica Ruzzolini, Silvia Peppicelli, Francesca Bianchini, Elena Andreucci and Chiara Nediani
Department of Experimental and Clinical Biomedical Sciences "Mario Serio", University of Florence, 50134 Florence, Italy

Silvia Urciuoli and Annalisa Romani
PHYTOLAB (Pharmaceutical, Cosmetic, Food Supplement Technology and Analysis)-DiSIA, Scientific and Technological Pole, University of Florence, 50019 Sesto Fiorentino (Florence), Italy

Katia Tortora and Giovanna Caderni
NEUROFARBA Department, Pharmacology and Toxicology Section, University of Florence, 50139 Florence, Italy

Lido Calorini
Department of Experimental and Clinical Biomedical Sciences "Mario Serio", University of Florence, 50134 Florence, Italy
Center of Excellence for Research, Transfer and High Education Deno THE University of Florence, 50134 Florence, Italy

Index

www.ingramcontent.com/pod-product-compliance
Lightning Source LLC
LaVergne TN
LVHW060551210926
848485LV00005B/1298